MW01243687

Mood Disorders in Later Life

MEDICAL PSYCHIATRY

1. Handbook of Depression and Anxiety: A Biological Approach, *edited by Johan A. den Boer and J. M. Ad Sitsen*
2. Anticonvulsants in Mood Disorders, *edited by Russell T. Joffe and Joseph R. Calabrese*
3. Serotonin in Antipsychotic Treatment: Mechanisms and Clinical Practice, *edited by John M. Kane, H.-J. Moller, and Frans Awouters*
4. Handbook of Functional Gastrointestinal Disorders, *edited by Kevin W. Olden*
5. Clinical Management of Anxiety, *edited by Johan A. den Boer*
6. Obsessive-Compulsive Disorders: Diagnosis • Etiology • Treatment, *edited by Eric Hollander and Dan J. Stein*
7. Bipolar Disorder: Biological Models and Their Clinical Application, *edited by L. Trevor Young and Russell T. Joffe*
8. Dual Diagnosis and Treatment: Substance Abuse and Comorbid Medical and Psychiatric Disorders, *edited by Henry R. Kranzler and Bruce J. Rounsaville*
9. Geriatric Psychopharmacology, *edited by J. Craig Nelson*
10. Panic Disorder and Its Treatment, *edited by Jerrold F. Rosenbaum and Mark H. Pollack*
11. Comorbidity in Affective Disorders, *edited by Mauricio Tohen*
12. Practical Management of the Side Effects of Psychotropic Drugs, *edited by Richard Balon*
13. Psychiatric Treatment of the Medically Ill, *edited by Robert G. Robinson and William R. Yates*
14. Medical Management of the Violent Patient: Clinical Assessment and Therapy, *edited by Kenneth Tardiff*

15. Bipolar Disorders: Basic Mechanisms and Therapeutic Implications, *edited by Jair C. Soares and Samuel Gershon*
16. Schizophrenia: A New Guide for Clinicians, *edited by John G. Csernansky*
17. Polypharmacy in Psychiatry, *edited by S. Nassir Ghaemi*
18. Pharmacotherapy for Child and Adolescent Psychiatric Disorders: Second Edition, Revised and Expanded, *David R. Rosenberg, Pablo A. Davanzo, and Samuel Gershon*
19. Brain Imaging In Affective Disorders, *edited by Jair C. Soares*
20. Handbook of Medical Psychiatry, *edited by Jair C. Soares and Samuel Gershon*
21. Handbook of Depression and Anxiety: A Biological Approach, Second Edition, *edited by Siegfried Kasper, Johan A. den Boer, and J. M. Ad Sitsen*
22. Aggression: Psychiatric Assessment and Treatment, *edited by Emil Coccaro*
23. Depression in Later Life: A Multidisciplinary Psychiatric Approach, *edited by James Ellison and Sumer Verma*
24. Autism Spectrum Disorders, *edited by Eric Hollander*
25. Handbook of Chronic Depression: Diagnosis and Therapeutic Management, *edited by Jonathan E. Alpert and Maurizio Fava*
26. Clinical Handbook of Eating Disorders: An Integrated Approach, *edited by Timothy D. Brewerton*
27. Dual Diagnosis and Psychiatric Treatment: Substance Abuse and Comorbid Disorders: Second Edition, *edited by Henry R. Kranzler and Joyce A. Tinsley*
28. Atypical Antipsychotics: From Bench to Bedside, *edited by John G. Csernansky and John Lauriello*
29. Social Anxiety Disorder, *edited by Borwin Bandelow and Dan J. Stein*
30. Handbook of Sexual Dysfunction, *edited by Richard Balon and R. Taylor Segraves*
31. Borderline Personality Disorder, *edited by Mary C. Zanarini*
32. Handbook of Bipolar Disorder: Diagnosis and Therapeutic Approaches, *edited by Siegfried Kasper and Robert M. A. Hirschfeld*
33. Obesity and Mental Disorders, *edited by Susan L. McElroy, David B. Allison, and George A. Bray*
34. Depression: Treatment Strategies and Management, *edited by Thomas L. Schwartz and Timothy J. Petersen*
35. Bipolar Disorders: Basic Mechanisms and Therapeutic Implications, Second Edition, *edited by Jair C. Soares and Allan H. Young*
36. Neurogenetics of Psychiatric Disorders, *edited by Akira Sawa and Melvin G. McInnis*
37. Attention Deficit Hyperactivity Disorder: Concepts, Controversies, New Directions, *edited by Keith McBurnett, Linda Pfiffner, Russell Schachar, Glen Raymond Elliot, and Joel Nigg*
38. Insulin Resistance Syndrome and Neuropsychiatric Disorders, *edited by Natalie L. Rasgon*

39. Antiepileptic Drugs to Treat Psychiatric Disorders, *edited by Susan L. McElroy, Paul E. Keck, Jr., and Robert M. Post*
40. Asperger's Disorder, *edited by Jeffrey L. Rausch, Marie E. Johnson, and Manuel F. Casanova*
41. Mood Disorders in Later Life, Second Edition, *edited by James M. Ellison, Helen H. Kyomen, and Sumer K. Verma*

MOOD DISORDERS IN LATER LIFE

Second Edition

Edited by

James M. Ellison

McLean Hospital

Belmont, Massachusetts, USA

Helen H. Kyomen

McLean Hospital

Belmont, Massachusetts, USA

Sumer Verma

McLean Hospital

Belmont, Massachusetts, USA

informa

healthcare

New York London

Informa Healthcare USA, Inc.
52 Vanderbilt Avenue
New York, NY 10017

Printed in the United States of America on acid-free paper
10 9 8 7 6 5 4 3 2 1

International Standard Book Number-10: 1-4200-5329-9 (Hardcover)
International Standard Book Number-13: 978-1-4200-5329-6 (Hardcover)

Library of Congress Cataloging-in-Publication Data

Mood disorders in later life / edited by James M. Ellison, Helen H. Kyomen,
Sumer K. Verma. – 2nd ed.
p. ; cm. – (Medical psychiatry series ; 41)
Rev. ed. of: Depression in later life. c2003.
Includes bibliographical references and index.
ISBN-13: 978-1-4200-5329-6 (hardcover : alk. paper)
ISBN-10: 1-4200-5329-9 (hardcover : alk. paper) 1. Depression in old age.
I. Ellison, James M., 1952– II. Kyomen, Helen. III. Verma, Sumer.
IV. Depression in later life. V. Series: Medical psychiatry ; 41.
[DNLM: 1. Mood Disorders–diagnosis. 2. Mood Disorders–therapy.
3. Aged. 4. Depression–diagnosis. 5. Depression–therapy. 6. Geriatric
Psychiatry–methods. W1 ME421SM v.41 2008 / WM 171 D42261 2008]
RC537.5.D457 2008
618.97′68527–dc22

2008039198

For Corporate Sales and Reprint Permission call 212-520-2700 or write to: Sales Department, 52 Vanderbilt Avenue, 7th floor, New York, Ny 10017.

Visit the Informa Web site at
www.informa.com

and the Informa Healthcare Web site at
www.informahealthcare.com

Preface

The high prevalence, frequent recurrence, and serious consequences of mood disorders among young and middle-aged adults are well recognized. The effects of mood disorders on older adults, however, have been less widely appreciated. Although demographic studies indicate a low-point prevalence of major depressive disorder and even lower prevalence of bipolar disorder among community-dwelling elderly cohorts, the clinical significance of mood symptoms is high among the elderly, especially in medical and institutional settings. Mood disorders represent a major disease burden in later life, contributing to suffering, functional impairment, medical disability, and excess mortality. Not only suicide risk but also morbidity and mortality appear to be increased in the presence of late-life mood disorders.

Given the aging of the American population and the enhanced survival of medically compromised elders, it is increasingly important that clinicians know how to evaluate and treat late-life mood disorders. At present, however, even recognition of these conditions is too limited. Seniors may minimize their psychologic distress and focus more directly on somatic or cognitive concerns, inadvertently obscuring the correct psychiatric diagnosis. Primary care clinicians—the health care providers likely to see the greatest number of affected elderly individuals and therefore most in need of evaluation and management skills cognizance—frequently miss the correct diagnosis. Even when the proper diagnosis is made, elderly patients who present mood symptoms to a primary care physician are less likely than younger ones to receive appropriate treatment and adequate follow-up care. Mental health specialists, too, have shown a limited degree of recognition of mood disorders among older patients. The need is apparent, therefore, for greater clinician awareness of the spectrum of unipolar and bipolar disorders in the elderly, from milder to more severe syndromes, as well as for education of the public, with particular focus on the family members and caregivers of older adults suffering from mood disturbances.

The literature on treatment of late-life depression has grown to include many treatment studies, while the literature on late-life bipolar disorder is still sparse. For both types of disorder, our therapeutic approaches still contain many areas of uncertainty. Treatments for mood disorders among the oldest old, the medically ill, or the demented, for example, have received much less attention than treatment of younger, medically healthier older adults. Beyond effects on symptom alleviation, we still know too little about how treatment affects quality of life. Furthermore, we need to understand more about how to integrate somatic therapies with psychotherapeutic approaches, now recommended by experts as an important treatment modality for late-life depression and bipolar disorder.

With invaluable contributions from noted experts, we have tried in this volume to present a comprehensive and current picture of late-life mood disorders. This collection of essays is intended for use by all clinicians who evaluate and treat elderly individuals with clinically significant mood symptoms. Psychiatrists and other mental health specialists as well as primary care clinicians should find in its pages information that is both up-to-date and practical. In addition, we along with the other contributing authors have attempted to present these important illnesses and their treatments in a larger context, highlighting currently available and evolving approaches to treatment and identifying areas in need of further investigation. It is our earnest hope, through the publication of this book, to increase professional and public awareness of late-life mood disorders, to disseminate the most current knowledge, to help identify areas for further inquiry, and ultimately to add our work to that of others dedicated to improving quality of life in the later years.

James M. Ellison, MD, MPH
Helen H. Kyomen, MD
Sumer K. Verma, MD

Acknowledgements

Edited books, at their best, incorporate expert contributions on a given topic into a broader view than any individual could achieve alone. Sometimes this breadth is achieved at the expense of ambiguities and stylistic inconsistencies introduced by a writing process that relies upon individual authors who separately shape and supply their portions of the final product. In the case of this book, however, we were fortunate to be working with a group of collaborators who in many cases not only contributed their own chapters but also generously advised us toward the overall goals of the book. The resulting volume, we hope, has enhanced the quality and value of each author's work. For their own chapters and their help in improving the entire book, the editors wish to express their gratitude to each of our contributing authors. Working with them has been a rewarding experience. In addition, two research assistants lent their editorial and writing skills, offering far more time and energy to this book than we ever expected. We predict a bright future for these young colleagues, Lauren Zeranski and Brittany Jordan.

The patients and staff of the McLean Hospital Geriatric Psychiatry Program, where the editors are privileged to work, also deserve our grateful recognition. They have helped us to understand both the devastating consequences of mood disorders and the remarkable benefits possible when treatment is effective. Our rich clinical experiences at McLean Hospital have, we hope, grounded this book clinically so as to increase its practical value to practitioners treating older adults.

Finally, we wish to thank our families. One never appreciates in advance the commitment of time that will be required to complete a project such as this, but it is always beyond any initial estimate. Our spouses and children have made a silent but absolutely necessary contribution to our work by sharing our conviction of its importance and by encouraging our continued writing even at times when they would have preferred our presence. For their love and support in the preparation of this book, as in so many other areas of our lives, we wish to dedicate our work to them.

James M. Ellison, MD, MPH
Helen H. Kyomen, MD
Sumer K. Verma, MD

Contents

Contributors

Iqbal Ahmed Professor of Psychiatry, John A. Burns School of Medicine, University of Hawaii, Honolulu, Hawaii, U.S.A.

George S. Alexopoulos Weill Medical College of Cornell University, New York, New York, U.S.A.

Francesca Cannavo Antognini Geriatric Psychiatry Program, McLean Hospital, Belmont, and Department of Psychiatry, Harvard Medical School, Boston, Massachusetts, U.S.A.

Ashok J. Bharucha Western Psychiatric Institute and Clinic, University of Pittsburgh School of Medicine, Pittsburgh, Pennsylvania, U.S.A.

Anna Burke Geriatric Psychiatry Program, McLean Hospital, Belmont, Massachusetts, U.S.A.

Yolonda Colemon Albert Einstein College of Medicine, Yonkers, New York, U.S.A.

Donald A. Davidoff Neuropsychological and Psychodiagnostic Testing Service, McLean Hospital, Belmont, and Department of Psychiatry, Harvard Medical School, Boston, Massachusetts, U.S.A.

James M. Ellison Geriatric Psychiatry Program, McLean Hospital, Belmont, and Department of Psychiatry, Harvard Medical School, Boston, Massachusetts, U.S.A.

Brent P. Forester Geriatric Psychiatry Program, McLean Hospital, Belmont, and Department of Psychiatry, Harvard Medical School, Boston, Massachusetts, U.S.A.

Gary L. Gottlieb Department of Psychiatry, Harvard Medical School, and Brigham and Women's Hospital, Boston, Massachusetts, U.S.A.

Ariel Gildengers Advanced Center for Interventions and Services Research for Late-Life Mood Disorders, Department of Psychiatry, University of Pittsburgh, School of Medicine, Pittsburgh, Pennsylvania, U.S.A.

Amber M. Gum Department of Aging and Mental Health, Louis de la Parte Florida Mental Health Institute, University of South Florida, St. Petersburg, Florida, U.S.A.

David S. Harnett Lawrence Memorial Hospital of Medford/Hallmark Health System, Medford, Massachusetts, U.S.A.

Brittany Jordan Geriatric Psychiatry Program, McLean Hospital, Belmont, Massachusetts, U.S.A.

Robert Emmett Kelly, Jr. Weill Medical College of Cornell University, New York, New York, U.S.A.

John S. Kennedy Department of Psychiatry, University of Alberta, Alberta, and Department of Neuroscience, Canadian Center for Behavioral Neuroscience, University of Lethbridge, Alberta, Canada

Bellinda King-Kallimanis Department of Aging and Mental Health, Louis de la Parte Florida Mental Health Institute, University of South Florida, St. Petersburg, Florida, U.S.A.

Julie A. Kmiec Advanced Center for Interventions and Services Research for Late-Life Mood Disorders, Department of Psychiatry, University of Pittsburgh, School of Medicine, Pittsburgh, Pennsylvania, U.S.A.

Robert Kohn Department of Psychiatry and Human Behavior, Miriam Hospital and The Warren Alpert Medical School of Brown University, Providence, Rhode Island, U.S.A.

Helen H. Kyomen McLean Hospital, Belmont, and Department of Psychiatry, Harvard Medical School, Boston, Massachusetts, U.S.A.

Helen Lavretsky Department of Psychiatry and Biobehavioral Sciences, David Geffen School of Medicine at UCLA, and Semel Institute for Neuroscience and Human Behavior at UCLA, Los Angeles, California, U.S.A.

Janet Lawrence McLean Hospital, Belmont, and Harvard Medical School, Boston, Massachusetts, U.S.A.

Benjamin Liptzin Department of Psychiatry, Baystate Health, Springfield, and Department of Psychiatry, Tufts University School of Medicine, Boston, Massachusetts, U.S.A.

Jeffrey M. Lyness Department of Psychiatry, University of Rochester Medical Center, Rochester, New York, U.S.A.

Vladimir Maletic Department of Neuropsychiatry and Behavioral Sciences, University of South Carolina School of Medicine, Greer, South Carolina, U.S.A.

Shunda M. McGahee Healthcare for the Homeless, Massachusetts General Hospital, and Department of Psychiatry, Harvard Medical School, Boston, Massachusetts, U.S.A.

Lianne K. Morris-Smith Health Sciences and Technology, Harvard Medical School, Boston, Massachusetts, U.S.A.

Christine Moutier Department of Psychiatry, University of California, San Diego, California, U.S.A.

Ronald Pies SUNY Upstate Medical University, Syracuse, New York, and Tufts University School of Medicine, Boston, Massachusetts, U.S.A.

Charles F. Reynolds III Advanced Center for Interventions and Services Research for Late-Life Mood Disorders and the John A. Hartford Center of Excellence in Geriatric Psychiatry, Department of Psychiatry, University of Pittsburgh, School of Medicine, Pittsburgh, Pennsylvania, U.S.A.

Carl Salzman Department of Psychiatry, Massachusetts Mental Health Center/Beth Israel Deaconess Hospital, and Department of Psychiatry, Harvard Medical School, Boston, Massachusetts, U.S.A.

Stephen Seiner ECT Clinic, McLean Hospital, Belmont, Massachusetts, U.S.A.

Benjamin C. Silverman MGH/McLean Adult Psychiatry Residency Training Program, Clinical Fellow in Psychiatry, Harvard University, Cambridge, Massachusetts, U.S.A.

E. Yusuf Sivrioglu Geriatric Psychiatry Unit, Department of Psychiatry, Uludag University Medical Faculty, Bursa, Turkey

Manjola Ujkaj Geriatric Psychiatry Program, McLean Hospital, Belmont, and Department of Psychiatry, Harvard Medical School, Boston, Massachusetts, U.S.A.

Kiran Verma Department of Accounting and Finance, University of Massachusetts Boston, Boston, Massachusetts, U.S.A.

E. Nalan Ward West End Clinic, Outpatient Addiction Services, Department of Psychiatry, Massachusetts General Hospital, and Department of Psychiatry, Harvard Medical School, Boston, Massachusetts, U.S.A.

Robert C. Young Department of Psychiatry, Weill Medical College of Cornell University, White Plains, New York, U.S.A.

Sidney Zisook Department of Psychiatry, University of California, San Diego, and Psychiatry Service, Veterans Affairs San Diego Healthcare System, San Diego, California, U.S.A.

1 Diagnosing Depression in Later Life

Janet Lawrence
McLean Hospital, Belmont, and Harvard Medical School, Boston, Massachusetts, U.S.A.

Donald A. Davidoff
Neuropsychological and Psychodiagnostic Testing Service, McLean Hospital, Belmont, and Harvard Medical School, Boston, Massachusetts, U.S.A.

John S. Kennedy
Department of Psychiatry, University of Alberta, Alberta, and Department of Neuroscience, Canadian Center for Behavioral Neuroscience, University of Lethbridge, Alberta, Canada

James M. Ellison
Geriatric Psychiatry Program, McLean Hospital, Belmont, and Department of Psychiatry, Harvard Medical School, Boston, Massachusetts, U.S.A.

INTRODUCTION: THE UNIQUE CHARACTERISTICS OF DEPRESSION IN LATER LIFE

The high prevalence, frequent recurrence, and serious consequences of depressive disorders among young and middle-aged adults are well recognized, yet the nature and consequences of depressive states in later life are less widely appreciated by health care providers and by the public. Although demographic studies indicate a low absolute prevalence of Major Depressive Disorder among community-dwelling elderly Americans, depressive symptoms and nonmajor depressive syndromes are common and debilitating in the elderly. The prevalence of major and nonmajor depressive states in medical and long-term care settings, moreover, is very high. In nursing homes, for example, depressive symptoms or syndromes are estimated to affect more than 40% of residents. These numbers take on alarming significance in light of the recent findings that link the presence of depression in later life with impaired functioning, diminished quality of life, excess use of nonpsychiatric medical services, and potentially dire health consequences including early mortality from suicide and other causes. Fortunately, the past decade has seen outstanding advances in our knowledge of depression's characteristic clinical manifestations in older adults as well as its pathophysiology and optimal treatments.

Recognition of late-life depression remains a prerequisite to treatment. Clinical awareness has improved in recent years, but even more aggressive case finding is needed. For a variety of reasons discussed in depth in chapter 5, treatment for late-life depression is typically first sought in the primary care setting. Many primary care clinicians consider the diagnosis and treatment of late-life depression as their responsibility, yet acknowledge their skills in this area to be inadequate (1). They discuss depression infrequently with their elderly patients (2) and may overlook its presence in the hustle of a busy primary care practice. Mental health professionals, too, miss the presence of significant depressive symptoms in older individuals, or mistakenly attribute them to the effects of adverse life events, medical illnesses, or cognitive impairments.

To aid recognition of late-life depression and suggest initial evaluative steps, this chapter will review the characteristics of late-life depression and discuss the usual process of assessment. The most commonly used diagnostic instruments, laboratory tests, and imaging studies will be reviewed. Many topics touched upon in this discussion are addressed in greater detail elsewhere in this book. Bipolar disorder, in particular, is reviewed comprehensively in chapter 4, although some of the issues associated with unipolar depression also apply to bipolar depression.

DIAGNOSTIC CRITERIA AND BRIEF ASSESSMENT INSTRUMENTS

Our most widely used clinical diagnostic system, the *Diagnostic and Statistical Manual of Mental Disorders* (DSM-IV TR) (3), helps clinicians arrive at a diagnosis by comparing an individual patient's presentation with a list of symptoms regarded as characteristic of a specific diagnostic entity. The symptom pattern chosen for major depressive disorder does not specifically take into account the ways in which older adults' depressions differ from those of younger adults. The diagnosis of a major depressive episode requires five or more of the specified nine symptoms, occurring during the same 2-week period, and causing clinically significant distress or impairment in social, occupational, or other important areas of functioning. The presence of either depressed mood or anhedonia is required (Table 1).

To a large extent, identification of these symptoms relies upon a patient's self-report unless a reliable informant is available. Self-report, in turn, depends upon the ability to recognize and name depressive experiences, an exercise in abstract thinking and communication that may become impaired in the context of depression or cognitive dysfunction. Whether older adults' observed tendency to under-report the presence of depressive phenomena reflects an actual absence of depressed mood, an inability to name the experience of depression accurately, a socioculturally based failure to acknowledge the presence of depression, or denial arising from altered biology remains unknown.

In the older population, it is believed that a major depressive disorder can occur in the absence of reported or observed "depressed mood," even though such a mood is considered a hallmark of depression in younger adults. This variant presentation, with greater focus on somatic concerns or changes in pleasure and

TABLE 1 DSM-IV TR Criteria for Major Depressive Episode

Symptom	DSM-IV TR diagnostic criteria for major depressive episode
Depressed mood	Depressed mood most of the day, on most days
Anhedonia	Markedly decreased interest or pleasure in most activities
Weight change	Substantial unintentional weight loss or gain
Sleep disturbance	Insomnia or hypersomnia most days
Psychomotor change	Psychomotor retardation or agitation most days
Lack of energy	Fatigue or loss of energy most days
Excessive guilt	Feelings of excessive guilt or worthlessness most days
Poor concentration	Diminished ability to think or concentrate most days
Suicidal ideation	Recurrent thought of death or suicide

Source: Adapted from Ref. 4.

engagement than on mood, has been described as "depression without sadness" (5). Going beyond a question about "depressed mood" and supplying common synonyms for depressed mood such as nervous, discouraged, hopeless, blue, or irritable may elicit a positive response that can lead to further and more revealing discussion about agitation, anhedonia, or dysphoria; some older patients, however, will endorse none of these adjectives while nonetheless appearing quite depressed as manifested by the non-mood depressive symptoms.

Beyond mood, other psychological dissimilarities between older and younger depressed adults have been described. Feelings of decreased self-esteem and worthlessness are more frequently reported in the elderly and ruminative thinking in which the individual dwells on particular themes or ideas may be prominent. Delusions, signifying the presence of a depression with psychotic features, are more commonly found in older than in younger patients. Hopelessness about the future and thoughts about death, however, may be more normative in the elderly and are not sufficient to indicate depression in the absence of other symptoms (6). Guilt and feelings of failure, by contrast, are more common depressive symptoms in younger patients (7).

The "neurovegetative" disturbances in sleep, appetite, and energy that constitute an important component of the DSM symptom list have some shortcomings as indicators of a depressive diagnosis in older adults. In the older adult, insomnia, anorexia, or fatigue may represent nonspecific findings associated with medical illness or the effects of medications. Apathy, on the other hand, can signal the presence of cerebrovascular small vessel disease and the so-called "vascular depression" that is discussed in detail in chapter 10.

Bodily experiences occupy a prominent role in the experience of late-life depression and must be taken into account during assessment. "Somatosensory amplification" (8), a term that describes the magnified perception of somatic symptoms as a result psychological distress, may further increase patients' focus on somatic complaints. An older, depressed patient may have difficulty in distinguishing the neurovegetative symptoms associated with depression, for example, disturbances of sleep, energy, and appetite, from those of feared or actual physical illness. A focus on physical functioning applied to the brain can give rise to a preoccupation with memory and cognitive performance, made all the more concerning because depression-associated impairments of attention, processing speed, and executive function can be mistakenly interpreted as primary difficulties with memory (see chap. 9 for a more extensive discussion). This worried focus on cognitive functioning can result in a misleading request for cognitive assessment when the actual problem is one of depression. Because of the frequency with which somatic complaints predominate in elderly depressives, an atypical presentation of a mood disorder should be included in the differential diagnosis of any patient whose physical symptoms or concerns about cognitive functioning cannot be explained on the basis of a nonpsychiatric illness. A diagnosis of depression may lead to appropriate intervention even when depressed mood is vehemently denied by a patient (9). Depression of this type, however, is a diagnosis of exclusion and the assignment of a diagnosis of depression should not curtail appropriate medical evaluation.

The burden of concurrent medical illnesses, common among the elderly, further confounds the diagnosis of depression in later life (10). Medical illnesses bear a complex and reciprocal relationship to depression. While certain disorders such as Parkinson's disease, for example, can produce a mood disorder responsive to antidepressants, others such as coronary artery disease are associated with symptoms that resemble depression (fatigue, insomnia) but must be addressed through treatment of the primary medical condition. The interrelationship between medical disorders and depression is discussed more fully in chapter 11. The effects on depression of substance abuse, a specific type of medical-psychiatric disturbance, are addressed in chapter 12.

The presence of mild or greater cognitive impairment, more frequent among elderly than among younger adults, can obstruct the assessment of depressive symptoms by reducing the memory or insight required to report depressive symptoms accurately. In significantly impaired individuals, furthermore, communication difficulties can exacerbate the difficulties of accurate evaluation. Recognition of depression in demented patients may require observation of signs of behavioral disturbance such as weeping, pacing, handwringing, social isolation, vocalization, failure to eat, aggression, or delusions. These may be combined with more typical depressive symptoms such as anorexia, sleep disturbance, or anhedonia. Depressive thought content may be expressed in a fragmented way owing to language impairment. When moderate-to-severe dementia is present, family members are often more aware than the patient of abnormal shifts in mood and affective expression. They are therefore essential informants during evaluation and monitoring (11). A modified set of DSM-IV TR criteria proposed for diagnosing depression in Alzheimer's disease patients stipulates the need for at least three of the following symptoms during the same 2-week period: depressed mood, anhedonia, social withdrawal, tearfulness (in less-verbal patients), or decreased positive affect or pleasure in response to social contacts or usual activities (12). The suggestion to require fewer symptoms in order to justify a diagnosis of major depressive disorder increases the sensitivity for detection of depression in dementia.

INSTRUMENTS FOR THE IDENTIFICATION OF DEPRESSION

Despite the complexities of diagnosing depression in later life, it is vitally important to identify affected individuals because effective treatments are readily available and because untreated depression has debilitating consequences. Much effort has been devoted, therefore, to the development of instruments suitable for case finding in various settings, for estimation of severity, and for assessment of treatment response (13). The available scales differ in several important ways. Some are used primarily as clinical tools while others are employed as research instruments. Some are self-report scales, while others are designed to be administered by a trained rater. Some are applicable to both older and younger individuals, while others validated primarily in older cohorts. The most important of these assessment scales will be reviewed here.

Geriatric Depression Scale (GDS)—15 and 30 Item (14,15)

The GDS is a very useful clinical assessment scale that can be completed within several minutes either as a self-report or as a verbal response to the series of questions. A trained rater is not necessary. The original 30-item GDS was developed by gathering 100 yes/no questions related to depression in the elderly and analyzing which 30 correlated best with the total score. The 15-item scale (GDS-S) correlates with the 30-item scale and can be used as a briefer screening instrument, with a cut off score of between five and seven suggesting depression. With a cut off score of 5/15, sensitivity of the GDS-S is reported to be 92% and specificity 81% (16). The value of the scale is limited by the quality of information provided by the patient. Studies in patients with dementia have suggested that it is not accurate in assessing demented individuals, especially those with a Mini-Mental State Examination (MMSE) score less than 15 (17).

Beck Depression Inventory (BDI) (18)

The BDI is a brief (20 minute), 21-item, self-report scale, which is widely used in older adults, though not specifically developed for the geriatric population. As with other self-report scales, its validity can be diminished by patients' denial or lack of awareness of depressive symptoms. Although other cutoff scores have been used, a common choice is 17, which has been shown to differentiate patients with moderate depression from those without depressive symptoms with a sensitivity of 87% and a specificity of 85% (7,18).

Zung Self-Rating Depression Scale (SDS) (19)

The SDS is a brief, self-administered instrument with 20 statements, each representing a different depressive symptom. For 10 of these statements, a positive response indicates the presence of depressive symptoms. A negative response to any of the other 10 statements indicates the presence of depressive symptoms. Responses are rated from 1 to 4, covering the range from "a little of the time" to "most of the time." A scoring key is provided. Low scores indicate a low likelihood of depression. The final score is expressed as an index derived by converting the sum of the raw score values to a percentage of the maximum score of 80, with percentages greater than 50% suggesting depression (20). Using this cutoff score among geriatric patients, the sensitivity and specificity of the SDS have been reported to be 76% and 82%, respectively (21).

Cornell Scale for Depression in Dementia (22)

In individuals whose Mini-Mental State Examination score falls in the range of 15/30 or below, self-report of depressive symptoms is apt to be rendered untrustworthy by cognitive impairment. The Cornell Scale is a 19-item instrument that allows the clinician to collect information by observation and interview with the patient and from an informant. By incorporating multiple sources of information, this scale overcomes some of the difficulties of an instrument based solely on self-report. The scale is correlated to the Hamilton Depression Rating Scale (HAMD) and thus is significantly affected by ratings of neurovegetative symptoms that are less specific for depression in older adults than in younger ones. A cutoff score of 7 has been reported to yield a sensitivity of 90% and specificity of 75% (23).

Brief Assessment Schedule Depression Cards (BASDEC) (24)

The BASDEC assessment tool is designed for use in hospitalized geriatric patients, where privacy might be an issue. The patient is handed a deck of 19 cards with statements about depressive symptoms and is asked to place each of the cards into one of two piles, "True" or "False." The positive predictive value of this test has been reported to be similar to that of the GDS, with sensitivity of 71% and specificity of 74% noted in hospitalized geriatric patients.

Minimum Data Set Depression Rating Scale (25)

This scale was developed by gathering results from the routine evaluation of nursing home patients using the Minimum Data Set of the Residential Assessment

Instrument, which includes ratings of mood symptoms. These results were correlated with the Hamilton and Cornell scales to identify seven mood items which could be used for case finding in this population and which compared favorably as an instrument with the 15-item GDS. With a cut off score of 3, sensitivity has been reported as 91% and specificity as 69% (25).

Center for Epidemiological Studies—Depression Scale (CES-D) (26)

The CES-D is a brief (5 minutes), 20-item, self-administered screen which has been used in large studies of the general population and has been found to be useful as well in assessing elderly adults. It compares favorably to the use of the GDS in terms of sensitivity and specificity in older adults, respectively, reported as 92% and 87% when using a cut off score of 21/60 (16).

Hamilton Depression Rating Scale (HAMD) (27,28)

The HAMD is familiar to many psychiatric clinicians and is the most commonly used and the best validated scale in the general adult population. Other newer scales are often compared to the HAMD for validation; however, its emphasis on somatic symptoms has the potential to result in over-diagnosis of depression when applied to older adults, especially those with medical illnesses. The HAMD also requires a trained clinician for administration, which limits its utility in nonpsychiatric settings. This scale and the Montgomery Asberg are often employed to establish the presence of depression and track its severity in a research cohort. Using a cutoff score of 16, the HAMD has been reported to have a sensitivity of 87.5% and a specificity of 99.1% in a community-dwelling geriatric population (29).

Montgomery Asberg Depression Rating Scale (MADRS) (30)

The MADRS was designed specifically to detect change in depression with great sensitivity. It is thus commonly used as an assessment tool in antidepressant treatment trials. The scale requires a trained interviewer and measures apparent and reported sadness, inner tension, changes in sleep, appetite and concentration, lassitude, inability to feel, and pessimistic and suicidal thoughts. Like the HAMD, it was not designed specifically to assess geriatric depression. In a geriatric population, the sensitivity and specificity have been reported to be 72% and 98.9%, respectively, using 21 as a cutoff score (29).

LABORATORY TESTING

To date, no practical biological markers of depression are used to establish a diagnosis of depression. With older patients, however, laboratory testing is quite useful in identifying remediable medical causes of depressive symptoms. This is true especially in patients presenting with an initial depressive episode in later life. Potentially useful tests include complete blood count and chemistry panel, thyroid function tests, B12 or methlmalonic acid, folate level or RBC folate, and urinalysis. When clinically indicated, laboratory testing may also be appropriate for the confirmation of other possible, but more unusual, causes of depression such as infectious diseases (VDRL, Lyme antibody titer, HIV), inflammatory or connective tissue diseases (ESR, ANA), endocrine disturbances (LH, FSH, testosterone, serum cortisol), drugs of abuse or heavy-metal poisoning (toxicology).

NEUROIMAGING

Similar to blood and urine testing, the role of neuroimaging in late-life depression is to identify treatable causes of secondary depressive symptoms rather than to positively establish a psychiatric diagnosis of depression. Findings from computed tomography (CT) or structural magnetic resonance imaging (MRI) studies have linked localized left hemisphere infarcts (31) and decreases in prefrontal volume (32) with the presence of depression, and other nonpsychiatric etiologies that may present with mood symptoms also include subdural hematomas, cerebrovascular disease, normal pressure hydrocephalus, mass lesions, or certain infectious conditions (33). MRI findings, too, can be considered along with other factors relevant to forecasting a patient's prognosis. The presence of extensive subcortical hyperintensities on MRI, for example, predicts a less robust response to treatment in some studies (34,35). The relationship of cerebrovascular disease to depressive states is explored at length in chapter 10.

Attempts to image markers of depression or prognostic indicators include promising new work with functional imaging, magnetic resonance spectroscopy (MRS), and electroencephalography (EEG). Depression in the elderly has been associated with reductions in whole brain glucose metabolic rate detectable on PET scanning (36,37). Increases in frontal myo-inositol/creatine and choline/creatine ratios on proton MRS are ushering in new investigations of energy metabolism in late-life mood disorders (38). EEG has been suggested to offer an inexpensive, noninvasive screen of general brain activity that may have the potential to be a useful secondary screening investigation in depressed patients with suspected cognitive impairment or other CNS pathology (39–42).

CASE FINDING FOR LATE-LIFE DEPRESSION IN PRIMARY CARE

While brief assessment instruments and rating scales for depression have been applied in many environments, case-finding is of particular importance in primary care, where many depressed older adults initially seek treatment (43). Unfortunately, as reviewed in greater detail in chapter 5, a variety of barriers impede the pathway to detection and treatment (44,45). Depression that falls short of DSM-IV TR major depressive disorder criteria is more common than major depression in the elderly (see chap. 2) and may be overlooked or considered insufficiently severe to merit a diagnosis. The presentation of depression is often obscured or confounded by the concurrent presence of medical problems, cognitive difficulties, or multiple medications. In addition, primary care physicians may not be sufficiently trained to recognize mood disturbances or may underestimate the value and importance of treatment in the elderly. They may feel that depression is of lesser importance than medical problems, or that depressive symptoms are fully explained as an acceptable and normative response to the losses associated with aging. In addition, the increasing time pressures and the rapid patient turnover in primary care make it more difficult to perform an in-depth interview and recognize changes in the patient's mood over time.

Brief assessment instruments would appear to be ideal as tools to increase case detection in primary care (46) and are known to perform better than a subjective clinical impression alone (47). A review by Schade et al. (48), however, notes that the benefit of "depression screening" is difficult to measure and remains controversial. Schade's data suggest that briefer tests, which have minimal costs in terms of time and personnel, perform as well as more complicated ones. Most brief tests, however, are based upon syndromal definitions of depression, which are more useful in hospital-based research. In primary care settings, by contrast, up to 50% of patients with depressive symptoms and functional impairment are not adequately classified by current psychiatric categories (49). The high prevalence in primary care populations of subsyndromal depressive states (described in detail in chap. 2 of this book) is of particular importance. The limitations of current brief assessment instruments, therefore, require that a clinician be prepared to override a score indicating the absence of depression when sufficient other clinical data suggest insensitivity of the test rather than a euthymic patient. Primary care providers can be educated in the use and limitations of currently available screening devices (50).

In recent years, efforts have been made to screen for depression in the elderly in a community setting, such as senior centers or libraries. National Depression Screening Day (NDSD), started in 1991, has become a large and successful program for screening and educating the public about depression in general (51). In addition, NDSD has helped to destigmatize the illness and its treatment. The initial programs used the Zung Self-Rating Scale (19) and it was reported that a relatively large proportion of individuals screening positive sought subsequent care (52). More recently, the specially developed Harvard Department of Psychiatry National Depression Screening Day Scale (HANDS) has been used. Since 1998, a modified version of the screening protocol has been available for older individuals and has used the 15-item GDS. The results of the elderly outreach effort have not been reported to date; however, based upon the authors' experience with large-scale community-based memory screening (53), the success of such an endeavor among older adults may be limited both by accessibility of the screening center and by the willingness of the older individual to seek treatment.

LATE ONSET DEPRESSION: A SUBSET OF DEPRESSION IN LATER LIFE

Discussion of the diagnosis of late-life depression requires acknowledgment that this heterogeneous classification lumps individuals with early onset recurrent depression along with those whose initial depressive episode occurred in the 60s or later. The distinction is often made in research studies, therefore, between these two very different depressive backgrounds. Earlier onset illness is more commonly associated with a positive family history of depression and substance abuse, while later onset depression is more commonly associated with observable brain abnormalities, especially microvascular changes visible with neuroimaging techniques. Studies have investigated whether late-onset depression differs from late-life depression in terms of course and prognosis. Although Reynolds et al. (54) suggested that response to treatment was similar in both groups, other than the observation that earlier age of onset may predict a slower remission, other studies have gathered data that support a different viewpoint (55,56). As reviewed in chapter 10, these studies have found that individuals with onset of depression after 60 may show a more intractable course of illness.

Some of the reported differences in outcome between late-onset and late-life depressions may be related to sample selection and whether a specific study included individuals who are more cognitively impaired or physically ill characteristics associated with a poorer prognosis. It appears well established, however, that late-onset illness is associated with more structural brain abnormalities, such as enlarged ventricles and white matter hyperintensities (57), and cognitive change. In a number of individuals, the cognitive changes develop into full-blown dementia of the vascular, Alzheimer, or mixed types (58). A worse outcome might intuitively be anticipated, therefore, in patients whose depression first began in later life.

DISTINGUISHING BETWEEN UNIPOLAR AND BIPOLAR DISORDERS

In order to provide optimal treatment, unipolar depression must be distinguished from depression occurring in the context of a bipolar disorder. Verification of a history of mania can be rendered more difficult in the elderly population, where mania sometimes presents with increased irritability and confusion rather than with the euphoria, increased energy, hyperactivity, and mental content reflecting increased sexual interest, religiosity, and grandiosity more typical of younger adults (59). Mania in the elderly can be difficult to distinguish from an agitated unipolar depression.

As with unipolar depression, a distinction can also be made between early- and late-onset bipolar disorder. Schurhoff and colleagues (60) found that earlier onset bipolar disorder was associated with more psychotic features, more mixed episodes, greater comorbidity with panic disorder and worse response to lithium prophylaxis than late-onset disorder. Late-onset bipolar disorder has also been associated in several studies with right hemisphere subcortical hyperintensities, which may represent vascular changes (61,62).

DEPRESSION AND DEMENTIA

The interface between depression and dementia is explored in chapter 9. This interface presents a vexing diagnostic problem when both cognitive and mood symptoms are present without a clear indication of which developed first. When depression is accompanied by cognitive symptoms that lead to a misdiagnosis of dementia, an elder may be subjected to the inappropriate and nihilistic attitude of "why bother doing anything?" and hence not receive treatment that might result in symptom remission and restoration of quality of life. By contrast, when depression is a prodrome for dementia (63–65), recognition and assessment can in some cases lead to an early diagnosis and more effective treatment approach. When depression reflects an introspective awareness of loss of function due to underlying organic pathology, it may be important to address both the cognitive impairment and the associated depressive reaction (66–68), suggesting the value of psychotherapy for such patients.

Even in the absence of dementia per se, the presence of depression is typically associated with some degree of cognitive inefficiency. Diagnostic criteria for major depressive disorder include difficulty in concentration (DSM-IV TR). A depressed individual who attends poorly to stimulus material, concentrates inadequately on the material to be processed, and lacks motivation will perform suboptimally on neuropsychological testing. Aging, too, contributes to cognitive inefficiency. The primary criteria for diagnosis of dementia in the elderly are cognitive in nature (DSM-IV TR, NINCDS) and require that there be a disturbance of memory (69). Yet memory appears impaired when information is not effectively perceived, attended to, ordered, and understood. Furthermore, assessment of memory requires that a subject be able to communicate what has been stored and retrieved (70). The apparent disturbance of memory seen in many older depressed patients may represent impairment of one of these associated cognitive functions rather than an inability to store or retrieve information. Precise characterization of a patient's cognitive difficulties by means of neuropsychological assessment, as described in chapter 9, can be diagnostically revealing.

DEMENTIA WITH DEPRESSION

Dementia is often accompanied by depression, requiring in assessment a sensitivity to the manner in which each disorder differentially impairs cognitive functioning. It is known, for example, that the prevalence of depression among elders with a primary degenerative dementia is markedly greater than in the general elderly population (71). Some studies (72) find major depressive disorder in 10% to 30% of individuals with dementia. This phenomenon of comorbidity occurs particularly in the earlier stages of dementia when the individual still retains a reflective sense of self, and can appreciate his or her own failing cognitive abilities (73,74). Furthermore, some studies (75) suggest that elders manifesting cognitive dysfunction are, in fact, more vulnerable to the cognitive sequelae of depression and may demonstrate apparent exacerbation of impairment in particular cognitive domains (e.g., memory).

SUMMARY

From the preceding discussion, it is evident that depression in the elderly is an important and heterogeneous disorder that can differ significantly from depression in younger adults. Older patients may present with fewer symptoms, or a different spectrum of symptoms, than are required when diagnosing major depressive disorder in younger adults. A patient's misleading emphasis on somatic or cognitive concerns can distract the clinician away from an accurate diagnosis. Life circumstances or losses, medical conditions, and cognitive dysfunction can further complicate the diagnosis of depression in the elderly by introducing confounding symptoms that may cause the depression itself to be overlooked, underdiagnosed or untreated. Current nosologic systems, such as the DSM-IV TR, do not adequately describe the range of presentations of depression in the elderly. Hence, use of such instruments as the GDS or application of the modified DSM diagnostic criteria for assessment of depression in Alzheimer's disease can increase the efficiency of case finding. Further efforts are suggested in training nonpsychiatric care providers, who provide the bulk of care to the depressed elderly, in the utilization of appropriate screening methods and instruments that may increase the rate of detection of depression and increase the opportunities for successful treatment. Furthermore, understanding the limitations of such screening instruments will encourage the care provider to make referrals in difficult or questionable cases. As our understanding of late-life depression increases, it is to be hoped that an increasing number of affected individuals will be correctly detected, diagnosed, and offered the potential benefits of appropriate treatment.

REFERENCES

1. Callahan C, Nienaber N, Hendrie H, et al. Depression of elderly outpatients: Primary care physicians' attitudes and practice patterns J Gen Intern Med 1992; 7:26–31.
2. Adelman R, Greene M, Friedmann E, et al. Discussion of depression in follow-up medical visits with older patients. J Am Geriatr Soc 2008; 56:16–22.

3. American Psychiatric Association. Diagnostic and Statistical Manual of Mental Disorders, 4th ed. Text Revision. Washington, D. C.: American Psychiatric Association, 2000.
4. Whooley MA, Simon GE. Managing depression in medical outpatients. N Engl J Med 2000; 343:1942–1950.
5. Gallo J, Rabins P. Depression without sadness: Alternative presentations of depression in late life Am Fam Physician 1999; 60:820–826.
6. Burkhart KS. Diagnosis of depression in the elderly patient. Lippincotts Prim Care Pract 2000; 4:149–162.
7. Burns A, Lawlor B, Craig S. Assessment Scales in Old Age Psychiatry. London, U. K.: Martin Dunitz, 1999.
8. Barsky AJ. Amplification, somatization, and the somatoform disorders. Psychosomatics 1992; 33:28–34.
9. Lyness JM, Cox C, Curry J, et al. Older age and the underreporting of depressive symptoms. J Am Geriatr Soc 1995; 43:216–221.
10. Lyness JM, Bruce ML, Koenig HG, et al. Depression and medical illness in late life: Report of a symposium J Am Geriatr Soc 1996; 44:198–203.
11. Ballard C, Bannister C, Oyebode F. Depression in dementia sufferers. Int J Geriatr Psychiatry 1996; 11:507–515.
12. Olin JT, Schneider LS, Katz IR, et al. Provisional diagnostic criteria for depression of Alzheimer disease. Am J Geriatr Psychiatry 2002; 10:125–128.
13. Blazer D. Depression in the elderly. N Engl J Med 1989; 320:164–166.
14. Yesavage JA, Brink TL, Rose TL, et al. Development and validation of a geriatric depression screening scale: A preliminary report J Psychiatr Res 1983; 17:37–49.
15. Sheikh J, Yesavage JA. Geriatric depression scale: Recent findings and development of a short version In: Clinical Gerontology: A Guide to Assessment and Intervention. New York, NY: Howarth Press, 1986.
16. Lyness JM, Noel TK, Cox C, et al. Screening for depression in elderly primary care patients. A comparison of the Center for Epidemiologic Studies—Depression Scale and the Geriatric Depression Scale Arch Intern Med 1997; 157:449–454.
17. McGivney SA, Mulvihill M, Taylor B. Validating the GDS depression screen in the nursing home. J Am Geriatr Soc 1994; 42:490–492.
18. Beck A, Ward C, Mendelson M, et al. An inventory for measuring depression. Arch Gen Psychiatry 1961; 4:53–63.
19. Zung W. A self-rating scale for depression. Arch Gen Psychiatry 1965; 12:63–70.
20. Zung W. Self-rating scales for psychopathology. In: Crook T, Ferris S, Bartus R, eds. Assessment in Geriatric Psychopharmacology. New Canaan, CT: Mark Powley Associates, 1983:145–151.
21. Okimoto JT, Barnes RF, Veith RC, et al. Screening for depression in geriatric medical patients. Am J Psychiatry 1982; 139:799–802.
22. Alexopoulos GS, Abrams RC, Young RC, et al. Cornell scale for depression in dementia. Biol Psychiatry 1988; 23:271–284.
23. Vida S, Des Rosiers P, Carrier L, et al. Depression in Alzheimer's disease: Receiver operating characteristic analysis of the Cornell scale for depression in dementia and the hamilton depression scale J Geriatr Psychiatry Neurol 1994; 7:159–162.
24. Adshead F, Cody DD, Pitt B. BASDEC: A novel screening instrument for depression in elderly medical inpatients BMJ 1992; 305:397.
25. Burrows AB, Morris JN, Simon SE, et al. Development of a minimum data set-based depression rating scale for use in nursing homes. Age Ageing 2000; 29:165–172.
26. Radloff L, Teri L. Use of the Center for Epidemiological Studies—Depression Scale in older adults. Clin Gerontol 1986; 5:119–137.
27. Hamilton M. A rating scale for depression. J Neurol Neurosurgery Psychiatry 1960; 23:56–62.
28. Hamilton M. Development of a rating scale for primary depressive illness. Br J Soc Clin Psychol 1967; 6:278–296.
29. Mottram P, Wilson K, Copeland J. Validation of the Hamilton Depression Rating Scale and Montgommery [sic] and Asberg Rating Scales in terms of AGECAT depression cases Int J Geriatr Psychiatry 2000; 15:1113–1119.

30. Montgomery SA, Asberg M. A new depression scale designed to be sensitive to change. Br J Psychiatry 1979; 134:382–389.
31. Robinson RG, Starr LB, Lipsey JR, et al. A two-year longitudinal study of post-stroke mood disorders: Dynamic changes in associated variables over the first six months of follow-up Stroke 1984; 15:510–517.
32. Kumar A, Jin Z, Bilker W, et al. Late-onset minor and major depression: Early evidence for common neuroanatomical substrates detected by using MRI Proc Natl Acad Sci U S A 1998; 95:7654–7658.
33. van Crevel H, van Gool WA, Walstra GJ. Early diagnosis of dementia: Which tests are indicated? What are their costs? J Neurol 1999; 246:73–78.
34. Simpson S, Baldwin RC, Jackson A, et al. Is subcortical disease associated with a poor response to antidepressants? Neurological, neuropsychological and neuroradiological findings in late-life depression. Psychol Med 1998; 28:1015–1026.
35. Lloyd AJ, Grace JB, Jaros E, et al. Depression in late life, cognitive decline and white matter pathology in two clinico-pathologically investigated cases. Int J Geriatr Psychiatry 2001; 16:281–287.
36. Meltzer CC, Smith G, DeKosky ST, et al. Serotonin in aging, late-life depression, and Alzheimer's disease: The emerging role of functional imaging Neuropsychopharmacology 1998; 18:407–430.
37. Kumar A. Functional brain imaging in late-life depression and dementia J Clin Psychiatry 1993; 54(Suppl.):21–25.
38. Kumar A, Thomas A, Lavretsky H, et al. Frontal white matter biochemical abnormalities in late-life major depression detected with proton magnetic resonance spectroscopy. Am J Psychiatry 2002; 159:630–636.
39. Kaszniak AW, Garron DC, Fox JH, et al. Cerebral atrophy, EEG slowing age, education, and cognitive functioning in suspected dementia. Neurology 1979; 29(9Pt 1):1273–1279.
40. Markand ON. Organic brain syndromes and dementias. In: Daly D, Pedley T, eds. Current Practice of Clinical Neurophysiology: Electroencephalography, 2nd ed. New York, NY: Raven Press, 1990:371–400.
41. Radermecker FJ. Degenerative diseases of the nervous system. In: Remond A, ed. Handbook of Electroencephalography and Clinical Neurophysiology, Vol 15 A. Amstrerdam, The Netherlands: Elsevier, 1977:162–191.
42. Robinson DJ, Merskey H, Blume WT, et al. Electroencephalography as an aid in the exclusion of Alzheimer's disease. Arch Neurol 1994; 51:280–284.
43. Gallo JJ, Marino S, Ford D, et al. Filters on the pathway to mental health care, II. Sociodemographic factors. Psychol Med 1995; 25:1149–1160.
44. Blank K, Cohen C, Cohen G. Failure to adequately detect suicidal intent in elderly patients in the primary care setting. Clinical Geriatrics 2001; 9:26–36.
45. Harman JS, Brown EL, Have TT, et al. Primary care physicians attitude toward diagnosis and treatment of late-life depression. CNS Spectr 2002; 7:784–790.
46. Oxman TE. New paradigms for understanding the identification and treatment of depression in primary care. Gen Hosp Psychiatry 1997; 19:79–81.
47. Mulrow CD, Williams JW Jr, Gerety MB, et al. Case-finding instruments for depression in primary care settings. Ann Intern Med 1995; 122:913–921.
48. Schade CP, Jones ER Jr, Wittlin BJ. A ten-year review of the validity and clinical utility of depression screening. Psychiatr Serv 1998; 49:55–61.
49. Barrett JE, Barrett JA, Oxman TE, et al. The prevalence of psychiatric disorders in a primary care practice. Arch Gen Psychiatry 1988; 45:1100–1106.
50. Gallo JJ, Coyne JC. The challenge of depression in late life: Bridging science and service in primary care JAMA 2000; 284:1570–1572.
51. Greenfield SF, Reizes JM, Magruder KM, et al. Effectiveness of community-based screening for depression. Am J Psychiatry 1997; 154:1391–1397.
52. Greenfield SF, Reizes JM, Muenz LR, et al. Treatment for depression following the 1996 national depression screening day Am J Psychiatry 2000; 157:1867–1869.
53. Lawrence JM, Davidoff DA, Katt-Lloyd D, et al. Is large-scale community memory screening feasible? Experience from a regional memory-screening day. J Am Geriatr Soc 2003; 51:1072–1078.

54. Reynolds CF III, Dew MA, Frank E, et al. Effects of age at onset of first lifetime episode of recurrent major depression on treatment response and illness course in elderly patients. Am J Psychiatry 1998; 155:795–799.
55. Caine E, Lyness J, King DA. Reconsidering depression in the elderly. Am J Geriatr Psychiatry 1993; 1:4–20.
56. Alexopoulos GS, Meyers BS, Young RC, et al. Recovery in geriatric depression. Arch Gen Psychiatry 1996; 53:305–312.
57. Krishnan K, Gadde K. The pathophysiologic basis for late-life depression—Imaging studies of the aging brain. Am J Geriatr Psychiatry 1996; 4(4 Suppl.):S22–S33.
58. Lebowitz BD, Pearson JL, Schneider LS, et al. Diagnosis and treatment of depression in late life. Consensus statement update JAMA 1997; 278:1186–1190.
59. Shulman KI, Herrmann N. The nature and management of mania in old age. Psychiatr Clin North Am 1999; 22:649–665.
60. Schurhoff F, Bellivier F, Jouvent R, et al. Early and late onset bipolar disorders: Two different forms of manic-depressive illness? J Affect Disord 2000; 58:215–221.
61. Berthier ML, Kulisevsky J, Gironell A, et al. Poststroke bipolar affective disorder: Clinical subtypes, concurrent movement disorders, and anatomical correlates J Neuropsychiatry Clin Neurosci 1996; 8:160–167.
62. McDonald WM, Krishnan KR, Doraiswamy PM, et al. Occurrence of subcortical hyperintensities in elderly subjects with mania. Psychiatry Res 1991; 40:211–220.
63. Raskind MA. The clinical interface of depression and dementia. J Clin Psychiatry 1998; 59(Suppl. 10):9–12.
64. Devanand DP, Sano M, Tang MX, et al. Depressed mood and the incidence of Alzheimer's disease in the elderly living in the community. Arch Gen Psychiatry 1996; 53:175–182.
65. Chen P, Ganguli M, Mulsant BH, et al. The temporal relationship between depressive symptoms and dementia: A community-based prospective study Arch Gen Psychiatry 1999; 56:261–266.
66. Geerlings MI, Schoevers RA, Beekman AT, et al. Depression and risk of cognitive decline and Alzheimer's disease. Results of two prospective community-based studies in the Netherlands. Br J Psychiatry 2000; 176:568–575.
67. Berger AK, Fratiglioni L, Forsell Y, et al. The occurrence of depressive symptoms in the preclinical phase of AD: A population-based study Neurology 1999; 53:1998–2002.
68. Dufouil C, Fuhrer R, Dartigues JF, et al. Longitudinal analysis of the association between depressive symptomatology and cognitive deterioration. Am J Epidemiol 1996; 144:634–641.
69. Kindermann SS, Brown GG. Depression and memory in the elderly: A meta-analysis J Clin Exp Neuropsychol 1997; 19:625–642.
70. Bassuk SS, Glass TA, Berkman LF. Social disengagement and incident cognitive decline in community-dwelling elderly persons. Ann Intern Med 1999; 131:165–173.
71. Bassuk SS, Berkman LF, Wypij D. Depressive symptomatology and incident cognitive decline in an elderly community sample. Arch Gen Psychiatry 1998; 55:1073–1081.
72. Cancellaro LA. Depression or dementia? South Med J 2001; 94:663.
73. Migliorelli R, Teson A, Sabe L, et al. Prevalence and correlates of dysthymia and major depression among patients with Alzheimer's disease. Am J Psychiatry 1995; 152:37–44.
74. Ott BR, Fogel BS. Measurement of depression in dementia: Self vs. clinical rating Int J Geriatr Psychiatry 1992; 7:899–904.
75. Veiel HO. A preliminary profile of neuropsychological deficits associated with major depression J Clin Exp Neuropsychol 1997; 19:587–603.

2 Geriatric Nonmajor Depressive Syndromes: Minor Depression, Dysthymia, and Subsyndromal Depression

Helen Lavretsky

Department of Psychiatry and Biobehavioral Sciences, David Geffen School of Medicine at UCLA, and Semel Institute for Neuroscience and Human Behavior at UCLA, Los Angeles, California, U.S.A.

Jeffrey M. Lyness

Department of Psychiatry, University of Rochester Medical Center, Rochester, New York, U.S.A.

INTRODUCTION

Depression of any severity in later life often carries with it serious health consequences, including increased mortality related to suicide and medical illness, amplification of disability associated with medical and cognitive disorders, and increased health care costs (1–3). Although major depressive disorder is the most studied and most clearly defined depressive syndrome, other depressive syndromes and subsyndromal conditions are also associated with significant functional impairment and disability. These so-called "lesser" or nonmajor clinical categories, which have received relatively scant attention in the psychiatric literature, are of considerable importance in the geriatric population.

Nonmajor depressive disorders such as dysthymic disorder, minor depression, and subsyndromal depression are thought to impact as many as 15% of community-dwelling elders (4) and as many as 70% of elders living in long-term care settings (5). Like major depressive disorder, these conditions contribute substantially to functional impairment and morbidity (6), yet the criteria for major depressive disorder outlined in the DSM-III and DSM-IV TR do not capture less severe symptomatology in depressed elders (8) and the presence of nonmajor depressive states often goes undetected. Blazer (10) observed that elderly patients rarely report depressed mood despite appearing to be depressed as determined by the presence of other depressive symptoms and measurable outcomes. Indeed research consistently reports the under-recognition of depressive symptomatology in elderly patients in both the primary care and nursing home settings, suggesting that greater attention must be paid to recognizing nonmajor depressive disorders (7). This chapter focuses on the identification, appreciation, and management of the clinically significant depressive states that do not meet established criteria for the *Diagnostic and Statistical Manual of Mental Disorders, 4th Edition* (DSM-IV) Major Depressive Disorder (MDD).

The disorders to be discussed here are categorized into several clinical subtypes differentiated by relatively subtle distinctions. We will discuss the clinical heterogeneity and nosologic complexities of these disorders, propose diagnostic criteria, and review the research data. We will highlight the phenomenological, neurobiological, and therapeutic evidence that characterize and support the validity of this category of disorders. Finally, we will examine the published evidence in support of the clinical utility of the nonmajor depressive syndromes.

DEFINITIONS AND CLINICAL FEATURES

Because the literature in this area is still in an evolving state, researchers and clinicians have not yet settled upon a universal definition of "less than major" depression. At present, minor and subsyndromal states are defined, as their names suggest, in terms of their differentiation from major depressive disorder, determined by differences in the severity, number, or duration of depressive symptoms.

The most important DSM-IV TR disorders that may present with nonmajor depressive symptoms are listed in Table 1 (11). Depression not otherwise specified (NOS) comprises a collection of disorders characterized by depressive symptoms but still in conceptual evolution, including such conditions as minor depressive disorder, premenstrual dysphoric disorder, recurrent brief depressive disorder, postpsychotic depressive disorder of schizophrenia, a major depressive episode superimposed on a psychotic disorder; and depressive states of unclear origin. In recognition of the need for more precise characterization of nonmajor depressive syndromes, the DSM-IV TR includes tentative criteria sets for minor depressive disorder, recurrent brief depressive disorder (RBD), and mixed anxiety-depressive disorder. Although this list indicates a move toward greater recognition of depressive spectrum disorders in all their complexity, it still does not cover all clinical presentations of persons suffering from clinically significant depressive symptoms.

One consequence of diagnostic imprecision and incompleteness is that the actual prevalence of nonmajor depressive states remains unclear. For example, the term "minor" depression is frequently used to encompass all cases of clinically significant depression failing to meet criteria for major depressive disorder rather than those cases that specifically conform to the criteria listed in DSM-IV TR as minor depression. The somewhat confusing term "subthreshold major depression," which has emerged as an alternative to the ambiguous term "minor depression," is used to indicate patients with fewer than the five depressive symptoms required in order to meet diagnostic criteria for major depressive disorder. These patients, despite falling short of a major depressive disorder diagnosis, have been shown in two epidemiologic surveys to have significant impairment in both social and occupational role functioning (12,13). Further research may help to clarify the

TABLE 1 DSM-IV TR Diagnostic Categories that may Present with Nonmajor Depressive Symptoms

major depressive episode in partial remission
depression NOS
minor depressive disorder
recurrent brief depressive disorder
mood disorder due to a general medical condition, with depressive features
dementia with depressed mood
adjustment disorder with depressed mood
substance induced mood disorder with depressive features
anxiety disorder with depressive features
dysthymic disorder

relationship of subthreshold major depression to minor depression and to explicate its course, outcome, and suicide risk.

NONMAJOR DEPRESSION'S PROMINENCE IN THE ELDERLY

Despite definitional ambiguity, the significance of geriatric nonmajor depressive disorders has been recognized by geriatric clinicians and researchers. (6,13–14). In medically ill older adults, for example, the identification of nonmajor depressive syndromes, achieved through an inclusive diagnostic method of counting depressive symptoms, has revealed that these syndromes have both a relatively high prevalence and an important predictive value (15). Awareness of the clinical significance of nonmajor depressive syndromes has also helped clinicians to understand what at first seems a paradoxical combination in the elderly of more prevalent depressive symptoms yet lower prevalence of DSM-IV TR major depressive disorder as compared to younger populations (16). Table 2 outlines proposed diagnostic criteria for nonmajor depression and Table 3 describes representative studies of nonmajor depression. Explanations of the difference in prevalence of minor

(*text continued on page 24*)

TABLE 2 Proposed Diagnostic Criteria for Clinically Significant Nonmajor Depression

1. Presence of low mood or loss of interest in all activities most of the day, nearly every day.
2. At least two additional symptoms from the DSM checklist,
   - Significant weight loss when not dieting or weight gain (a change of more than 5% in body weight in a month) or a decrease or increase in appetite nearly every day;
   - Insomnia or hypersomnia nearly every day;
   - Psychomotor retardation or agitation nearly every day (observable by others, not merely subjective feelings of restlessness or slowness);
   - Fatigue or loss of energy nearly every day;
   - Feelings of worthlessness or excessive or inappropriate guilt (which may be delusional) nearly every day (not merely self-reproach or guilt about being sick);
   - Diminished ability to think or concentrate, or indecisiveness, nearly every day (either by subjective account or as observed by others);
   - Recurrent thoughts of death (not just fear of dying), recurrent suicidal ideation without a specific plan, or a suicide attempt, or a specific plan for committing suicide.
3. The symptoms cause clinically significant distress or impairment in social and occupational functioning.
4. A score of at least 10 on the 17-item Hamilton depression scale or at least 12 on the geriatric depression scale (GDS) (or a GDS score of at least 5 on the 15-item scale).
5. Duration of at least one month; duration subtypes are, 1 to 6 months, 6 to 24 months, and more than 24 months.
6. The symptoms may be associated with precipitating events, such as the loss of a significant other.
7. Organic criteria based on comorbid conditions are as follows:
   - objective evidence from physical and neurologic examination and laboratory tests or history of cerebral disease, damage, or dysfunction or of systemic physical disorder known to cause cerebral dysfunction, including hormonal disturbances and drug effects.
   - a presumed relationship between the development or exacerbation of the underlying disease and clinically significant depression.
   - the disturbance is confined to the direct psychological effect of alcohol or drug use.
   - recovery or significant improvement in the depressive symptoms after removal of or improvement in the underlying presumed cause.
8. Exclusion criteria: No lifetime history of an episode of mania or hypomania, or a chronic psychotic disorder, such as schizophrenia or delusional disorder. History of major depressive episode is not an exclusion criterion.

Source: Adapted from Ref. 83.

TABLE 3 Representative Studies of Nonmajor Clinically Significant Depression

Area of research	Authors	Study design	Sample	Depressive subtype	Results
Epidemiology 1. Community samples	(60)	Literature review by the level of casesness	Review of 16 community studies of geriatric depression in 22,794 patients	Major depression, Minor depression, Depressive symptoms	Weighted average prevalence of major depression, 1.8%; minor depression, 9.8%; depressive symptoms, 13.5%
	(44)	A community sample- 86 subjects age 60 and older	Prevalence rates of life-time prevalence	Minor, major, and subthreshold depression	4.9% had a life-time diagnosis of major depression and 31.8% either minor or recurrent brief depression
	(66)	90% of Cache county (Utah) elderly community sample	4,559 individuals, aged 65–100 years	Major, minor, subclinical depression	Prevalence of major depression was 4.4% in women and 2.7% in men. Lifetime prevalence was 20.4% in women and 9.6% of men decreasing with age. Only 35.7% with MDD were treated with antidepressants
	(61)	A community survey in Edmonton, Canada	1119 community residents aged 65 years and older were administered the Geriatric Mental State (GMS) questionnaire and compared to the DSM-III R diagnoses	Major and Minor depression	Prevalence of GMS-AGECAT depression (11.4%) was higher than the DSM-III R diagnosis of major (0.86%) or minor depression (3.6%), which was determined mainly by proportion of dysphoric symptoms of the instrument
	(58)	Cross-sectional prevalence and clinical correlates study of depression	ICD-10 and DSM-III R depressive diagnoses	Depressive disorder versus symptoms	Elderly had many depressive symptoms, which did not increase with age. The number of depressive symptoms correlated with neuroticism, poor physical health, disability, and prior depression

2. Medical illness	(54)	Prevalence of depression in patients with congestive heart failure	542 consecutive medical patients	Major and minor depression	Major depression rate was 36.5% in patients with CHF compared to 25.5% in patients without CHF. The rate of minor depression was 21.5% in patients with CHF compared to 17% in patients without CHF
	(25)	Prevalence of depression in primary care patients and associated functional disability	224 outpatients age 60 and older in the outpatient family medicine and internal medicine practices	Major, minor subsyndromal depression	31.7% of patients had a diagnosis of a mental disorder. Major depression-6.5%, minor depression-5.2%, subsyndromal-9.9%, 0.9% for dysthymia. Subsyndromal depression is associated with functional disability and medical comorbidity, and often treated with antidepressants
3. Neurological illness	(85)	Risk factors for minor and major depression in 15 month follow-up	164 poststroke and 100 control subjects	Major and Minor depression	Major or minor depression was present in 20.7% at follow-up. Depression was associated with dementia and functional impairment at follow-up
	(94)	Risk factors for poststroke depression in 4 months follow-up	191 first ever stroke patients were followed for 4 months	Major and minor depression	17% had major and 11%had minor depression at 4 months poststroke. Predictors of depression included functional impairment, living in a nursing home, being divorced
	(95)	Cross-sectional study	33 patients with Alzheimer disease	Depressive symptoms	Frequency ranged 6–33% depending on definition of depression and instruments used
	(96)	Cross-sectional comparison of patients with Parkinson disease and Progressive Supranuclear Palsy (PSP)	19 patients with PSP and 42 with Parkinson disease	Depressive symptoms	42% of the PSP group had mild-to-moderate depression. 52% of patients had some degree of dementia

(*Continued*)

TABLE 3 Representative Studies of Nonmajor Clinically Significant Depression (*Continued*)

Area of research	Authors	Study design	Sample	Depressive subtype	Results
	(97)	Four diagnostic systems for dementia and depression were compared by using Latent Trait Ananlysis	274 community dwelling elderly	Depression and dementia	DSM-III, Gurland's system and AGECAT, and clinician's ratings were used. Two distinct clusters of symptoms were identified and the levelof severity (threshold) was identified
Phenomenology	(98)	Epidemiological Berlin Aging Study (BASE)	Community sample	Subthreshold depression, Dysthymia, Major depression	Subthreshold depression had fewer symptoms with less continuity; with fewer suicidal ideations, thoughts of guilt or worthlessness
	(99)	Cross-sectional comparison of older and younger adults	193 outpatients in the internal medicine and family practices	Minor depression	No differences were observed between older and younger adults with minor depression
	(100)	2-year follow-up	20 bereaved elderly	Subsyndromal depression	Subsyndromal depression was associated with greater functional impairment, worse sleep quality, less perceived interpersonal support, and more intense grieving, than nondepressed bereaved subjects
Outcomes	(18)	Cross-sectional association study of depression and disability	646 community-dwelling older adults aged 55–85 years	Major and minor depression	Associations of major and minor depression with disability and well-being remained significant after controlling for chronic disease and functional limitations. Adequate treatment was often not administered, even in subjects with major depression. Major and minor depression were associated with an excessive use of nonmental health services

	(101)	A longitudinal follow-up of the community sample	2847 community-dwelling persons aged 55–85; 450 subjects with and 2397 subjects without cardiac disease	Major depression (DSM-III) and minor depression (CES-D > 16)	Depression increased the risk of cardiac mortality in subjects with and without cardiac disease. The excess cardiac mortality was more than twice as high for major depression as for minor depression
	(102)	Longitudinal follow-up of a community sample (4.5 years)	3107 older persons (55–85 years old)	Major depression (DSM-III) and minor depression (CES-D > 16)	At baseline, 12.8% had minor depression, and 2% had major depression. Minor depression was associated with a significantly greater decline in functional status and performance, as well as with increased risk of death in men. Major depression increased risk of functional decline and death in men and women
	(103)	Epidemiologic follow-up of community samples (the established populations for epidemiologic studies of the elderly)	4825 persons aged 71 years and older followed up at 3 and 6 years	Chronic depression (CES-D) based on cutoff criteria	When present for at least 6 years, depression was associated with a generally increased risk of cancer, after controlling for age, sex, race, disability, hospital admissions, alcohol intake, and smoking
Neuroimaging	(62)	Cross-sectional quantitative MRI study: whole brain volumes and normalized measures of prefrontal and temporal volumes	18 subjects with minor depression, 35 patients with late-onset major depression, and 30 normal controls	Major and minor depression	Normalized prefrontal lobe volumes show a significant linear trend with severity of depression, with volumes decreasing with volume severity
Genetics	Anderson et al., 1996 (104)	A family study of subaffective-character spectrum and primary dysthymia	97 early-onset dysthymic outpatients received diagnostic interview and family history interviews	Dysthymia, subaffective disorder	Subaffectives had had higher rates of major depression, depressive symptoms, and depressive personality features, as well as higher rate of alcoholism in families

(*Continued*)

TABLE 3 Representative Studies of Nonmajor Clinically Significant Depression (*Continued*)

Area of research	Authors	Study design	Sample	Depressive subtype	Results
	(60)	Family study	Examined first degree relatives of probands with depressive-spectrum diagnosis	Probands with minor depression, major depression, dysthymia, and "double" depression	When morbidity risks were calculated for the first-degree relatives using the maximum likelihood approach, the results showed no significant differences in morbidity risk calculations to first-degree relatives
Cognition	(86)	Cross-sectional sample of minor- and major depressed patients and nondepressed volunteers	95 elderly subjects with minor- and major depression and 71 control volunteers	Executive function was a mediator for depressed patients verbal learning scores.	Verbal memory deficits result from impaired executive functioning Patients with minor depression performed in the impaired range between patients with depression and normal controls
Interventions	(87)	16 weeks of randomized trial of sertraline, exercise, or usual care	37 elderly outpatients with minor depression	Minor depression	Sertraline and exercise were superior to usual care in improving depression and mental health. Exercise improved physical health
	(77)	Meta-analysis of 89 studies of depressive disorders	5328 older adults received pharmaco- or psychotherapy	Nonmajor depressive disorders	Clinician-rated depression scores improved by 0.80 standard deviation (SD) units, and by 0.69 SD units in pharmacotherapeutic studies compared to 1.09 SD units in studies of psychotherapy
	(82)	138 elderly minor depression	Subjects received citalopram 20mg/day (66) or sertraline 50mg/day (72) for 1 year.	Minor and subsyndromal depression	Sertraline and citalopram improved depressive and cognitive symptoms. Nearly 50% achieved remission
	(17)	6-week open-label study of sertraline treatment of minor depression	12 nursing home residents	Minor depression	75% achieved remission and all tolerated medication well

(105)	Cognitive-behavioral intervention for minor depression	Elderly Chinese Americans were assigned to intervention versus controls	Minor depression	The experimental group showed an improvement and the control group did not
(76)	Randomized 11-week effectiveness trial	Comparing paroxetine to placebo, and Problem Solving Therapy in primary care (PST-PC).	Minor depression, Dysthymia	The paroxetine group showed greater symptoms resolution than the placebo group in patient with dysthymia and minor depression. Patients treated with PST-PC did not show more improvement than placebo, but their symptoms improved more rapidly than those of placebo patients
(78), PROSPECT	Randomized controlled trial in primary care	Based on a clinical algorithm, including antidepressants or IPT	Major or "clinically significant" minor depression with outcome suicidal ideations	Did not find a treatment effects for minor depression unless with suicidalitiy
(88) IMPACT	Randomized controlled trial in primary care	Depression care manager, psychotherapy, or antidperessants	1801 elderly with major depression (17%), dysthymic disorder (30%), or both (53%)	Treatment improved depression and function
(79), PEARLS	Home-based program	PST and depression care manager	138 elderly with minor depression (51.4%) or dysthymia (48.6%)	Treatment improved depression and function

Representative studies of late-life major and nonmajor depression, as well as genetic studies addressing depressive spectrum have been included in the Table.
Source: Adapted from Ref. 1.

depressive syndromes between older and younger populations have been suggested and some of these are discussed in detail also, in chapter 3 of this book. While it is possible that there is indeed a true decline in the prevalence of major depressive disorder and emergence of more frequent minor depressive states in the elderly, an alternative possibility is that "major depression" in the elderly expresses itself with fewer identifiable symptoms or a different set of symptoms, creating a false semantic distinction between major and minor disorders in this group. Other possibilities are that the differences in prevalence of major and minor depressive diagnoses among age groups can be explained by cohort effects (due to an increasing rate of depression in successive generations), nonparticipation of more depressed elders in studies, selective forgetting of major depressive symptoms or past episodes in the elderly, or validity problems with diagnostic instruments used to determine the presence of depression in the elderly. The setting in which an elderly population is studied, furthermore, affects the measured prevalence of depressive symptoms. The importance of setting is shown by studies of long-term care facility residents, up to 50% of whom can be diagnosed with nonmajor depressive states. Up to 25% of individuals assessed in a primary care setting meet diagnostic criteria for these conditions as well.

DSM-IV TR DEFINITIONS: DYSTHYMIC DISORDER AND MINOR DEPRESSIVE DISORDER

Dysthymic disorder is defined as a mild chronic depression of at least two years duration, though it has often been present even longer, with no extended remission during that period and no prior major depressive disorder or other explanatory diagnosis. DSM-IV TR specifies early-onset as before age 21, late-onset as 21 or older. The research literature uses the term "double depression" to indicate that a patient with preexisting dysthymic disorder has subsequently experienced one or more major depressive episodes. Concomitant personality disorders are common among young adults with dysthymic disorder (19,20) and further studies are needed in order to assess the level of comorbidity of depressive disorders with personality disorders among older adults.

Minor depressive disorder is a DSM-IV TR "category under consideration" with a set of diagnostic research criteria proposed for further studies (11). The essential criterion for diagnosis of minor depression is one or more episodes that resemble major depressive episodes in duration 2 weeks or longer, but manifest fewer symptoms and less impairment. Symptoms meeting research criteria for minor depression can be difficult to distinguish from periods of sadness that are an inherent part of everyday life; however, the minor depressive disorder diagnosis requires that these depressive symptoms cause clinically significant distress or impairment. Minor depression is considered to be a residual category and is not to be used if there is a history of a major depressive episode, manic episode, mixed episode, or hypomanic episode, or if the presentation meets the criteria for dysthymic or cyclothymic disorder. This definition places minor depression within a depressive disorders spectrum in which diagnoses can be conceptualized as differing in number of episodes, severity, and duration of symptoms ranging from least to most severe.

AN ADDITIONAL SUGGESTED DIAGNOSTIC CATEGORY: SUBSYNDROMAL DEPRESSIVE SPECTRUM DISORDERS

To introduce consistency into a confusing nosology and to avoid use of the ambiguous term "minor depression," Lavretsky and Kumar have proposed that the term *subsyndromal depressive spectrum disorder* be used to describe a group of states (7) operationally defined by the presence of any two or more concurrent symptoms of depression that persist for at least two weeks, are associated with evidence of social dysfunction, and occur in patients who do not meet criteria for a diagnosis of DSM-IV-defined major depression, dysthymic disorder, or minor depression (21). Besides providing a more inclusive category for nonmajor depressive syndromes, the use of this "subsyndromal" category facilitates the differential characterization of a clinically significant nonmajor depression's longitudinal course (22–23). Prospective longitudinal data from studies of young adults reveal that major depressive disorders are frequently both antecedent to and sequelae of subsyndromal states, providing evidence for the validity of the spectrum concept of depression in major and nonmajor forms (22).

Several investigators involved in longitudinal studies of large populations of adult and geriatric patients have reported evidence that supports the validity of a subsyndromal depressive spectrum. Angst and colleagues (23), for example, found very little stability for the specific types of depression presented at baseline by patients who remained symptomatic during a follow-up period; 51% of those initially diagnosed with major depressive disorder and 44% of those with recurrent brief depression (RBD) also met criteria for another subtype of during a follow up period. Among subjects diagnosed with a single subtype, symptom severity was actually the greatest among those with dysthymic disorder. These researchers concluded that symptom threshold and recurrence were better predictors of illness outcome than the distinction between minor and major depression (2) in this cohort of adults. In research on geriatric subjects, Lyness and colleagues have explored the predictive value of depressive symptoms and varying definitions of subsyndromal depression forecasting outcome. When defined simply as a low score ($\leq$10) on the Hamilton Rating Scale for Depression (Ham-D) (24), the prevalence of subsyndromal depression in a geriatric population was 9.9% (25), while alternate definitions yielded higher prevalence estimates; the presence of any two threshold symptoms from the proposed SSD definition in Table 2, for example, lifted the prevalence to 16.2%, while requiring the presence of depressed mood or decreased interest along with one other threshold or subthreshold symptom increased the prevalence estimate to 28.1%. (14). Each of these SSD definitions identified a group of elders that were more symptomatic and more functionally impaired than a nondepressed group but not quite so impaired as those with DSM-IV TR minor or major depressive disorders. Analyses comparing the outcomes of these three SSD groups are currently in progress.

Interestingly, Lyness and colleagues found that patients with subsyndromal depression were being treated with antidepressant medications by their primary care physicians at rates comparable to those for minor and major depressive disorders (25). This finding highlights the need for further research addressing the efficacy and safety of pharmacotherapy of SSD, which may well be effective but is not at present evidence based.

DIFFERENTIAL DIAGNOSIS OF NONMAJOR GERIATRIC DEPRESSIVE DISORDERS

In the differential diagnosis of nonmajor clinically significant depression (10), three syndromes of particular importance are Adjustment disorder with depressed mood, complicated bereavement, and substance induced mood disorder. Adjustment disorder with depressed mood is diagnosed if the depressive symptoms occur in response to a psychosocial stressor. Depressive disorder NOS, the DSMIVTR category that currently includes minor depressive disorder, encompasses a spectrum of syndromes, many with fewer than the 4 depressive symptoms required for a diagnosis of major depressive disorder. Criteria under consideration for the diagnosis of minor depressive disorder suggest that 2 to 4 depressive symptoms be required.

Depressive symptoms developed in response to the loss of a loved one are generally attributed to bereavement, discussed in Chapter 14 of this book. In studies of spousal bereavement, prior history of depression predicted future depression throughout the unipolar depressive spectrum (40). Subsyndromal and minor depression stood between major depression and no depression in terms of their effect on overall adjustment to widowhood, reinforcing the "spectrum" concept. Prigerson and colleagues identified distinct patterns of symptoms in complicated grief and bereavement-related depression (41). Seven symptoms characterized complicated grief, which are, searching, yearning, preoccupation with thoughts of the deceased, crying, disbelief regarding the death, feeling stunned by the death, and the lack of acceptance of the death. These symptoms were associated with enduring functional impairment.

Substance-induced mood disorder is due to the direct physiologic effects of a drug of abuse, or due to the side effects of a medication (e.g., steroids). Mood disorder due to a general medical condition is diagnosed when depression is considered due to the direct effect of a general medical condition.

THE IMPORTANCE OF COMORBIDITY

Comorbid personality disorder traits or axis I psychiatric disorders can affect the clinical course and prognosis of a nonmajor depressive disorder and may diminish functional capacity in late-life major depression. Overall, however, the research database on comorbidity of such conditions in major and nonmajor late-life depression is relatively sparse. We will summarize data relative to comorbid personality disorders or traits, alcohol-use disorders, and anxiety.

Personality disorders occur in 10% to 30% of patients with late-life major depression or dysthymic disorder, particularly in patients with early onset depressive illness. Cluster C disorders, including the avoidant, dependent, and obsessive-compulsive subtypes predominate, while Cluster B diagnoses, including borderline, narcissistic, histrionic, and antisocial, are rare (42). Subsyndromal depression in adult patients, often co-occurs with character traits such as neuroticism or "existential depression" (31). Longitudinal studies of what has been termed "characterological" depression, unsurprisingly, describe common transformations into moderate to melancholic or psychotic depressive, and even bipolar, disorders. Concurrent neuroticism, a well-characterized personality trait with demonstrated stability across the adult life span (32–33), has been associated with poor outcome in young adults with major depression (34–36), but has received relatively little investigation in older adults with major or nonmajor depression (37). Neuroticism, however, may moderate the important relationship between medical illness burden and major depression (38), and in one study independently predicted 1-year depression outcome (including both major and nonmajor depression) (39).

Generally, in late-life depression, common comorbid psychiatric disorders are alcohol use, anxiety, and personality disorders (42). Elderly depressed patients are three to four times more likely to have an alcohol-use disorder compared with nondepressed elderly subjects, with a prevalence of 15% to 30% in patients with late-life major depression. While the presence of a comorbid alcohol–use disorder may worsen the prognosis for geriatric depression, limited data suggest that successful treatment of depression combined with reducing alcohol use leads to the best possible outcomes.

Most studies show that the overall prevalences of anxiety disorders, particularly panic disorder and obsessive-compulsive disorder, are low in geriatric depression, but generalized anxiety disorder may be more common. It remains unclear if the presence of a comorbid anxiety disorder impacts on the treatment and prognosis of late-life major depression. Angst (27) examined coexisting depression and anxiety at both threshold and subthreshold levels. He attempted to improve diagnostic precision and clarify treatment needs by exploring a classification based on number of symptoms as well as their duration, frequency, and associated functional impairment (22,27). Comorbid anxiety, seen frequently with geriatric depression, presents an additional challenge to providing adequate treatment and achieving remission (28–30).

NONMAJOR DEPRESSION IN MEDICAL SETTINGS

In all settings, the prevalence of significant late-life depressive symptoms is 2- to 4-fold higher than the prevalence of major depression (5). Furthermore, the rates of both late-life symptoms and disorders in the elderly vary by setting. Among the institutionalized elderly, up to 70% acknowledge feeling "depressed, sad, or blue" at least enough to cause minor problems in their day-to-day activities. Many of the studies of nonmajor depression have been carried out in these institutional settings or in primary care, since these are the settings associated with a higher prevalence of nonmajor depression. Epidemiologic studies, in fact, have found that most older patients with mental illness are seen exclusively in primary care medicine (42–45). Between 3% and 16% of medical outpatients suffer from nonmajor depression, and up to 64% of medical outpatients acknowledge depressed mood (46). These patients often present with medically unexplained somatic symptoms and utilize at least twice as many health visits as those without depressive symptoms. In medical patients, depressive symptoms are likely to affect length of hospitalization and functional outcomes of the medical illness.

Depressive States in Medically Ill Older Adults

Studies of depression in the medically ill usually report depression's negative impact on the rates and speed of recovery as well as the overall outcome of medical illnesses, often producing additional disability as well as increased cost of care (46,52,53). In 542 patients aged 60 years and older, Koenig reported an increased risk for major or minor depression (OR 1.5–2) associated with the presence of congestive heart failure (CHF) (54). Compared with nondepressed CHF patients, those with depression were more likely to have comorbid psychiatric disorders, severe medical illness, and severe functional impairment. The depressed CHF patients characteristically remained depressed for a prolonged period, and more than 40% failed to remit during the year following their discharge. The majority of depressed CHF patients did not receive treatment for their depression with either antidepressants or psychotherapy.

Etiology and Pathogenesis of Nonmajor Depression

There is no etiologically based classification of depression, which is recognized as a truly multifactorial disorder (55–57). The antecedents to depression will differ even among individuals with similar symptoms and similar levels illness severity. Family or personal history of depression, psychosocial factors (e.g., marital status, social supports, life events) and physiologic influences (e.g., hormonal changes and increased inflammation with aging) reduce resilience to stress and increased vulnerability to developing depression in late life (58). The heterogeneous etiologic nature of depression may be all the more relevant to nonmajor depressive syndromes, and we will review some of the emerging data related to genetics, neuroimaging, and neuropsychological assessment.

Genetics

Genetic data, in the future, may shed light on nosologic and etiologic issues related to major and nonmajor depressive syndromes. To date, however, the results of association studies in behavioral genetics have been inconsistent. This is usually explained by the observation that some significant-appearing relationships between marker allele frequencies and psychiatric conditions prove to be artifactual, generated not be true differences in the predisposition to depression but rather by population heterogeneity, statistical errors introduced through unequal stratification of a population, or other confounding factors. Sher suggested that a major problem with association studies in psychiatric disorders is that analyses have been predicated on psychiatric diagnoses that represent theoretical rather than biological constructs; in other words, a syndromal psychiatric diagnosis such as depression includes etiologically, pathologically, and prognostically heterogeneous disorders (59).

Genetic studies have only minimally addressed subsyndromal depressive spectrum disorders and, when they do, will need to address the very significant confounding factors associated with the evolving diagnostic categorizations of these disorders. One initial foray into this complex area was reported by Remick and colleagues, who examined first-degree relatives of probands with diagnoses of minor depression, major depression, dysthymia, and "double" depression (60). When morbidity risks were calculated for the first-degree relatives using the maximum likelihood approach, the results for these relatives showed no significant differences. From the genetic perspective employed in this study, there was no way to demonstrate familial aggregation of single depression, recurrent depression, minor depression, or double depression. This finding could raise some doubt concerning the validity of a biologic differentiation among these clinically differentiated depressive spectrum disorders.

Neuroimaging

Both computerized tomography (CT) and magnetic resonance imaging (MRI) studies have shown that late-life major depressive disorder is associated with widespread neuroanatomic changes in neocortical areas and subcortical nuclei. Neuroimaging studies of geriatric nonmajor depressed patients, however, are very limited at present. One recent report demonstrated that patients with late-life minor depression had smaller prefrontal lobe volumes compared to age-matched, nondepressed controls (61). The findings indicate that patients with minor depression may present with specific neuroanatomic abnormalities that are similar to those in the major depression group but significantly different from controls (62). Normalized prefrontal lobe volumes showed a significant linear correlation between decreased volume and increased depression severity. Whole brain volumes did not differ significantly among groups. These findings are consistent with the hypothesis of common neurobiological substrates across a spectrum of depressive disorders. Neuroanatomic abnormalities may represent one aspect of a broader neurobiological diathesis to late-life mood disorders. Additional studies combining neuroimaging with focused postmortem and other neurochemical studies are required to further elucidate the biologic basis of late-life mood disorders. Research is just beginning to examine the extent to which structural abnormalities of the brain, such as white matter hyperintensities on MRI, covary with functional deficits. Furthermore, among depressed patients, continued memory decline is associated with lower baseline hippocampal volume but not with the hypercortisolemia that is considered a correlate of depression severity (63).

Functional neuroimaging correlates have been identified for late-life major depressive disorder and include widespread reductions in glucose metabolism and cerebral blood flow on positron emission tomography (PET) and single photon emission-computed tomography (SPECT). Cerebral blood flow and metabolism are reduced in prefrontal cortical regions, superior temporal and anterior–parietal areas in major depressive disorder (64). Matsui et al. studied patients with Parkinson disease with and without minor depression using SPECT (65). They reported hypoperfusion of the left superior and inferior frontal gyrus in depressed patients. Other functional imaging studies of subsyndromal mood disorders in late life are lacking to date, but could provide information about the pathophysiology of these conditions compared to syndromal depression. Postmortem tissue from well-characterized samples will better elucidate the pathways to depression and to cognitive impairment, especially if the samples can be integrated with antemortem neuroimaging findings.

Neuropsychological Assessment

Patients with minor depression show functional and cognitive deficits similar in many ways to those demonstrated by patients with major depressive disorder (66–68). One study demonstrated that both patients with minor and major depression differed similarly from controls on an executive composite score that includes visuospatial construction, complex attention, and visual naming, but those with minor depressions were not so impaired as those with major depression on a verbal learning and recall composite score (66). Verbal recall scores across both major and minor patients correlated negatively with depression severity as measured by the Hamilton Depression Scale. The relationship between cognitive impairment and late-life minor depressive syndromes is of clinical significance and bears further investigation.

TREATMENT

Studies evaluating the treatment of nonmajor depressive disorders are limited to date. Most of the available studies have focused on dysthymia and minor depression, and have been sited in primary care settings (6,72–75). Descriptive studies have established that in treating depression primary care providers use one or more of following three modalities. Watchful waiting, medication, and referral to specialists (48). Used most commonly, watchful waiting entails monitoring return visits, providing sympathetic listening and a show of interest, and in some cases brief "common sense" counseling and tension-reducing suggestions (48).

Several recent randomized trials have compared different strategies for management of nonmajor depression. In one U.S. randomized 11-week effectiveness trial comparing paroxetine to placebo and problem solving therapy in primary care (PST-PC), the paroxetine group showed greater symptom resolution than the placebo group. Paroxetine showed moderate benefit for depressive symptoms and mental health functioning in elderly patients with dysthymia and more severely impaired elderly patients with minor depression. The benefits of PST-PC were smaller, slower to manifest, and more vulnerable to site differences than those of paroxetine. Patients treated with PST-PC did not show more improvement than placebo, but their symptoms improved more rapidly than those of placebo patients during the latter treatment weeks. PST-PC/placebo differences were more pronounced in the minor depression group than in patients with dysthymia (76).

In a recent meta-analysis, Pinquart and colleagues integrated the results of 89 controlled studies of treatments for acute major depression (37 studies) and other depressive disorders (52 studies conducted with mixed diagnostic groups, including patients with major depression, minor depression, and dysthymia) (77). A total of 5328 older adults received pharmacotherapy or psychotherapy in these studies. The authors reported that for those studies including less severe forms of depression, psychosocial treatments had larger effect sizes than do pharmacologic treatments. Unfortunately, there were not enough studies focusing specifically on less-than-major depression, or studies with well-operationalized less-than-major patients, to allow separate analyses of these groups.

Several recent collaborative trials have addressed the effectiveness of antidepressant treatment in patients with depressive syndromes treated in primary care settings. Two of these are the NIMH-supported Prevention of Suicide in the Primary Care Elderly Collaborative Trial (PROSPECT) study, (73) and the Hartford Foundation-supported Improving Mood: Promoting Access to Collaborative Treatment for Late Life Depression (IMPACT) study. Both evaluated the effectiveness of Depression Care Management models that supplemented primary care with the involvement of a nurse health specialist (74). IMPACT's on-site collaborative care model, using a depression care manager to support antidepressant medication treatment or brief psychotherapy, was effective in improving symptomatic and functional outcomes for older primary care patients with major depression or dysthymic disorder treated in the primary care setting (74). The PROSPECT study evaluated a program in which the intervention group received care based on a clinical algorithm that offered depressed participants antidepressant medication or, for those declining medication, the offer of a brief individual psychotherapy called interpersonal therapy. Depression care managers located on site in the various primary care practices implemented the treatment management. Patients were recruited if they had either major depression or "clinically significant" minor depression. The PROSPECT intervention substantially reduced suicidal ideation at rates comparable with that seen in prior efficacy studies and in specialty mental health clinical settings. However, the reduction in overall depressive symptoms for the minor depression subgroup did not differ significantly from that in the control group, save for the relative few whose initial symptoms included suicidal ideation. It is possible that improvement in the minor depression usual care group resulted from improved physician recognition of depression, but other factors may also have been involved, such as a tendency for milder types of depression to improve even under study control conditions, which in effect often amount to a nonspecific supportive psychosocial intervention (79)

Further collaborative treatment data come from the report by Ciechanowski and colleagues of findings from a randomized controlled trial of a home-based program called PEARLS (Program to Encourage Active, Rewarding Lives for Seniors) that offered treatment for minor depression or dysthymic disorder in seniors recruited through community agencies (80). The intervention group received problem-solving therapy, modified to emphasize physical activity and increased socialization. For participants who did not improve during the first few weeks, a depression care management team made recommendations to the primary care physician about diagnostic evaluation and antidepressant medication therapy. These interventions improved symptomatic and functional states substantially, with outcomes comparable to those from primary care–based studies that included patients with major depression. The PEARLS intervention, while different from PROSPECT, similarly lends itself to adaptation and implementation across a variety of settings, including community agencies in the case of PEARLS.

Only a few recent trials among outpatients and nursing home residents find promise in alleviating depressive symptoms through pharmacotherapy alone. In an open label study of fluvoxamine, patients with minor depression and subthreshold depression associated with dysfunction and disability demonstrated improvement in depression and functioning (81). In an open trial of sertraline, involving 12 nursing home residents who met the DSM-IV description for minor depressive disorder, 75% of patients reached remission by week six. All patients were able to tolerate sertraline (17). Kaskow and associates reported that citalopram was well tolerated and effective in the treatment of minor depression in ten elderly subjects (82). Rocca and colleagues reported that both sertraline and citalopram improved depressive symptoms and cognitive function in elderly nondemented patients with minor depressive disorder or subsyndromal depressive symptomatology (83).

Existing treatments help many of our patients, but also leave many unimproved (79). Interventional research on depression in later life, therefore, must continue to rigorously test the application of existing treatment strategies for patients in a variety of medical and community settings while also exploring new somatic therapies, integration of treatment modalities, lifestyle and psychosocial interventions, and collaborative care approaches. At the same time, studies of risk factors and potential moderating factors will help identify patients with less-than-major depressions who might benefit most with specific treatment interventions or who are at highest risk for persistent or worsening symptoms and disability.

SUMMARY

We have identified differences and similarities in the clinical presentation of clinically significant minor depressive disorders. There is evidence stemming from epidemiologic, longitudinal, neuroimaging, cognitive, and genetic studies supporting the idea of a continuum of depressive disorders, ranging from the very mild "subthreshold" disorders to major unipolar and bipolar depression. The current approaches to studying affective illness strictly by nosologic groups or by settings may not be sufficient for improving our understanding of this group of disorders. On the other hand, including patients with various degrees of depression severity, following them longitudinally, studying them with the modern tools of neuroimaging and neurogenetics, and, studying treatment response in these patients would provide more information about the neurobiology of these conditions. Studies testing pathogenetic models involving factors across the biopsychosocial systems continuum have the goal of defining etiologically distinct subgroups that might respond preferentially to specific existing or future treatments.

ACKNOWLEDGMENT

This work was supported by the NIH grants R01 MH077650 and R-21 AT003480 to Dr Lavretsky and NIMH grants R01 MH61429 & K24 MH071509 to Dr Lyness.

REFERENCES

1. Lavretsky H, Kumar A. Methylphenidate augmentation of citalopram in elderly depressed patients. Am J Geriatr Psychiatry 2001; 9:298–303.
2. Cole MG, McCusker J, Ciampi A, et al. The prognosis of major and minor depression in older medical inpatients. Am J Geriatr Psychiatry 2006; 14(11):966–975.
3. Schneider LS, Reynolds CF III, Lebowitz BD, et al. Diagnosis and Treatment of Depression in Late Life: Results of the NIH Consensus Development Conference. Washington, D.C.: American Psychiatric Press, 1994.
4. Blazer DG. Is depression more frequent in late life? An honest look at the evidence. Am J Geriatr Psychiatry 1994; 2(3):193.
5. Mulsant BH, Ganguli M. Epidemiology and diagnosis of depression in late life. J Clin Psychiatry 1999; 60(20):9–15.
6. Rollman BL, Reynolds CF III. Minor and subsyndromal depression: Functional disability worth treating [editorial; comment]. J Am Geriatr Soc 1999; 47:757–758.
7. Lavretsky H, Kumar A. Clinically significant non-major depression: Old concepts, new insights. Am J Geriatr Psychiatry 2002; 10:239–255.
8. Flint AJ. The complexity and challenge of non-major depression in late life. Am J Geriatr Psychiatry 2002; 10(3):229–232.
9. Tannock C, Katona C. Minor depression in the aged: Concepts, prevalence and optimal management. Drugs Aging 1995; 6:278–292.
10. Blazer D, Woodbury M, Hughes DC, et al. A statistical analysis of the classification of depression in a mixed community and clinical sample. J Affect Disord 1989; 16:11–20.
11. American Psychiatric Association. Diagnostic and Statistical Manual of Mental Disorders, 4th ed. Text Revision. Washington, D.C.: American Psychiatric Association, 2000.
12. Broadhead WE, Blazer DG, George LK, et al. Depression, disability days, and days from work in a prospective epidemiological survey. JAMA 1990; 264:2524–2528.
13. Wells KB, Stewart A, Hays RD, et al. The functioning and well-being of depressed patients: Results from the medical outcomes study. JAMA 1989; 262:914–919.
14. Lyness JM, Kim J, Tang W, et al. The clinical significance of subsyndromal depression in older primary care patients. Am J Geriatr Psychiatry 2007; 51(11):1554–1562.
15. Koenig HG, George LK, Peterson BL, et al. Depression in medically ill hospitalized older adults: Prevalence, characteristics, and course of symptoms according to six diagnostic schemes. Am J Psychiatry 1997; 154:1376–1383.
16. Blazer DG. Epidemiology of late-life depression. In: Schneider LS, Reynolds CF, Lebowitz BD, Friedhoff AJ, eds. Diagnosis and Treatment of Depression in Late-life. Results of the NIH Consensus Development Conference. Washington, D.C.: American Psychiatric Press, 1994; 9–20.
17. Rosen J, Mulsant BH, Pollock BG. Sertraline in the treatment of minor depression in nursing home residents: A pilot study. Int J Geriatr Psychiatry 2000; 15(2):177–180.

18. Beekman AT, Deeg DJ, Braam AW, et al. Consequences of major and minor depression in later life: A study of disability, well-being and service utilization. Psychol Med 1997; 27:1397–1409.
19. Devanand DP, Nobler MS, Singer T, et al. Is dysthymia a different disorder in the elderly? Am J Psychiatry 1994; 151:1592–1599.
20. Devanand DP, Adorno E, Cheng J, et al. Late onset dysthymic disorder and major depression differ from early onset dysthymic disorder and major depression in elderly outpatients. J Affect Disord 2004; 78(3):259–267.
21. Judd LL, Akiskal HS, Maser JD, et al. A prospective 12-year study of subsyndromal and syndromal depressive symptoms in unipolar major depressive disorders. Arch Gen Psychiatry 1998; 55:694–700.
22. Angst J, Merikangas K. The depressive spectrum: Diagnostic classification and course. J Affect Disord 1997; 45:31–39, discussion 39–40.
23. Angst J, Sellaro R, Merikangas KR. Depressive spectrum diagnoses. Compr Psychiatry 2000; 41(2 suppl 1):39–47.
24. Hamilton M. A rating scale for depression. J Neurol, Neurosurg Psychiatry 1960; 23:56–62.
25. Lyness JM, Caine ED, King DA, et al. Psychiatric disorders in older primary care patients. J Gen Intern Med 1999; 14:249–254.
26. Chopra MP, Zubritsky C, Knott K, et al. Importance of subsyndromal symptoms of depression in elderly patients. Am J Geriatr Psychiatry 2005; 13:597–606.
27. Angst J. Depression and anxiety: Implications for nosology, course, and treatment. J Clin Psychiatry 1997; 58(suppl 8):3–5.
28. Flint AJ, Rifat SL. Anxious depression in elderly patients. Response to antidepressant treatment. Am J Geriatr Psychiatry 1997; 5:107–115.
29. Lenze EJ, Mulsant BH, Shear MK, et al. Comorbid anxiety disorders in depressed elderly patients. Am J Psychiatry 2000; 157:722–728.
30. Prigerson HG, Bierhals AJ, Kasl SV, et al. Complicated grief as a disorder distinct from bereavement-related depression and anxiety: A replication study. Am J Psychiatry 1996; 153:1484–1486.
31. Akiskal HS, Judd LL, Gillin JC, et al. Subthreshold depressions: Clinical and polysomnographic validation of dysthymic, residual and masked forms. J Affect Disord 1997; 45:53–63.
32. Costa PT, McCrae RR. The NEO Personality Inventory: Revised Professional Manual. Odessa, FL: Psychological Assessment Resources, 1992.
33. Costa PT, McCrae RR. From catalog to classification: Marray's needs and the five-factor model. J Pers Soc Psycho 1988; 58:258–265.
34. Duggan CF, Lee AS, Murray RM. Does personality predict long-term outcome in depression? Br J Psychiatry 1990; 157:19–24.
35. Hirschfeld RM, Klerman GL, Andreasen NC, et al. Psycho-social predictors of chronicity in depressed patients. Br J Psychiatry 1986; 148:648–654.
36. Katon W, Lin E, Von Korff M, et al. The predictors of persistence of depression in primary care. J Affect Disord 1994; 31:81–90.
37. Duberstein PR, Lyness JM, Conwell Y, et al. Dimensional measures and the five factor model. Clinical implications and research directions. In: Rosowsky E, Abrams RC, Zweig RA, eds. Personality Disorders in Older Adults: Emerging Issues in Diagnosis and Treatment. Hillsdale, NJ: Lawrence Erlbaum Associates, 1999.
38. Lyness JM, Duberstein PR, King DA, et al. Medical illness burden, trait neuroticism, and depression in older primary care patients. Am J Psychiatry 1998; 155:969–971.
39. Lyness JM, Caine ED, King DA, et al. Depressive disorders and symptoms in older primary care patients: One-year outcomes. Am J Geriatr Psychiatry 2002; 10:275–282.
40. Zisook S, Paulus M, Shuchter SR, et al. The many faces of depression following spousal bereavement. J Affect Disord 1997; 45(1–2):85–94.
41. Prigerson HG, Frank E, Kasl SV, et al. Complicated grief and bereavement-related depression as distinct disorders: Preliminary empirical validation in elderly bereaved spouses. Am J Psychiatry 1995; 152:22–30.

42. Devanand DP. Comorbid psychiatric disorders in late life depression. Biol Psychiatry 2002; 52(3):236–242.
43. Regier DA, Hirshfield RMA, Goodwin FK, et al. The NIMH Depression Awareness, Recognition, and Treatment Program: Structure, aims, and scientific basis. Am J Psychiatry 1988; 45:1351–1357.
44. Eisenberg L. Treating depression and anxiety in primary care: Closing the gap between knowledge and practice. N Engl J Med 1992; 326:1080–1084.
45. Brody DS, Larson DB. The role of primary care physicians in managing depression J Gen Intern Med 1992; 7:243–247.
46. Beck DA, Koenig HG. Minor depression: A review of the literature. Int J Psychiatry Med 1996; 26:177–209.
47. Unutzer J, Patrick DL, Simon G, et al. Depressive symptoms and the cost of health services in HMO patients aged 65 years and older. A 4-year prospective study. JAMA 1997; 277:1618–1623.
48. Barrett JE, Williams JW, Oxman TE, et al. The treatment effectiveness project. A comparison of the effectiveness of paroxetine, problem-solving therapy, and placebo in the treatment of minor depression and dysthymia in primary care patients: Background and research plan. Gen Hosp Psychiatry 1999; 21:260–273.
49. Harm WJ, van Marwijk HW, de Bock GH, et al. Prevalence of depression and clues to focus diagnosis. A study among dutch general practice patients 65+ years of age. Scand J Prim Health Care 1996; 14:142–147.
50. Callahan CM, Hendrie HC, Dittus RS, et al. Improving treatment of late-life depression in primary care: A randomized clinical trial. J Am Geriatr Soc 1994; 42:839–846.
51. Katon E, Von Korff M, Lin E, et al. Collaborative management to achieve treatment guidelines. JAMA 1995, 273:1026–1031.
52. Lyness JM, Bruce ML, Koenig HG, et al. Depression and medical illness in late life: Report of symposium. J Am Geriatr Soc 1996; 44:198–203.
53. Rovner BW, Ganguli M. Depression and disability associated with impaired vision: The Movies project. J Am Geriat Soc 1998; 46:617–619.
54. Koenig HG. Depression in hospitalized older patients with congestive heart failure. Gen Hosp Psychiatry 1998; 20:20–43.
55. Jorm AF. Does old age reduce the risk of anxiety and depression? A review of epidemiological studies across the adult life span. Psychol Med 2000; 30:11–22.
56. Beekman AT, de Beurs E, van Balkom AJ, et al. Anxiety and depression in later life: Co-occurrence and communality of risk factors. Am J Psychiatry 2000; 157:89–95.
57. Snowdon J. Epidemiologic questions on mood disorders in old age. Clin Neurosci 1999; 4:3–7.
58. Lavretsky H. Irwin MR. Resilience and aging. Aging Health 2007; 3(3):309–323.
59. Sher L. Psychiatric diagnoses and inconsistent results of association studies in behavioral genetics. Med Hypotheses 2000; 54:207–209.
60. Remick RA, Sadovnick AD, Lam RW, et al. Major depression, minor depression, and double depression: are they distinct clinical entities. Am J Med Genet 1996; 67:347–353.
61. Kumar A, Schweizer E, Zhisong J, et al. Neuroanatomical substrates of late-life minor depression. A quantitative magnetic resonance imaging study. Arch Neurl 1997; 54:613–617.
62. Kumar A, Jin Z, Bilker W. Late-onset and major depression: Early evidence for common neuroanatomical substrates detected by using MRI. Proc Natl Sci 1998; 95:7654–7658.
63. O'Brien JT, Lloyd A, McKeith I, et al. A longitudinal study of hippocampal volume, cortisol levels, and cognition in older depressed subjects. Am J Psychiatry 2004; 161:2081–2090.
64. Nobler MS, Pelton GH, Sackeim HA. Cerebral blood flow and metabolism in late-life depression and dementia. J Geriatr Psychiatry Neurol 1999; 12:118–127.
65. Matsui H, Nishinaka K, Oda M, et al. Minor depression and brain perfusion images in Parkinson's disease. Mov Disord 2006; 21(8):1169–1174.

66. Elderkin-Thompson V, Kumar A, Bilker WB, et al. Neuropsychological deficits among patients with late-onset minor and major depression. Arch Clin Neuropsychol. 2003; 18(5):529–549.
67. Elderkin-Thompson V, Mintz J, Haroon E, et al. Executive dysfunction and memory in older patients with major and minor depression. Arch Clin Neuropsychol 2006; 21(7):669–676.
68. Rapaport MH, Judd LL, Schettler PJ, et al. A descriptive analysis of minor depression. Am J Psychiatry 2002; 159(4):637–643.
69. Devanand DP, Sano M, Tang MX, et al. Depressed mood and the incidence of Alzheimer's disease in the elderly living in the community. Arch Gen Psychiatry 1996; 53:175–182.
70. Jorm AF. History of depression as a risk factor for dementia: An updated review. Aust N Z J Psychiatry 2001; 35:776–781.
71. Lavretsky H, Ercoli L, Siddarth P, et al. Apolipoprotein epsilon4 allele status, depressive symptoms, and cognitive decline in middle-aged and elderly persons without dementia. Am J Geriatr Psychiatry 2003; 11:667–73.
72. Katz IR. What should we do about undertreatment of late life psychiatric disorders in primary care? J Am Geriatr Soc 1998; 46:1573–1575.
73. Bruce ML, Pearson JL. Designing an intervention to prevent suicide: Prospect (Prevention of Suicide in Primary Care Elderly Collaborative Trial). Dialogues Clin Neurosci 1999; 1:100–112.
74. Katz IR, Coyne JC. The public health model for mental health care for the elderly. JAMA 2000; 283:1–6.
75. Baldwin RC, Anderson D, Black S, et al. Guideline for the management of late-life depression in primary care. Int J Geriatr Psychiatry 2003; 18(9):829–838.
76. Williams JW, Barrett J, Oxman T, et al. Treatment of dysthymia and minor depression in primary care. A randomized controlled trial in older adults. JAMA 2000; 284:1519–1526.
77. Pinquart M, Duberstein PR, Lyness JM. Treatment for later-life depressive conditions: a meta-analytic comparison of pharmacotherapy and psychotherapy. AM J Psychiatry 2006; 163(9):1493–501.
78. Bruce ML, Ten Have TR, Reynolds CF III, et al. Reducing suicidal ideation and depressive symptoms in depressed older primary care patients: A randomized controlled trial. JAMA 2004; 291:1081–1091.
79. Lyness JM. Naturalistic outcomes of minor and subsyndromal depression in older primary care patients. Int J Geriatr Psychiatry 2008, Jan 16; [Epub ahead of print].
80. Ciechanowski P, Wagner E, Schmaling K, et al. Community-integrated home-based depression treatment in older adults: A randomized controlled trial. JAMA 2004; 291:1569–1577.
81. Rappoport MH, Judd LL. Minor depressive disorder and subsyndromal depressive symptoms: Functional impairment and response to treatment. J Affect Disord 1998; 48:227–232.
82. Kasckow JW, Welge J, Carroll BT, et al. Citalopram treatment of minor depression in elderly men: an open pilot study. Am J Geriatr Psychiatry 2002; 10(3):344–347.
83. Rocca P, Calvarese P, Faggiano F, et al. Citalopram versus sertraline in late-life nonmajor clinically significant depression: A 1-year follow-up clinical trial. J Clin Psychiatry 2005; 66(3):360–369.
84. Lavretsky H, Kumar A. Practical geriatrics: Clinically significant nonmajor geriatric depression. Psychiatr Serv 2003; 54(3):297–299.
85. Brodaty H, Withall A, Altendorf A, et al. Rates of depression at 3 and 15 months post-stroke and their relationship with cognitive decline: the Sydney Stroke Study. Am J Geriatr Psychiatry 2007; 15(6):477–486.
86. Elderkin-Thompson V, Mintz J, Haroon E, et al. Executive dysfunction and memory in older patients with major and minor depression. Arch Clin Neuropsychol 2007; 22(2):261–270.
87. Brenes GA, Williamson JD, Messier SP, et al. Treatment of minor depression in older adults: a pilot study comparing sertraline and exercise. Aging Ment Health 2007; 11(1):61–68.

88. Unützer J, Katon W, Callahan CM, et al. Improving mood-promoting access to collaborative treatment. Collaborative care management of late-life depression in the primary care setting: a randomized controlled trial. JAMA 2002; 288(22):2836–2845.
89. Beekman AT, Copeland JR, Prince MJ. Review of community prevalence of depression in later life. Br J Psychiatry 999; 174:307–311.
90. Heun R, Papassotiropoulos A, Ptok U. Subthreshold depressive and anxiety disorders in the elderly. Eur Psychiatry 2000; 15 :173–182.
91. Steffens DC, Skoog I, Norton MC, et al. Prevalence of depression and its treatment in an elderly population: the Cache County study. Arch Gen Psychiatry 2000; 57:601–607.
92. Newman Sc, Sheldon CT, Bland RC. Prevalence of depression in an elderly community sample: a comparison of GMS-AGECAT and DSM-IV diagnostic criteria. Psychol Med 1998; 28:1339–1345.
93. Henderson AS, Jorm AF, MacKinnon A, et al. The prevalence of depressive disorders and the distribution of depressive symptoms in later life: a survey using Draft ICD-10 and DSM-III-R. Psychol Med 1993; 23(3):719–729.
94. Burvill P, Johnson G, Jamrozik K, et al. Risk factors for post-stroke depression. Int J Geriatr Psychiatry 1997; 12(2):219–226.
95. Cummings JL, Ross W, Absher J, et al. Depressive symptoms in Alzheimer disease: assessment and determinants. Alzheimer Dis Assoc Disord 1995; 9(2):87–93.
96. Menza MA, Cocchiola J, Golbe LI. Psychiatric symptoms in progressive supranuclear palsy. Psychosomatics 1995; 36(6):550–554.
97. Grayson DA, Henderson AS, Kay DW. Diagnoses of dementia and depression: a latent trait analysis of their performance. Psychol Med 1987 Aug; 17(3):667–675.
98. Geiselmann B, Bauer M. Subthreshold depression in the elderly: qualitative or quantitative distinction? Compr Psychiatry 2000 Mar–Apr; 41(2 Suppl 1):32–38.
99. Oxman TE, Barrett JE, Barrett J, et al. Symptomatology of late-life minor depression among primary care patients. Psychosomatics 1990; 31:174–180.
100. Pasternak RE, Reynolds CF 3rd, Houck PR, et al. Sleep in bereavement-related depression during and after pharmacotherapy with nortriptyline. J Geriatr Psychiatry Neurol 1994; 7(2):69–73.
101. Penninx BW, Beekman AT, Honig A, et al. Depression and cardiac mortality: results from a community-based longitudinal study. Arch Gen Psychiatry 2001; 58(3):221–227.
102. Penninx BW, Deeg DJ, van Eijk JT, et al. Changes in depression and physical decline in older adults: a longitudinal perspective. J Affect Disord 2000; 61(1–2):1–12.
103. Penninx BW, Guralnik JM, Pahor M, et al. Chronically depressed mood and cancer risk in older persons. J Natl Cancer Inst 1998; 90(24):1888–1893.
104. Anderson RL, Klein DN, Riso LP, et al. The subaffective-character spectrum subtyping distinction in primary early-onset dysthymia: a clinical and family study. J Affect Disord 1996; 38(1):13–22.
105. Dai Y, Zhang S, Yamamoto J, et al. Cognitive behavioral therapy of minor depressive symptoms in elderly Chinese Americans: a pilot study. Community Ment Health J 1999; 35(6):537–542.

3 The Epidemiology of Major Depression in Geriatric Populations

Robert Kohn

Department of Psychiatry and Human Behavior, Miriam Hospital and The Warren Alpert Medical School of Brown University, Providence, Rhode Island, U.S.A.

Amber M. Gum and Bellinda King-Kallimanis

Department of Aging and Mental Health, Louis de la Parte Florida Mental Health Institute, University of South Florida, St. Petersburg, Florida, U.S.A.

INTRODUCTION

The worldwide burden of major depression is considerable among the elderly population. Based on 2002 estimates, for those aged 60 and older, major depression accounts for 5.2% of all the years lived with disability (YLD). Of all YLD, major depression accounts for 6.1% among older females and 3.9% among older males. Only cataracts, Alzheimer disease, and other dementias, adult-onset hearing loss, cerebrovascular disease, age-related vision disorders, and osteoarthritis result in more YLDs for elderly individuals. In high-income countries major depression is the fifth most common cause of YLD out of 136 other disorders, accounting for 4.7% of all YLDs (1). Although the amount of YLD accounted for by major depression in the elderly population is tremendously high, this is in contrast to younger adults where major depression is ranked either first or second. Among the elderly population, major depression was noted to result in 9.3 days of disability in the past four weeks, in which they were completely unable to carry out their usual activities or had to cut down. This was more than days of disability for anxiety disorders, substance use disorders, or personality disorders (2). At least half of those with major depression have impairment in work and social roles, and over two-thirds are unable to perform household functions (3). Clearly, the degree of disability associated with major depression makes it a major public health issue in geriatrics.

THE PREVALENCE OF MAJOR DEPRESSION

There is a considerable debate as to whether elderly individuals are at a higher risk for major depression than younger persons. Prior to the advent of community-based diagnostic epidemiologic studies, the prevailing attitude was summed with the following quote by De Beauvoir from 1977 (4), "Old people are physically fragile. Socially they are outcasts, and this has serious effects upon their mental state. Both their existential situation and their sexual state are favourable to the development of neuroses and psychoses." The belief that the elderly were at high risk is bolstered by studies that examined depressive symptoms in the community suggesting high rates among those older than 50 years, with the highest rates among the very old, those older than 80 years (5,6). However, not all studies using symptom scales have found an increase with age (7). In addition, the fact that suicide rates are highest among those older than 65 years(8), further argues for the notion that there should be an increased vulnerability toward mood disorders in later life.

With the advent of community-based diagnostic epidemiologic surveys utilizing DSM or ICD-10 diagnostic criteria, a different picture emerged. Many of these studies found an inverse linear relationship between the rates of major depression and age, with those older than 65 years having the lowest rates. This inverse relationship found for both lifetime prevalence and prevalence; periods other than lifetime is counterintuitive, as the risk for a disorder should increase with longevity. When this was first noted, Blazer (9) at that time called this an "epidemiologic dilemma."

The Epidemiological Catchment Area (ECA) study in the 1980s was the first diagnostic community-based psychiatric epidemiologic survey using a structured diagnostic interview across all age groups conducted in the United States. The ECA study used the Diagnostic Interview Schedule (DIS) to produce DSM-III diagnoses (10). The population studied consisted of 19182 individuals in five catchment areas—Los Angeles, CA; New Haven, CT; Baltimore, MD; St. Louis, MO; Durham, NC. Over one-fourth or the sample was over the age of 65 ($N = 5723$). This study noted a markedly lower rate among elderly respondents for major depression compared to younger cohorts for both lifetime (2.0% vs. 6.3%) and 1-year prevalence (1.4% vs. 3.7%) (11).

The Cache County study conducted in the early 1990s, which was limited to individuals older than 65 years, found markedly higher rates of major depression than the ECA. The Cache County study also used the DIS, and produced DSM-IV diagnoses. This population study, however, was limited to a community from Utah (12). The 1-year prevalence rate was 4.3% and the lifetime rate 15.8%. In 1996, the first of three waves of The Health and Retirement study (HRS) was conducted using the Composite International Diagnostic Interview–Short Form (CIDI-SF) to produce DSM-III R diagnoses (13). The HRS is a longitudinal study of a nationally representative sample of community-dwelling adults in the United States. The study had 9748 participants, of which 1538 were older than 65 years. The HRS, similar to the Cache County study, also found an estimated 1-year prevalence rate for major depression of 4.0% among adults aged 65 years and older (14). The most current study conducted in the United States, The National Comorbidity Survey Replication (NCS-R), a household psychiatric survey in a probability sample from the 48 contiguous states, also suggested that the rates from the earlier ECA study may be low (15,16). The NCS-R used the Composite International Diagnostic Interview (CIDI) to make DSM-IV diagnoses in 9090 individuals in the community, of which 1461 were 65 years or older (17). Although the rates for older adults were higher than what was found in the ECA study, the NCS-R also confirmed that the rates for major depression among the elderly population were markedly lower than the rest of the population (1-year prevalence 2.3% vs. 6.7% and lifetime prevalence 9.3% vs. 16.6%).

Several other studies have been conducted in the United States that produced rates for major depression in the elderly population. Weissman and Myers (18) conducted one of the earliest psychiatric epidemiologic investigations that used DSM-III diagnostic criteria and included the full age spectrum. They reported a 5.4% 1-month prevalence rate and a 20.0% lifetime rate for major depression among elderly respondents. The DIS study by Brown et al. (19) was limited to 865 urban African-American respondents. A 1-year prevalence rate of 3.2% was noted among those older than the age of 65 years. Turvey et al.'s (20) report is based on an earlier wave of the HRS utilizing the CIDI-SF in those 70 years and older. This survey evaluated 5449 individuals in the community and found that 3.6% had 1-year prevalent major depression.

This markedly lower rate of major depression in older cohorts has been noted worldwide (Tables 1 and 2), although a number of exceptions do exist (18,21–27). The lifetime prevalence rate for major depression among individuals aged 65 years and older varies widely across studies and nations from 1.4% in the Untied States (11) to 27.7% in Ethiopia (21).

Unfortunately, many studies that examine age as a risk factor for major depression do not publish rates specific to the elderly population; instead they collapse rates across mood disorders and often report odds ratios by age. For example, the European Study of the Epidemiology of Mental Disorders (ESEMeD) found that, for mood disorders, those older than 64 years had a 1-year prevalence rate of 3.2% in contrast to a rate of 4.2% for the entire sample of 21425 respondents (27). The ESEMeD is part of the World Mental Health (WMH) initiative and utilized the Composite International Diagnostic Interview (CIDI) (28,29). A number of the current international reports of rates in the elderly population are from the WMH surveys and have the advantage of utilizing similar methodology and diagnostic instrument (Table 3). Of the five studies presenting data only on mood disorders, only the ESEMeD and the study conducted in Japan from the WMH survey showed statistical significance between those older than 64 years and the other age groups. Another example comes from Finland in a study of persons older than 30 years that published odds ratios for mood disorders found lower rates among those 65 years and older; for ages 30 to 44 OR = 2.1, 95% CI (1.5, 3.0); ages 45 to 54 OR = 2.2, 95% CI (1.6, 3.1); ages 55 to 64 OR = 1.6, 95% CI (1.1–2.4); and ages 65+ OR = 1.0, reference group) (30). The National Survey of American Life (NSAL) limited to African-Americans in the United States reported a lifetime rate for mood disorders of 5.8% for individuals between the ages of 64 and 74 and a rate of 1.5% for those older than 74 (31). The NSAL found a significantly lower rate of lifetime mood disorders for those older than 74 years (55–64 OR = 5.0 , 95% CI (2.0, 12.7); 64–74 OR = 3.6, 95% CI (1.5, 8.7); 75 ≥, OR = 1.0, reference group).

A small number of studies have examined the distribution of major depression among those older than age 65 years (Table 4). Interestingly, half of these reports suggest that the prevalence rate of major depression once again begins to rise after age of 65 years. However, the rates do not achieve those of younger age groups. This perhaps reflects that proportion of females in the population increases due to earlier mortality in males.

INCIDENCE OF MAJOR DEPRESSION IN THE ELDERLY

A few studies have examined the incidence of major depression among older populations. The Cache County study examined the incidence of new onset of depression over a period of three years using three different sources of data namely diagnosis on follow-up using the DIS only; DIS and new onset antidepressant use; and DIS, antidepressant, and postmortem data (32). The investigators found an incident rate of using the DIS only of 16.4 per 1000, males 13.1 and females 16.4; for the DIS plus medications 19.5 per 1000, males 15.6 and females 23.3; and for all three sources of data 26.3 per 1000, males 20.7 and females 26.3. In addition, an increasing incidence

TABLE 1 Lifetime Prevalence Rates (%) of Major Depression in Community-Based Surveys Published Since 1980

Country	Reference	Interview	Diagnosis	Age	Total	Male	Female	Overall
São Paulo, Brazil	(126)	CIDI	DSM-III R	60	10.7	11.5	10.3	16.6
CCHS 1.2, Canada	(127)	WMH-CIDI	DSM-IV	65	6.4			12.2
Edmonton, Canada	(128)	DIS	DSM-III	65	4.1			8.6
Sterling County, Canada	(129)	DIS	DSM-III	65	4.1			7.9
Chile	(113)	CIDI	DSM-III R	65	5.1	5.6	4.8	9.4
Beijing, China	(130)	WMH-CIDI	DSM-III R	60	7.8	4.7	10.7	N/A
Kumming, China	(25)	WHM-CIDI	DSM-IV	65	3.6	2.1	5.3	2.0
Shanghai, China	(131)	WMH-CIDI	DSM-III R	65	2.6			3.5
Colombia	(27)	CIDI	DSM-IV	61	25.2			19.6
Addis Ababa, Ethiopia	(23)	SRQ/CIDI	ICD-10	60	15.4			5.0
Butajira, Ethiopia	(21)	SRQ/CIDI	ICD-10	60	27.7			6.2
Montpellier, France	(112)	MINI	DSM-IV	65	26.5	16.6	33.6	N/A
Japan	(132)	UM-CIDI	DSM-III R	65	2.2			2.9
Rural, Mexico	(133)	CIDI	ICD-10	60	4.2	2.1	7.5	6.2
New Zealand	(134)	WMH-CIDI	DSM-IV	65	9.8			16.0
Ibadan, Nigeria	(3)	WMH-CIDI	DSM-IV	65	26.2	20.6	33.4	N/A
South Africa	(135)	WMH-CIDI	DSM-IV	65	6.5			9.8
Taiwan, P.R. China	(22)	DIS	DSM-III	65	1.5			1.2
ECA, U.S.A.	(11)	DIS	DSM-III	65	1.4			4.9
NCS-R, U.S.A.	(15)	WMH-CIDI	DSM-IV	65	9.3	4.9	12.6	16.6
New Haven, U.S.A.	(18)	SADS	RDC	65	20.0			14.4
Utah, U.S.A.	(12)	DIS	DSM-IV	65	15.8	9.6	20.4	N/A

Age = age cut-off used for the elderly population; Overall = refers to the rate in the total population sample for studies not limited to geriatric samples.
Abbreviations: CIDI, Composite Diagnostic Interview; DIS, Diagnostic Interview Schedule; MINI, Mini International Neuropsychiatric Interview; RDC, Research Diagnostic Criteria; SADS, Schedule for Affective Disorders and Schizophrenia; SRQ, Symptom Rating Questionnaire; UM, University of Michigan; WMH, World Mental Healt.

TABLE 2 Prevalence Rates (%) of Major Depression in Community Based Surveys Published Since 1980 in Elderly Other Than Lifetime

Country	Reference	Interview	Diagnosis	Age	Total	Male	Female	Overall
Australia	(2)	CIDI	ICD-10	65+	2.4	1.4	3.1	5.1
São Paulo, Brazil	(126)	CIDI	DSM-III R	60+	4.0	4.5	3.7	6.7
Edmonton, Canada	(128) (6 months)	DIS	DSM-III	65+	1.2	0.9	1.4	3.2
CCHS 1.2, Canada	(135)	WMH-CIDI	DSM-IV	65+	1.9			4.0
NPHS, Canada	(136)	CIDI-SF	DSM-III R	60+	2.5			5.6
Sterling County, Canada	(129) (1 month)	DIS	DSM-III	65+	0.9			2.6
Chile	(113)	CIDI	DSM-III R	15+	2.9	1.4	3.9	5.5
Beijing, China	(130)	WMH-CIDI	DSM-III R	60+	4.3	2.1	6.2	N/A
Kumming, China	(25)	WHM-CIDI	DSM-IV	65+	2.1	1.6	2.6	1.1
Colombia	(27)	CIDI	DSM-IV	61+	1.8			1.9
Finland	(137) (6 months)	CIDI	DSM-III R	60+	2.4	2.0	2.8	4.1
FINHCS, Finland	(138)	CIDI-SF	DSM-III R	65+	6.7	4.1	8.4	9.3
Montpellier, France	(112)	MINI	DSM-IV	65+	1.8	4.0	3.1	N/A
Athens, Greece	(139) (1 month)	PEF	DSM-III	65+	1.6	2.1	1.2	N/A
Lari, Italy	(24)	PSE	ICD-9	60+	18.1			11.0
Sardina, Italy	(140)	PSE	ICD-9	65+	10.1	5.4	13.5	10.2
Japan	(132) (6 months)	UM-CIDI	DSM-III R	65+	1.1			1.2
Netherlands	(141)	DIS		65+	2.0			N/A
New Zealand	(142)	WMH-CIDI	DSM-IV	65+	1.7			5.7
Norway	(26) (2 weeks)	HSCL-25/CIDI	ICD-10	60+	4.2	1.2	7.9	2.6
Ibadan, Nigeria	(3)	WMH-CIDI	DSM-IV	65+	7.1	6.2	9.3	N/A
Taiwan, P.R. China	(22)	DIS	DSM-III	65+	1.0			0.9
ONS, U.K.	(143) (1 month)	CIS-R/SCAN	ICD-10	60+	0.6–1.1	0.2–0.5	1.0–1.7	2.6
United Kingdom	(144) (1 month)	Sleep Eval	DSM-IV	15+	4.7	2.6	6.2	5.0

(*Continued*)

TABLE 2 Prevalence Rates (%) of Major Depression in Community Based Surveys Published Since 1980 in Elderly Other Than Lifetime (*Continued*)

Country	Reference	Interview	Diagnosis	Age	Total	Male	Female	Overall
African-American, U.S.A.	(19)	DIS	DSM-III	65+	3.2			3.1
ECA, U.S.A.	(11)	DIS	DSM-III	65+	0.9	0.4	1.4	2.7
HRS, U.S.A.	(20)	CIDI-SF	DSM-III R	70+	3.6	2.5	4.2	N/A
HRS, U.S.A.	(14)	CIDI-SF	DSM-III R	65+	4.0			6.6
NCS-R, U.S.A.	(15)	WMH-CIDI	DSM-IV	65+	2.3	0.9	3.4	6.7
New Haven, U.S.A.	(18) (1 month)	SADS	RDC	65+	5.4			4.3
Utah, U.S.A.	(12)	DIS	DSM-IV	65+	4.3	3.2	5.1	N/A

Unless stated otherwise prevalence periods are one year. Age = age cut-off used for the elderly population; Overall = refers to the rate in the total population sample for studies not limited to geriatric samples.

Abbreviations: CIDI, Composite Diagnostic Interview; CIS-R, Clinical Interview Schedule; DIS, Diagnostic Interview Schedule; HSCL-25, Hopkins Checklist 25; MINI, Mini International Neuropsychiatric Interview; PSE, Present State Examination; RDC, Research Diagnostic Criteria; SADS, Schedule for Affective Disorders and Schizophrenia; SCAN, Schedules for Clinical Assessment in Neuropsychiatry; SF, Short Form; SRQ, Symptom Rating Questionnaire; UM, University of Michigan; WMH, World Mental Health.

TABLE 3 One-Year Prevalence of Selected WMH Studies of Mood Disorders Not Represented in Table 2; Odds Ratios and 95% Confidence Intervals

Age	Europe (ESEMeD)[a]	China[b]	Japan[c]	Lebanon[d]	Israel[e]
18–24	1.0				
25–34	0.7 (0.5–1.1)	2.0 (0.8–4.8)[f]	2.3 (0.3–17.2)	1.8 (0.8–3.8)[f]	1.5 (0.9–2.4)[g]
35–49	0.6 (0.4–0.9)	0.9 (0.4–1.9)	2.7 (0.4–21.2)	2.8 (1.2–6.5)	1.5 (0.9–2.3)
50–64	0.7 (0.5–1.0)	–	4.6 (0.7–29.7)	2.4 (1.3–4.7)	1.3 (0.9–2.1)
65+	0.5 (0.4–0.7)	1.0	1.0	1.0	1.0

[a] Alonso et al. 2004 (144)
[b] Shen et al. 2006 (146)
[c] Kawakami et al. 2005 (147)
[d] Karam et al. 2006 (148)
[e] Levinson et al. 2007 (149)
[f] age: 18–34
[g] age 21–34

rate was seen with age; those individuals from 70 to 79 years had an incidence rate of 17 per 1000 and older than 79 years had an incidence rate of 44 per 1000.

The Baltimore ECA followed the original population sample from 1981 to 2004 permitting evaluation of the incidence of major depression across different age groups at baseline (33). Those who were 65 or older had an incidence rate of 0.9 per 1000, males 0.7 per 1000 and females 1.0 per 1000, for the years 1981—to 1993. The incidence rate was lower among those who were elderly in contrast to other age groups; for the entire sample the incidence rate was 3.2 per 1000. There were no new cases among those aged 65 and older at baseline from 1993 to 2004; however, those who had entered old age from 1983 to 2004 had a similarly low incidence rate of 1.9 per 1000, males 0.9 per 1000 and females 2.6 per 1000.

The Stirling County study from Canada followed a cohort population using the DIS on average 2.8 years to determine the incidence of DSM-IV major depression (34). The incidence rate per 1000 of those 65 and older was 8.8, males 6.7 and females 10.4; this was lower than the 11.0 for the 40- to 64-year old age group.

In a representative Swedish sample of 392 individuals followed from age 70 to 85 the incidence rate for DSM-III major depression was 12 per 1000 in men and 30 per 1000 in women (35). The Lundby study also conducted in Sweden followed a population cohort for more than 50 years (36). From 1947 to 1972, the incidence rate for those from age 70 to 99 years was 2.3 per 1000 in contrast to 3.3 per 1000 for the whole sample. Those individuals between 70 and 99 years during the period from 1972 to 1997 had a higher incidence rate of 3.6 per 1000, and higher than the rest of the population that is, 2.8 per 1000. Another Swedish study followed 865 individuals between the age of 78 and 102 for three years. In this study from the Kungsholmen district of Stockholm, the incidence of depression was 1.4% per person per year (0.8% per person per year for males and 1.5% per person per year for females) (37). Magnússon (38) in Iceland conducted one of the earliest incidence studies. Among those from 74 to 85 years, the incidence rate of affective disorders was 0.6 per 100 per year for males and about 1.1 per 100 per year for females.

These seven studies suggest that the incidence rate for major depression decreases with age. The one exception is a study conducted in Munich; in a 1-year follow-up of individuals 85 years and older, the incidence rate was very high—133.5 per 1000 (39). In addition, these studies also suggest that incident or new

TABLE 4 Prevalence Rates (%) Across Age Groups for Major Depression in Community-Based Surveys Published Since 1980

Country	Reference	Prevalence Period	Interview	Diagnosis	65–69	70–74	75–79	80+
Australia	(90)	1 yr	CIDI	DSM-IV	2.3	1.7	0.2	0.2
Canada–males	(150)	1 yr	WMH-CIDI	DSM-IV	2.0	1.7	2.4	
Canada–females	(150)	1 yr	WMH-CIDI	DSM-IV	2.8	1.6	1.3	
Chile	(113)	1 yr	CIDI	DSM-III R	1.6	5.0		
Beijing, China	(130)	1 yr	WMH-CIDI	DSM-IV	8.9	7.3		3.2[a]
Netherlands	(141)	1 mo	DIS	DSM-III	1.8	2.1	2.5	2.7
Baltimore, U.S.A.	(151)	6 mo	DIS	DSM-III	0.7	0.7	1.3	1.3
NCS-R, U.S.A.	(15)	1 yr	WMH-CIDI	DSM-IV	2.3	1.3		
Utah, U.S.A.	(12)	1 mo	DIS	DSM-IV	3.8	3.8	4.4	4.4[b]

[a] age breakdown was 60–69, 70–79, 80+.
[b] after age 85 the rate falls to 4.0.

onset cases among individuals older than 65 years are more common in females than males. It had been suggested that the gender difference in the rates of major depression would no longer be pronounced after menopause (40); however, these studies suggest otherwise.

POTENTIAL REASONS FOR THE LOWER PREVALENCE RATES

Up to 15% to 20% of older adults have significant depressive symptoms (41), yet the lifetime prevalence rates for the elderly population is markedly lower than those who are younger. The reasons for the lower rates in the elderly could be attributed to a number of methodological explanations, (*i*) the current cohort of older adults may truly be at decreased risk; (*ii*) older adults may under-report depressive symptoms for past as well as current episodes; (*iii*) older adults with major depression may be unavailable for interview due to differential mortality, disability, or institutionalization; (*iv*) the structured interviews may not capture depressive symptoms that are ascribed to physical causes; (*v*) some diagnostic instruments may be more sensitive than others; and (*vi*) diagnostic instruments may not be sensitive to depressive symptoms in older adults. These hypotheses will be examined in turn.

One, there may be a cohort effect, in which the elderly truly are at a decreased risk (42). Using the ECA data, Wickramaratne et al. (43) modeled the possibility that a cohort effect exists, that major depression is on the rise in younger populations, and showed a sharp rise in major depression among males and females born during the years 1935 to 1945. Klerman and Weissman (42) argued that artifacts in reporting, recall, mortality, or labeling could not explain the cohort effect; however, others have argued otherwise. In recent studies the rates for major depression in the elderly are higher; however, this is attributable to differing methodology, e.g., NCS-R compared to the ECA. The rates in recent studies are higher across all age groups and continue to remain lowest in the oldest age groups suggesting that a cohort effect may still be a factor explaining the differential rates across ages.

Two, the elderly may have poorer recall of past episodes or may minimize their present symptoms (44,45); this includes both age-related forgetting and post-dating of episodes. This may be consistent with the hypothesis that the elderly do not easily assent to feelings of sadness (46). Gallo showed that the elderly were less likely to report sadness or anhedonia than younger adults, a requirement for the diagnosis of the disorder of major depression. Several investigators have tested this hypothesis and demonstrated that recall failure can explain a flat or declining lifetime major prevalence across age groups (47,48). In the longitudinal Baltimore ECA, psychiatric symptoms were assessed twice, once in 1981 and again in 1994 (49). Periods when an episode of depressed mood was not present were more consistently recalled than when a prior episode of a depressed mood had occurred. Other reports suggest that memory effects alone cannot explain this phenomenon (50); by demonstrating that using interviews blinded to their earlier diagnoses, older respondents were no more likely than younger ones to omit diagnoses nor to postdate their ages of first major depression. Andrews and colleagues tested the validity of lifetime diagnoses by following up with patients hospitalized 25 years earlier to assess whether they could recall enough information to meet diagnostic criteria; only half could do so (51). Other investigators have suggested that older respondents are less likely to recognize major depression based on a study using vignettes, and as a result less likely to recall prior depressive episodes (52). Taken together, these findings suggest that older adults may be less likely than younger adults to recognize depressive symptoms, but both groups seem to have similar accuracy in recalling past self-reports.

Similarly, there may be an underestimation of older individuals with lifetime rates of major depression, as they may be at increased risk of developing memory disorders and dementia and be less likely to provide accurate self-report. Results from the NCS-R suggest an association between a lifetime history of depression and self-reported memory problems (53). The relationship between depression and cognitive decline has also been examined in the HRS (54). Elevated depressive symptoms were associated with declines in episodic learning and memory over time, with little influence from demographic or medical conditions. Similar finding was noted in a 7-year longitudinal study of older Mexican-Americans (55). The results suggest that learning and memory decline may be a long-term feature associated with depressive symptoms among the older adult population. Earlier the Longitudinal Aging Study Amsterdam (LASA) found that depression unlike anxiety was negatively associated with cognitive performance (56). Depressive symptoms in the Monongahela Valley Independent Elders Survey accessed longitudinally over 12 years were noted to be a precursor for the development of dementia (57). Longitudinal community–based studies have also found an association between depressed mood and manifestation of Alzheimer disease (58). Major depression present even 25 years prior to the advent of Alzheimer disease may be a risk factor (59). A 2001 meta-analysis of seven case-control and six prospective studies supported the association between depression and the risk of developing dementia (60). In addition to recall bias, those who are cognitively impaired also are not available to provide information on their psychiatric status.

Thus, a third possibility is that individuals who develop or are at risk of developing major depression are unavailable for interview due to differential mortality, disability due to physical illness or dementia, or increased risk of institutionalization. Any of these explanations would result in household studies underestimating the prevalence among the aged. As shown in Table 5 nearly all longitudinal community–based investigations of older populations have found that there is a modest increase in mortality due to depression, that is not a result of external causes, such as suicide or homicide, and not limited to cardiovascular disease. Some of these reports have suggested that the increased risk may be more pronounced in males compared to females (61,62). An earlier, more extensive review found that 43% of studies found a gender effect with an increased risk for mortality among males and 36% found no gender relationship (63). Similarly, a recent report confirmed that although elderly females are more susceptible to depression and have more persistent illness, older males are more prone to mortality from depression (64). This 6-year follow-up of depressed and nondepressed individuals found that men were more than four times as likely to die from depression.

The relationship between physical illness and major depression in older populations is unclear. A meta-analysis of prospective studies found no relationship between having a new medical illness or poor health status and the subsequent development of depression in the elderly (65). An epidemiologic study of elderly individuals, conducted in Australia, supported this conclusion (2). Other researchers using cross-sectional studies have argued that an increased risk for depression exists for coronary artery disease, cancer, Parkinson disease, and stroke (66), as well as lung disease and arthritis (67). An association between depression in the elderly population and asthma has been recently confirmed in a

TABLE 5 Depression and Mortality Ratios in Community-Based Surveys of Populations Limited to Populations Aged 65 years and older

Country	Reference	Diagnostic	Years	Age	Total	Male	Female
Japan	(152)	RDC	15	65	1.5[a]	1.3	1.6[a]
Netherlands	(62)	GMS-AGECAT	10	65	1.4[a]	2.4[a]	1.3[a]
Israel	(153)	CES-D	12	75	0.9		
Finland, Italy, Netherlands	(154)	Zung	5	70	1.4[a]		
Sweden	(155)	GDS	1	85	2.2[a]		
United Kingdom	(156)	GDS	3	75	1.5[a]		
U.S.A.	(157)	CES-D	10	65	1.1[a]		
Netherlands	(158)	GDS	3.2	85	1.8[a]		
Sweden	(159)	HSCL-25	6	65	2.5[a]		
New Zealand	(61)	SelfCARE-D	11	65	1.4[a]	2.1[a]	1.1
Netherlands	(160)	GMS-AGECAT	6	65		2.9[a]	1.3[a]
Spain	(161)	GMS-AGECAT	4.5	65	3.0[a]		
Finland	(162)	DSM-III	6	65	2.0[a]		
Norway	(163)	GMS	3	75	1.6[a]		

Years, Years of follow-up.
[a] statistically significant risk ratios.

community-based sample (68). However, the relationship with stroke and depression has been recently questioned in one prospective study (69). Depression as a predisposing factor for stroke in the most recent study was confirmed only among men but not women (70). Furthermore, there is no evidence from community-based studies to support a relationship between depression in old age and increased risk for cerebral atrophy (71). There is no clear evidence to support a relationship between hypertension and diabetes and depression in older individuals (69,72). However, meta-analysis does support an association between depression and a broad range of cardiovascular disease (73). Community-based studies do confirm that loss of hearing is associated with an increased risk for depression (74). A linear association between depressive symptoms and disability, as well as a dose relationship with chronic disease may exist (75). The relationship between chronic medical conditions and major depression in the elderly may be less clear than with younger age groups. This is highlighted in findings from the NCS-R (15). In the NCS-R, the rates for comorbidity with medical illness and major depression were lower for those older than 65 years, compared to those between ages 18 and 64. Unlike those who were younger, the older age group with and without major depression frequently had indistinguishable rates for many of the medical conditions.

The long-term care setting has a disproportionate number of individuals with major depression compared to the community. The current prevalence of major depression in nursing homes ranges from 5% to 31% (76). The 1-year incidence rate for depressive disorders ranges from 12% to 25%. However, is the increased prevalence in the long-term care setting due to the high rate of new development of depression upon long–term care placement, or are community-dwelling older adults who are depressed more likely to be placed in long-term care, raising the prevalence rate? Individuals who are depressed apparently are at higher risk for nursing home admission. A longitudinal study of 11 European countries found that depressed individuals admitted into homecare were at higher risk than those who were not depressed to be placed in a nursing home (77). A study of Medicare +

Choice enrollees who identified themselves as feeling sad or depressed much of the time over the previous year were at significantly higher risk of placement (78). However, long-term care facilities appear to place the residents at risk for developing depression, as noted in a longitudinal follow-up study of individuals from the community admitted into such facilities (79). Residents in these institutions where the prevalence of depression is very high are excluded from community-based surveys.

Fourth, the structured diagnostic interview schedules, such as the ECA and the NCS-R, used a probe flow chart that questions whether or not psychiatric symptoms are explained by physical causes. The possibility that older individuals might ascribe symptoms to physical rather than psychological causes cannot be ignored as a source of variance (80). The additional probe questions designed to identify the degree to which symptoms were caused by factors other than psychological revealed that in an analysis of the Munich Follow-up Study that older subjects more often attribute such symptoms to physical illnesses or conditions. This resulted in the exclusion of the reported symptoms as a basis for diagnosing depression. A reanalysis of the ECA data by Heithoff (81) to account for this problem did not substantially result in higher prevalence among the elderly, however. These findings, Heithoff argued, supported the original prevalence estimates obtained for late-life depression in the ECA. Another test was conducted using medically ill patients with lay interviewers using the CIDI compared to physician diagnoses obtained with the SCID; overall agreement was good, although discordant cases were due to difficulties in attribution of symptoms to medical illness (82). Thus, attribution of symptoms to physical causes in older adults may contribute to differential rates, although the degree of this influence is not clear.

Fifth, it is possible that the diagnostic instruments themselves are responsible for the rates being lower in the elderly. The impact of instruments on prevalence rates was highlighted by a study that compared prevalence rates in the ECA, which used the DIS for case ascertainment, and the National Comorbidity Survey (NCS), which used the CIDI (83,84). The prevalence rates in the NCS were considerably higher than ECA, suggesting that the CIDI diagnoses might be overinclusive or, alternatively, DIS diagnoses may be too restrictive. There is some evidence that CIDI-SF may be even more permissive than CIDI. A comparative study of CIDI-SF against CIDI found that 25% of participants who met criteria for major depression on CIDI-SF did not meet such criteria on CIDI (85). On the other hand, a recent study found that the DIS missed more than 70% of the cases of major depression identified by a semistructured interview administered by psychiatrists (86), thus grossly underestimating the prevalence of major depression. However, this argument should result in uniform bias across all age groups, as seen with the NCS-R, resulting in higher rates in for all age groups, yet the prevalence rates continue to have an inverse relationship with age.

Six, another argument for the low rates among the elderly population is that diagnostic instruments used are inappropriate for older populations, and that the criteria should be adjusted for this age group. Several diagnostic interview schedules have been developed specifically for the elderly population. These have mainly been used in European epidemiologic studies. The two most commonly used ones are the Comprehensive assessment and Referral Evaluation (CARE) (87) and the Geriatric Mental State–AGECAT (GMS-AGECAT) (88). Table 6 summaries the results of community-based studies using GMS-AGECAT. In those studies that

TABLE 6 Current Prevalence Rates (%) of Depression in Community-Based Surveys Elderly Using GMS-AGECAT

Country	Reference	Age	Total	Male	Female
Hobart, Australia	(164)	70	16.1		
Edmonton, Canada	(165)	65	11.4	7.3	14.1
Beijing, China	(166)	60		0.2	0.5
Shanghai, China	(166)	60		1.5	2.0
China	(167)	65	2.3	2.1	2.3
Berlin, Germany	(168)	70	16.5		
Munich, Germany	(169)	85	23.6		
Korea	(170)	65	13.3	8.1	17.0
AMSTEL, Netherlands	(171)	65	12.7	6.8	16.4
Nigeria	(172)	60	18.3	16.5	21.8
Singapore	(173)	65	5.7		
Singapore	(174)	65	5.5		
Taiwan	(175)	65	21.2		
United Arab Emirates	(176)	60	20.2		
Bradford, U.K.	(177)	65	20.0	20.0	20.0
Liverpool, U.K.	(178)	65	10.0		
Liverpool, U.K.	(179)	65	11.3	7.6	13.6
London, U.K.	(180)	65	19.4	13.1	22.8
MRC CFAS, U.K.	(181)	65	8.7	6.5	10.4
New York, USA	(180)	65	16.2	13.0	18.3
Zaragoza, Spain	(182)	65	7.4		
EURODEP	(183)	65	12.3	8.6	14.1
Berlin, Germany			16.5		
Munich, Germany			23.6		
Iceland			8.8		
Dublin, Ireland			11.9		
Verona, Italy			18.3		
Amsterdam, Netherlands			12.0		
Liverpool, U.K.			10.0		
London, U.K.			17.3		
Zaragoza, Spain			10.7		

Age, age cut-off used for the elderly population.

apply DSM criteria using the GMS-AGECAT, DSM criteria consistently produces markedly lower rates in older adults than the GMS-AGECAT. This difference was highlighted when individuals who participated in the DIS study in Edmonton, Canada were reinterviewed with the GMS-AGECAT (89). The AGECAT depression rate was 11.4% while the DSM-IV rate was 4.5%. There is a difference in the two diagnostic systems with respect to the handling of somatic symptoms of depression. In DSM-IV, dysphoria is an entry criterion for the diagnosis of major depression. Subsequently, somatic symptoms are important in determining case status. In AGECAT, the algorithm for depression uses dysphoric symptoms alone to decide on caseness; somatic symptoms only play a role in determining the subtype of depression. The higher rates found in the GMS-AGECAT studies also counter an argument that the low rates of depression using DSM or ICD-10 criteria could be due to psychological immunization, that exposure to earlier adversity engenders a protective effect to older individuals from events that occur late in life that may increase the risk for developing major depression.

O'Connor (90) provided a summary of the reasons that depression rates are lower for older adults, (*i*) aged care facilities were excluded from the survey despite robust evidence of high rates of anxiety and depression in these settings; (*ii*) mentally disordered older people decline to participate in surveys or are shielded by carers; (*iii*) complex diagnostic interviews place an undue burden on cognitively frail respondents; (*iv*) older people falsely attribute anxiety and depression to medical illness; and (*v*) diagnostic glossaries like ICD- 10 or DSM-IV fail to capture important psychological morbidity. Therefore, potential causes include measurement bias, sampling bias, and differential reporting by respondents of different ages. Although some degree of sampling bias is likely across all ages (i.e., younger adults with more severe mental disorders also are less likely to participate in community-based epidemiologic studies), mental disorders may particularly interfere with older adults' ability to participate in research, particularly when they are more likely to also be burdened by physical and cognitive impairments.

PSYCHIATRIC COMORBIDITY

Data on comorbidity of major depression in the elderly with psychiatric disorders other than dementia from community-based studies are sparse. Most reports on the prevalence of major depression fail to examine this issue. Two reviews on the topic have been conducted to date (91,92). The Amsterdam study of the elderly (AMSTEL) argued that depression and anxiety were on a continuum rather than categorical (93). They argued this to be the case as the higher severity of each disorders was associated with a higher co-occurrence of comorbidity. Generalized anxiety was found in 14.5% of the depressed subjects diagnosed using the GMS-AGECAT and alternatively 60.4% of those with generalized anxiety had depression. In addition, an increased risk along a gradient of severity for both disorders was noted. In the LASA using the DIS after screen with the CES-D, 47.5% of those with 6-month prevalent major depressive disorder also met criteria for anxiety disorders, whereas 26.1% of those with anxiety disorders also met criteria for major depressive disorder (94). As for specific anxiety disorders, major depressive disorder was comorbid in 30.3% of those with generalized anxiety disorder; 25.0% with social phobia; 50.0% with panic disorder; and 44.4% with obsessive-compulsive disorder.

Comorbid cases appeared to represent more severe disorders. The group with anxiety disorders plus major depressive disorder had a distinct risk factor profile and may represent those with a more severe disorder. In another analysis from the LASA slightly different 6-month prevalence rates for comorbidity were published (95). Of the respondents with major depression, 36% also had any anxiety disorder, while 13% of the subjects with any anxiety disorder also were diagnosed with major depression. The proportion of individuals with comorbid major depression was significantly greater than those without comorbidity or pure major depression. Significant comorbid relationships were present with each of the specific anxiety disorders; 39% with panic disorder, 13% with phobic disorders, 29% with obsessive-compulsive disorder, and 15% with generalized anxiety disorder. As in the two earlier reports severity was associated with comorbidity as noted by higher scores on the Hamilton Depression Scale-A and the CES-D. An earlier study using the Comprehensive Assessment and Referral Examination (CARE) found a significant association between anxiety and depression as well (96).

The Canadian WMHS (97) examined comorbidity between major depression and anxiety, but only with social phobia, agoraphobia, and panic disorder among individuals older than 55 years. Generalized anxiety disorder was excluded. 12-month prevalence of social phobia was present in 14.5% of individuals with major depression, while agoraphobia and panic disorder were present in 5.3% and 9.0% of respondents, respectively. Among those with an anxiety disorder major depression was highly prevalent, social phobia 31.0%; agoraphobia 25.1%, and panic disorder 29.5%.

More recently, the NCS-R has provided an opportunity to examine comorbidity among those of 65 years and older (15). Approximately half, 51.8%, of the sample aged 65 years and older who were diagnosed with major depressive disorder had a 12-month diagnosis of another disorder, in contrast to a slightly higher rate, 60.6%, for respondents aged from 18 to 64 years. For older adults, the most prevalent comorbidity was social phobia, 25.0%, whereas specific phobia, 25.1%, was the most prevalent comorbidity for the younger respondents. Comorbidty is as much of an issue for the elderly population as in younger individuals.

RISK FACTORS OTHER THAN MEDICAL COMORBIDITY

In addition to medical comorbidity, several other important risk factors have been identified in older adults with major depression. A meta-analysis of 20 studies with a prospective design examined risk factors for depression among elders living in the community (65); significant risk factors for major depression in later life included female physical disability, bereavement, sleep disturbance, and prior episodes of depression. The meta-analysis did not find being older, less educated, unmarried, lower social class, poor health status, cognitive impairment, living alone, and having a new medical illness to be statistically significant. Since this seminal article, however, the relationship between socioeconomic status and depression has been revisited (98). Both low education and low income placed older subjects at increased risk for depression in a European study. This relationship was in part explained by physical and psychosocial status (99). However, in Nigeria, lifetime major depression was more prevalent in those of higher socioeconomic status (3), a finding the authors attributed either to artifact or to protective factors from retention of traditional social networks. In an earlier review of the literature based on longitudinal studies life events and ongoing difficulties; death of a spouse or other loved one; disability and functional decline; and lack of social contact; as well as presence of medical illness were associated with the risk of developing depression (100). Cigarette smoking among older persons has been shown to be associated with depression (99); as has excessive use of alcohol (101). This association with smoking was not substantiated in a more recent study (69). Physical exercise has been shown to be protective in a longitudinal study (101). Personality factors, in particular neuroticism, appear to be an important risk factor for the development of depression later in life (102). In the Longitudinal Aging Study Amsterdam, neuroticism was a more important predictor for the onset of depression than situational or health-related factors.

In a large community-based study of men in Australia a number of biologic risk factors for depression using the Geriatric Depression Scale were examined. The relationship between C-reactive protein and late-life depression although initially significant prior to controlling for confounders among men, was no longer significant once physical comorbidity was accounted for (103). Low testosterone, however, was found to be associated with depression (104). Those with depression also had higher plasma homocysteine, an amino acid, and triglycerides (105), both of which are risk factors for cardiovascular disease and the former also possibly for dementia.

Vink and colleagues (106) summarized the findings of 71 longitudinal and cross-sectional studies that explored risk factors in old age. Their results are summarized in Table 7. In general, a number of risk factors for depression were identified, including poor health and chronic physical conditions, vascular factors, disability, personality traits, maladaptive coping, poor self-image, poor social support, and stressful events. Results were more mixed across studies in terms of age, education, gender, and socioeconomic status.

EARLY- VS. LATE-ONSET DISORDERS

Although most individuals with major depression have had an episode of depression prior to reaching late age, a substantial number have late-onset depression. Late-onset depression in most studies has been defined as a first episode of depression that occurs at the age of 60 or later. Data on the age of onset of depression in prevalence studies are sparse. A few studies in respondents of age 65 and older have reported the mean age of onset of major depression, age 51 in Nigeria (3) and age 44.8 in France (107). In Chile, 36.4% of those older than 65 years were noted to have an age of onset after age 59 (108). These studies suggest that a considerable proportion of older individuals have late-onset disorders.

Community-based epidemiologic samples have not been able to consistently find a distinction in risk factors between late-onset depression and early-onset major depression. In a study from the Netherlands other than those with late-onset disorder being older and more likely to be widowed, there was no distinction in family psychiatric history, vascular pathology, and stressful early- and late-life events. This study found that individuals with early onset had more often double depression, major depression and dysthymia, and more anxiety (109). In a prospective study limited to women, few differences again emerged between late-onset and early-onset disorders (110). There were no differences between the groups on marital conflict and social support. Those with early-onset depression scored higher than those with late-onset disorder on neuroticism. However, the late-onset group reported poorer health.

GENETICS

Late-life-onset depression appears to have less of a genetic risk, less familial aggregation, than early-onset depression (111). A study of late-life depression in a sample of elderly reared-apart and reared-together Swedish twins found evidence of only limited heritability, that is 16% (112). In contrast, in a sample of Danish twins of 75 years and older depression was moderately heritable, approximately 35% (113). Clinical samples that have examined the association between depression in the elderly and Apo E genotype have had variable findings. A community-based study conducted in Taiwan has suggested that Apo E ε4 was correlated with severe depression in the elderly (114); however, like the clinical literature this association was less clear in the Cache County study conducted in the United States (115). Although no overall association was noted with Apo E ε4 in the Cache county study, there was an association with late-onset depression and increasing age.

TABLE 7 Risk Factors for Depressive Symptoms and Depressive Disorders in the Elderly Population from Cross-Sectional and Longitudinal Community-Based Studies (Number of Positive Studies by Number of Total Studies Based on Review by Vink et al., 2008

		Depressive symptoms	Depressive disorders
Chronic Disease			
	Number of Chronic Health Conditions	7/8	10/13
	Parkinsonism	1/1	
	Cognitive impairment/dementia	3/3	3/4
Vascular factors			
	Cardiovascular factors		1/1
	Cerebrovascular factors	1/2	2/3
	White matter hyperintensities	3/3	
	Atherosclerosis		1/1
	High blood pressure	0/1	1/1
	Low blood pressure	1/1	
	Fetal undernutrition	1/1	
Health			
	Poor health status	2/2	2/3
	New medical illness	1/1	1/2
	Sleep disturbance		2/2
	Low exercise level/lower number of activities	4/6	2/2
Medicine use			
	Use of psychotropic and somatic medication	2/2	1/1
	Drug misuse		1/1
Self-perceived health			
	Pain		3/3
	Poor self-perceived health	3/3	3/3
Disability			
	Functional limitations	11/12	15/17
	Vision or hearing loss	0/1	1/2
Genetic factors			
	APOE-E4 allele	1/3	0/1
	Family history of psychiatric disorder		1/1
Habits			
	Alcohol problem	1/1	1/1
	Smoking	1/1	2/2
	Obesity		1/1
Personality traits			
	External locus of control/lower level of mastery	2/2	3/4
	Neuroticism	3/3	5/5
	Lower level of extraversion		1/1
	Impulsivity	1/1P	
Coping			
	Dysfunctional coping	1/1	
	Lack of self-efficacy	2/2	2/2
Self-image			
	Low self-esteem	1/1	2/2
	Ego-strength	1/1P	
Psychopathology			
	More symptoms at baseline	3/3	
	Psychiatric history	1/1	10/10

(*Continued*)

TABLE 7 Risk Factors for Depressive Symptoms and Depressive Disorders in the Elderly Population from Cross-Sectional and Longitudinal Community-Based Studies (Number of Positive Studies by Number of Total Studies Based on Review by Vink et al., 2008 (*Continued*)

		Depressive symptoms	Depressive disorders
Quantitative aspects of social network			
	Low contact frequency	2/2	1/2
	Smaller network size	1/2	6/6
	Church attendance religious	3/3PPP	2/2PP
	Unmarried	3/4	6/7
	Marital status	0/4	2/8
	Being childless		0/1
Qualitative aspects of social network			
	Lack of social support	5/5	5/9
	Loneliness	2/2	3/3
	Not satisfied with friendship		1/1
	Problems with spouse		1/1
Stressful event			
	Serious event WWII		1/1
	Negative life events in childhood	1/1	1/1
	Bereavement	2/2	4/5
	Recent negative life events	3/3	8/9
	Care-giving status		1/1
	Depressive symptoms in spouse	1/1	
	Traumatic events		1/1
	Long-term difficulties		3/3
Social demographics			
	Being older	4/9PP	5/10PP
	Lower level of education	4/8P	5/9
	Female gender	7/13	10/16
	Urbanization		1/3
	Ethnic Minority	1/3	1/4
	Lower income	1/3	2/4
Living conditions			
	Living alone		1/2
	Living in a kibbutz	1/1P	
	Institutionalized		1/1

P = number of positive studies where the risk factor is protective.
Source: Adapted from Ref. (106).

COURSE OF DEPRESSION

Only a small number of community-based studies have examined the course and natural history of depression in elderly individuals. A meta-analysis of studies conducted between 1955 and 1994 examined the prognosis of depression in the elderly and revealed an overall poor outcome (116). Five studies based on community samples were included in that review and found that more than 27% remained ill during the course of follow-up, which ranged from one to three years. Since that review, a community-based longitudinal study in Islington found 53.3% of the 45 depressed subjects followed for 2.6 years, remained ill (117). The Longitudinal Aging Study

Amsterdam followed 277 subjects aged 55 years and older from a community-based sample over six years (118). Only a minority had a good outcome, with 32% having a severe chronic course, and 44% with a fluctuating course. In a 4-year follow-up of 64 subjects from the Health and Retirement study, 37.8% had persistent depressive symptoms (14). In contrast to this group of studies with generally poor outcomes, a community-based study of Australians aged 70 years and older, followed for 3.6 years, found that 57% recovered (119). However, 10.4% were lost to follow-up and 21.7% died which may have accounted for the better outcome among those available for follow-up. The Leiden study of individuals older than 85 years found an annual remission rate of only 14%. In more than half of the participants with a remission of depression, a relapse occurred during follow-up (120). The AMSTEL study reported that pure depression in contrast to comorbid depression with anxiety was associated with worse outcomes including mortality (62). In elderly persons, generalized anxiety has been shown to progress to depression or to the mixed condition. These comorbid conditions have a poorer prognosis than non-comorbid generalized anxiety (121). Clinical-based samples equally have shown a poor prognosis for depression in the elderly (121–123).

CONCLUSIONS

Over 15 years ago, an NIH consensus conference was held that was extremely critical of the state of psychiatric epidemiology of the elderly population (125). This report pointed out that elderly subjects were frequently excluded from studies, that current knowledge of rates were felt to be underestimated, age appropriate diagnostic criteria did not exist, and the rates of disorders did not reflect the degree of symptomatology with its resulting poor outcomes. Concern was raised that reports of relatively low prevalence of psychiatric illnesses among elderly persons could contribute to a dismissive neglect of these conditions.

Since the ECA study, steady advances in the knowledge base of the epidemiology of major depression in the elderly population have been seen, including recent prevalence estimates for the United States from the publications of results from the Cache County study and the NCS-R. The longitudinal follow-up study from the Baltimore ECA site has provided much valuable information on the course and incidence of depression in old age. The NCS-R has provided data on comorbidity with specific psychiatric disorders. However, much of what has been learned in the past 10 years comes from research conducted on populations outside the United States, in particular regarding risk factors and course of illness. The prevalence rates in studies around the world remain low in elderly cohorts and the reasons continue to be debated. Instruments that presumably are more specific for geriatric populations have done little to resolve these issues, as they remain untested in younger cohorts. Diagnostic instruments designed for the elderly, if tested in younger adults, should yield similar rates as structured diagnostic instruments designed for the general adult population, and subsequently diverge in prevalence rates when administered in older populations if the argument that diagnostic tools used in the general adult population are unsuited for the elderly respondents is true. Such studies have not been done.

Nonetheless, we have learned much about the epidemiology of depression in the elderly during the last decade. The disorder carries a high burden. That comorbidity is highly prevalent, although comorbidity with medical issues may be lower than in younger cohorts. At least from an epidemiologic perspective, the distinction between late- and early-onset disorder remains controversial. The course of illness is poor, although studies are few. Major depression in the elderly, despite its low prevalence, is a major public health issue.

REFERENCES

1. World Health Organization. Global burden of disease estimate. Available from: http://www.who.int/healthinfo/bodestimates/en/index.html.
2. Trollor JN, Anderson TM, Sachdev PS, et al. Prevalence of mental disorders in the elderly: The Australian national mental health and well-being survey. Am J Geriatr Psychiatry 2007; 15:455–466.
3. Gureje O, Kola L, Afolabi E. Epidemiology of major depressive disorder in elderly nigerians in the ibadan study of ageing: A community-based survey. Lancet 2007; 370:957–964.
4. De Beauvoir S. Old Age. Harmondsworth: Penguin, 1977.
5. Kessler RC, Foster C, Webster PS, et al. The relationship between age and depressive symptoms in two national surveys. Psychol Aging 1992; 7:119–126.
6. Mirowsky J, Ross CE. Age and depression. J Health Soc Behav 1992; 3:187–205.
7. Jorm AF. Does old age reduce the risk of anxiety and depression? A review of epidemiological studies across the adult life span. Psychol Med 2000; 30:11–22.
8. Friedmann H, Kohn R. Mortality in the suicidal population. Suicide and Life Threat Behav 2008; 38:287–301.
9. Blazer D, Burchett B, Service C, et al. The association of age and depression among the elderly: An epidemiologic exploration. J Gerontol 1991; 46:M210–M215.
10. Robins LN, Helzer JE, Croughan J, et al. National institute of mental health diagnostic interview schedule: Its history, characteristics, and validity. Arch Gen Psychiatry 1981; 38:381–389.
11. Weissman MM, Bruce ML, Leaf PJ, et al. Affective disorders. In: Robins LN, Regier DA, eds. Psychiatric Disorders in America: The Epidemiologic Catchment Area Study. New York, NY: Free Press, 1991:53–80.
12. Steffens DC, Skoog I, Norton MC, et al. Prevalence of depression and its treatment in an elderly population: The Cache County study. Arch Gen Psychiatry 2000; 57:601–607.
13. Kessler RC, Andrews G, Mroczek D, et al. The World Health Organization Composite International Diagnostic Interview Short-Form (CIDI-SF). Intern J Methods Psychiatr Res 1998; 7:171–185.
14. Mojtabai R, Olfson M. Major depression in community-dwelling middle-aged and older adults: Prevalence and 2- and 4-year follow-up symptoms. Psychol Med 2004; 34:623–634.
15. Gum AM, King-Kallimanis B, Kohn R. Prevalence and predictors of mood, anxiety, and substance abuse disorders for older Americans in the National Comorbidity Survey–Replication. Am J Geriatr Psychiatry 2008; 46(suppl 1):A119.
16. Kessler RC, Berglund P, Demler O, et al. National Comorbidity Survey Replication. The epidemiology of major depressive disorder: Results from the National Comorbidity Survey Replication (NCS-R). JAMA 2003; 289:3095–3105.
17. Robins LN, Wing J, Wittchen HU, et al. The Composite International Diagnostic Interview: An epidemiologic instrument suitable for use in conjunction with different diagnostic systems and in different cultures. Arch Gen Psychiatry 1988; 45:1069–1077.
18. Weissman MM, Myers JK. Psychiatric disorders in a U. S. community. The application of research diagnostic criteria to a resurveyed community sample. Acta Psychiatr Scand 1980; 62:99–111.
19. Brown DR, Ahmed F, Gary LE, et al. Major depression in a community sample of African Americans. Am J Psychiatry 1995; 152:373–378.
20. Turvey CL, Carney C, Arndt S, et al. Conjugal loss and syndromal depression in a sample of elders aged 70 years or older. Am J Psychiatry 1999; 156:1596–1601.

21. Awas M, Kebede D, Alem A. Major mental disorders in Butajira, southern Ethiopia. Acta Psychiatr Scand Suppl 1999; 397:56–64.
22. Hwu HG, Chang IH, Yeh EK, et al. Major depressive disorder in Taiwan defined by the Chinese Diagnostic Interview Schedule. J Nerv Ment Dis 1996; 184:497–502.
23. Kebede D, Alem A. Major mental disorders in Addis Ababa, Ethiopia, II. Affective disorders. Acta Psychiatr Scand Suppl 1999; 397:18–23.
24. Morosini PL, Coppo P, Veltro F, et al. Prevalence of mental disorders in Tuscany: A community study in Lari (Pisa). Annali Ist super sanità 1992; 28:547–52.
25. Lu J, Ruan Y, Huang Y, et al. Major depression in Kunming: Prevalence, correlates and co-morbidity in a south-western city of China. J Affect Disord 2008; Mar 28 [Epub ahead of print].
26. Sandanger I, Nygård JF, Ingebrigsten G, et al. Prevalence, incidence and age at onset of psychiatric disorders in Norway. Soc Psychiatry Psychiatr Epidemiol 1999; 34:570–579.
27. Torres de Galvis Y, Montoya ID. Segundo Estudio Nacional de Salud Mental y Consumo de Sustancias Psicoactivas, Colombia 1997. Bogata, TX: Ministerio de Salud, 1997.
28. Demyttenaere K, Bruffaerts R, Posada-Villa J, et al. WHO World Mental Health Survey Consortium. Prevalence, severity, and unmet need for treatment of mental disorders in the World Health Organization World Mental Health Surveys. JAMA 2004; 291:2581–2590.
29. Kessler RC, Ustün TB. The World Mental Health (WMH) Survey initiative version of the World Health Organization (WHO) Composite International Diagnostic Interview (CIDI). Int J Methods Psychiatr Res 2004; 13:93–121.
30. Pirkola SP, Isometsä E, Suvisaari J, et al. DSM-IV mood-, anxiety- and alcohol use disorders and their comorbidity in the Finnish general population—Results from the Health 2000 Study. Soc Psychiatry Psychiatr Epidemiol 2005; 40:1–10.
31. Ford BC, Bullard KM, Taylor RJ, et al. Lifetime and 12-month prevalence of diagnostic and statistical manual of mental disorders, 4th ed. Disorders among older African Americans: Findings from the National Survey of American Life. Am J Geriatr Psychiatry 2007; 15:652–659.
32. Norton MC, Skoog I, Toone L, et al. Cache County investigators. Three-year incidence of first-onset depressive syndrome in a population sample of older adults: The Cache County study. Am J Geriatr Psychiatry 2006; 14:237–245.
33. Eaton WW, Kalaydjian A, Scharfstein DO, et al. Prevalence and incidence of depressive disorder: The Baltimore ECA follow-up, 1981–2004. Acta Psychiatr Scand 2007; 116:182–188.
34. Murphy JM, Nierenberg AA, Laird NM, et al. Incidence of major depression: Prediction from subthreshold categories in the Stirling County Study. J Affect Disord 2002; 68:251–259.
35. Pálsson SP, Ostling S, Skoog I. The incidence of first-onset depression in a population followed from the age of 70 to 85. Psychol Med 2001; 31:1159–1168.
36. Mattisson C, Bogren M, Nettelbladt P, et al. First incidence depression in the Lundby Study: A comparison of the two time periods, 1947–1972 and 1972–1997. J Affect Disord 2005; 87:151–160.
37. Forsell Y, Winblad B. Incidence of major depression in a very elderly population. Int J Geriatr Psychiatry 1999; 14:368–372.
38. Magnússon H. Mental health of octogenarians in Iceland. An epidemiological study. Acta Psychiatr Scand Suppl 1989; 349:1–112.
39. Meller I, Fichter MM, Schroppel H. Incidence of depression in octo- and nonagenerians: Results of an epidemiological follow-up community study. Eur Arch Psychiatry Clin Neurosci. 1996;246(2):93–99.
40. Bebbington P, Dunn G, Jenkins R, et al. The influence of age and sex on the prevalence of depressive conditions: Report from the National Survey of Psychiatric Morbidity. Int Rev Psychiatry 2003; 15:74–83.
41. Gallo JJ, Lebowitz BD. The epidemiology of common late-life mental disorders in the community: Themes for the new century. Psychiatr Serv 1999; 50:1158–1166.
42. Klerman GL, Weissman MM. Increasing rates of depression. JAMA 1989; 261:2229–2235.

43. Wickramaratne PJ, Weissman MM, Leaf PJ, et al. Age, period and cohort effects on the risk of major depression: Results from five United States communities. J Clin Epidemiol 1989; 42:333–343.
44. Parker G. Are the lifetime prevalence estimates in the ECA study accurate? Psychol Med 1987; 17:275–282.
45. Rogler LH, Malgady RG, Tryon WW. Evaluation of mental health. Issues of memory in the Diagnostic Interview Schedule. J Nerv Ment Dis 1992; 180:215–222.
46. Gallo JJ, Anthony JC, Muthén BO. Age differences in the symptoms of depression: A latent trait analysis. J Gerontol 1994; 49:P251–P264.
47. Giuffra LA, Risch N. Diminished recall and the cohort effect of major depression: A simulation study. Psychol Med 1994; 24:375–383.
48. Patten SB. Recall bias and major depression lifetime prevalence. Soc Psychiatry Psychiatr Epidemiol 2003; 38:290–296.
49. Thompson R, Bogner HR, Coyne JC, et al. Personal characteristics associated with consistency of recall of depressed or anhedonic mood in the 13-year follow-up of the Baltimore Epidemiologic Catchment Area survey. Acta Psychiatr Scand 2004; 109:345–354.
50. Warshaw MG, Klerman GL, Lavori PW. Are secular trends in major depression an artifact of recall? J Psychiatr Res 1991; 25:141–151.
51. Andrews G, Anstey K, Brodaty H, et al. Recall of depressive episode 25 years previously. Psychol Med 1999; 29:787–791.
52. Hasin D, Link B. Age and recognition of depression: Implications for a cohort effect in major depression. Psychol Med 1988; 18:683–688.
53. Sachs-Ericsson N, Joiner T, Blazer DG. The influence of lifetime depression on self-reported memory and cognitive problems: Results from the National Comorbidity Survey-Replication. Aging Ment Health 2008; 12:183–192.
54. González HM, Bowen ME, Fisher GG. Memory decline and depressive symptoms in a nationally representative sample of older adults: The Health and Retirement Study (1998–2004). Dement Geriatr Cogn Disord 2008; 25:266–271.
55. Raji MA, Reyes-Ortiz CA, Kuo YF, et al. Depressive symptoms and cognitive change in older Mexican Americans. J Geriatr Psychiatry Neurol 2007; 20:145–152.
56. Bierman EJ, Comijs HC, Jonker C, et al. Effects of anxiety versus depression on cognition in later life. Am J Geriatr Psychiatry 2005; 13:686–693.
57. Ganguli M, Du Y, Dodge HH, et al. Depressive symptoms and cognitive decline in late life: A prospective epidemiological study. Arch gen Psychiatry 2006; 63:153–160.
58. Devanand DP, Sano M, Tang MX, et al. Depressed mood and the incidence of Alzheimer's disease in the elderly living in the community. Arch Gen Psychiatry 1996; 53:175–182.
59. Green RC, Cupples LA, Kurz A, et al. Depression as a risk factor for Alzheimer disease: The MIRAGE Study. Arch Neurol 2003; 60:753–79.
60. Jorm AF. History of depression as a risk factor for dementia: An updated review. Aust N Z J Psychiatry 2001; 35:776–781.
61. Abas M, Hotopf M, Prince M. Depression and mortality in a high-risk population. 11-Year follow-up of the Medical Research Council Elderly Hypertension Trial. Br J Psychiatry 2002; 181:123–128.
62. Holwerda TJ, Schoevers RA, Dekker J, et al. The relationship between generalized anxiety disorder, depression and mortality in old age. Int J Geriatr Psychiatry 2007; 22:241–249.
63. Schulz R, Drayer RA, Rollman BL. Depression as a risk factor for non-suicide mortality in the elderly. Biol Psychiatry 2002; 52:205–255.
64. Barry LC, Allore HG, Guo Z, et al. Higher burden of depression among older women: The effect of onset, persistence, and mortality over time. Arch Gen Psychiatry 2008; 65:172–178.
65. Cole MG, Dendukuri N. Risk factors for depression among elderly community subjects: A systematic review and meta-analysis. Am J Psychiatry 2003; 160:1147–1156.
66. Krishnan KR, Delong M, Kraemer H, et al. Comorbidity of depression with other medical diseases in the elderly. Biol Psychiatry 2002; 52:559–588.

67. Bisschop MI, Kriegsman DM, Deeg DJ, et al. The longitudinal relation between chronic diseases and depression in older persons in the community: The Longitudinal Aging Study Amsterdam. J Clin Epidemiol 2004; 57:187–194.
68. Ng TP, Chiam PC, Kua EH. Mental disorders and asthma in the elderly: A population-based study. Int J Geriatr Psychiatry 2007; 22:668–674.
69. Austey KJ, von Sanden C, Sargent-Cox K, et al. Prevalence and risk factors for depression in a longitudinal, population-based study including individuals in the community and residential care. Am J Geriatr Psychiatry 2007; 15:497–505.
70. Bos MJ, Lindén T, Koudstaal PJ, et al. Depressive symptoms and risk of stroke: The Rotterdam Study. J Neurol Neurosurg Psychiatry 2008 Jan 21 [Epub ahead of print].
71. Pálsson S, Aevarsson O, Skoog I. Depression, cerebral atrophy, cognitive performance and incidence of dementia. Population study of 85-year-olds. Br J Psychiatry 1999; 174:249–253.
72. Engum A. The role of depression and anxiety in onset of diabetes in a large population-based study. J Psychosom Res 2007; 62:31–38.
73. Van der Kooy K, van Hout H, Marwijk H, et al. Depression and the risk for cardiovascular diseases: Systematic review and meta analysis. Int J Geriatr Psychiatry 2007; 22:613–626.
74. Woodcock K, Pole JD. Health profile of deaf Canadians: Analysis of the Canada Community Health Survey. Can Fam Physician 2007; 53:2140–2141.
75. Braam AW, Prince MJ, Beekman AT, et al. Physical health and depressive symptoms in older Europeans. Results from EURODEP. Br J Psychiatry 2005; 187:35–42.
76. Teresi J, Abrams R, Holmes D, et al. Prevalence of depression and depression recognition in nursing homes. Soc Psychiatry Psychiatr Epidemiol 2001; 36:613–620.
77. Onder G, Liperoti R, Soldato M, et al. Depression and risk of nursing home admission among older adults in home care in Europe: Results from the Aged in Home Care (AdHOC) study. J Clin Psychiatry 2007; 68:1392–1398.
78. Harris Y, Cooper JK. Depressive symptoms in older people predict nursing home admission. J Am Geriatr Soc 2006; 54:593–597.
79. Pot AM, Deeg DJ, Twisk JW, et al. The longitudinal relationship between the use of long-term care and depressive symptoms in older adults. Gerontologist 2005; 45:359–369.
80. Knäuper B, Wittchen HU. Diagnosing major depression in the elderly: Evidence for response bias in standardized diagnostic interviews? J Psychiatr Res 1994; 28:147–164.
81. Heithoff K. Does the ECA underestimate the prevalence of late-life depression? J Am Geriatr Soc 1995; 43:2–6.
82. Booth BM, Kirchner JE, Hamilton G, et al. Diagnosing depression in the medically ill: Validity of a lay-administered structured diagnostic interview. J Psychiatr Res 1998; 32:353–360.
83. Regier DA, Kaelber CT, Rae DS, et al. Limitations of diagnostic criteria and assessment instruments for mental disorders. Implications for research and policy. Arch Gen Psychiatry 1998; 55:109–115.
84. Narrow WE, Rae DS, Robins LN, et al. Revised prevalence estimates of mental disorders in the United States: Using a clinical significance criterion to reconcile 2 surveys' estimates. Arch Gen Psychiatry 2002; 59:115–123.
85. Patten SB, Brandon-Christie JD, Sedmark B. Performance of the Composite International Diagnostic Interview Short Form for major depression in a community sample. Chronic Dis Can 2000; 21:68–72.
86. Eaton WW, Neufeld K, Chen L, et al. A comparison of self-report and clinical diagnostic interviews for depression. Arch Gen Psychiatry 2000; 57:217–222.
87. Gurland B, Kuriansky J, Sharpe L, et al. The Comprehensive assessment and Referral Evaluation (CARE)—Rationale, development and reliability. Int J Aging Hum Dev 1977–1978; 8:9–42.
88. Copeland JR, Kelleher MJ, Kellett JM, et al. A semi-structured clinical interview for the assessment of diagnosis and mental state in the elderly: The geriatric mental state schedule. I. Development and reliability. Psychol Med 1976; 6:439–449.

89. Newman SC, Sheldon CT, Bland RC. Prevalence of depression in an elderly community sample: A comparison of GMS-AGECAT and DSM-IV diagnostic criteria. Psychol Med 1998; 28:1339–1345.
90. O'Connor DW. Do older Australians truly have low rates of anxiety and depression? A critique of the 1997 National Survey of Mental Health and Wellbeing. Aust N Z J Psychiatry 2006; 40:623–631.
91. Devanand DP. Comorbid psychiatric disorders in late life depression. Biol Psychiatry 2002; 52:236–242.
92. Gum AM, Cheavens JS. Psychiatric comorbidity and depression in older adults. Curr Psychiatry Rep 2008; 10:23–29.
93. Schoevers RA, Beekman AT, Deeg DJ, et al. Comorbidity and risk-patterns of depression, generalised anxiety disorder and mixed anxiety-depression in later life: Results from the AMSTEL study. Int J Geriatr Psychiatry 2003; 18:994–1001.
94. Beekman AT, de Beurs E, van Balkom AJ, et al. Anxiety and depression in later life: Co-occurrence and communality of risk factors. Am J Psychiatry 2000; 157:89–95.
95. van Balkom AJ, Beekman AT, de Beurs E, et al. Comorbidity of the anxiety disorders in a community-based older population in The Netherlands. Acta Psychiatr Scand 2000; 101:37–45.
96. Lindesay J, Briggs K, Murphy E. The Guy's/Age Concern Survey. Prevalence rates of cognitive impairment, depression and anxiety in an urban elderly community. Br J Psychiatry 1989; 155:317–329.
97. Cairney J, Corna LM, Velhuizen S, et al. Comorbid depression and anxiety in later life: Patterns of association, subjective well-being, and impairment. Am J Geriatr Psychiatry 2008; 16:201–208.
98. Koster A, Bosma H, Kempen GI, et al. Socioeconomic differences in incident depression in older adults: The role of psychosocial factors, physical health status, and behavioral factors. J Psychosom Res 2006; 61:619–627.
99. van Gool CH, Kempen GI, et al. Relationship between changes in depressive symptoms and unhealthy lifestyles in late middle aged and older persons: Results from the Longitudinal Aging Study Amsterdam. Age Ageing 2003; 32:81–87.
100. Bruce ML. Psychosocial risk factors for depressive disorders in late life. Biol Psychiatry 2002; 52:175–184.
101. van Gool CH, Kempen GI, Bosma H, et al. Associations between lifestyle and depressed mood: Longitudinal results from the Maastricht Aging Study. Am J Public Health 2007; 97:887–894.
102. Steunenberg B, Beekman AT, Deeg DJ, et al. Personality and the onset of depression in late life. J Affect Disord 2006; 92:243–251.
103. Almeida OP, Norman P, Hankey GJ, et al. The association between C-reactive protein concentration and depression in later life is due to poor physical health: Results from the Health in Men Study (HIMS). Psychol Med 2007; 37:1775–1786.
104. Almeida OP, Yeap BB, Hankey GJ, et al. Low free testosterone concentration as a potentially treatable cause of depressive symptoms in older men. Arch Gen Psychiatry 2008; 65:283–289.
105. Almeida OP, Flicker L, Norman P, et al. Association of cardiovascular risk factors and disease with depression in later life. Am J Geriatr Psychiatry 2007; 15:506–513.
106. Vink D, Aartsen MJ, Schoevers RA. Risk factors for anxiety and depression in the elderly: A review. J Affect Disord 2008; 106:29–44.
107. Ritchie K, Artero S, Beluche I, et al. Prevalence of DSM-IV psychiatric disorder in the French elderly population. Br J Psychiatry 2004; 184:147–152.
108. Kohn R, Vicente B, Saldivia S, et al. Psychiatric epidemiology of the elderly population in Chile. Am J Geriatr Psychiatry 2008; 46(suppl 1):A115.
109. Janssen J, Beekman AT, Comijs HC, et al. Late-life depression: The differences between early- and late-onset illness in a community-based sample. Int J Geriatr Psychiatry 2006; 21:86–93.
110. Sneed JR, Kasen S, Cohen P. Early-life risk factors for late-onset depression. Int J Geriatr Psychiatry 2007; 22:663–667.

111. Heun R, Hein S. Familial aggregation of depression, but no familial aggregation of individual depressive symptoms. Eur Psychiatry 2007; 22:16–21.
112. Gatz M, Pedersen NL, Plomin R, et al. Importance of shared genes and shared environments for symptoms of depression in older adults. J Abnorm Psychol 1992; 101:701–708.
113. McGue M, Christensen K. Genetic and environmental contributions to depression symptomatology: Evidence from Danish twins 75 years of age and older. J Abnorm Psychol 1997; 106:439–448.
114. Yen YC, Rebok GW, Gallo JJ, et al. ApoE4 allele is associated with late-life depression: A population-based study. Am J Geriatr Psychiatry 2007; 15:858–868.
115. Steffens DC, Norton MC, Hart AD, et al. Cache County Study Group. Apolipoprotein E genotype and major depression in a community of older adults. The cache county study. Psychol Med 2003; 33:541–547.
116. Cole MG, Bellavance F, Mansour A. Prognosis of depression in elderly community and primary care populations: A systematic review and meta-analysis. Am J Psychiatry 1999; 156:1182–1189.
117. Livingston G, Watkin V, Milne B, et al. The natural history of depression and the anxiety disorders in older people: The Islington community study. J Affect Disord 1997; 46:255–262.
118. Beekman AT, Geerlings SW, Deeg DJ, et al. The natural history of late-life depression: A 6-year prospective study in the community. Arch Gen Psychiatry 2002; 59:605–611.
119. Henderson AS, Korten AE, Jacomb PA, et al. The course of depression in the elderly: A longitudinal community-based study in Australia. Psychol Med 1997; 27:119–129.
120. Stek ML, Vinkers DJ, Gussekloo J, et al. Natural history of depression in the oldest old: Population-based prospective study. Br J Psychiatry 2006; 188:65–69.
121. Schoevers RA, Deeg DJ, van Tilburg W, et al. Depression and generalized anxiety disorder: Co-occurrence and longitudinal patterns in elderly patients. Am J Geriatr Psychiatry 2005; 13:31–39.
122. Mueller TI, Kohn R, Leventhal N, et al. The course of depression in elderly patients. Am J Geriatr Psychiatry 2004; 12:22–29.
123. Mitchell AJ, Subramaniam H. Prognosis of depression in old age compared to middle age: A systematic review of comparative studies. Am J Psychiatry 2005; 162:1588–1601.
124. Kohn R, Epstein-Lubow G. Course and outcomes of depression in the elderly. Curr Psychiatry Rep 2006; 8:34–40.
125. Schneider LS, Reynolds CF, Lebowitz BD, et al., eds. Diagnosis and Treatment of Depression in Late Life: Results of the NIH Consensus Development Conference. Washington, DC: American Psychiatric Press; 1994.
126. Andrade LH, Lolio CA, Gentil V, et al. Epidemiologia dos transtornos mentais em uma área definida de captação da cidade de São Paulo, Brazil. Rev Psiquiatr Clin 1999; 26:257–262.
127. Patten SB, Wang JL, Williams JV, et al. Descriptive epidemiology of major depression in Canada. Can J Psychiatry 2006; 51:84–90.
128. Bland RD, Newman SC, Orn H. Prevalence of psychiatric disorders in the elderly in Edmonton. Acta Psychiatr Scand Suppl 1988; 338:57–63.
129. Murphy JM, Laird NM, Monson RR, et al. A 40-year perspective on the prevalence of depression. The Stirling County Study. Arch Gen Psychiatry 2000; 57:209–215.
130. Ma X, Xiang YT, Li SR, et al. Prevalence and sociodemographic correlates of depression in an elderly population living with family members in Beijing, China. Psychol Med 2008; 26:1–8 [Epub ahead of print].
131. Lee S, Tsang A, Zhang MY, et al. Lifetime prevalence and inter-cohort variation in DSM-IV disorders in metropolitan China. Psychol Med 2007; 37:61–71.
132. Kawakami N, Shimizu H, Haratani T, et al. Lifetime and 6-month prevalence of DSM-III-R psychiatric disorders in an urban community in Japan. Psychiatry Res 2004; 121:293–301.
133. Salgado de Snyder VN, Diaz-Pérez M. Los trastornos afectivos en la población rural [Affective disorders in the rural population]. Salud Mental 1999; 22:68–74.

134. Browne MA, Wells JE, Scott KM, et al. New Zealand Mental Health Survey Research Team. Lifetime prevalence and projected lifetime risk of DSM-IV disorders in Te Rau Hinengaro: The New Zealand Mental Health Survey. Aust N Z J Psychiatry 2006; 40:864–874.
135. Stein DJ, Seedat S, Herman A, et al. Lifetime prevalence of psychiatric disorders in South Africa. Br J Psychiatry 2008; 192:112–117.
136. Patten SB, Charney DA. Alcohol consumption and major depression in the Canadian population. Can J Psychiatry 1998; 43:502–506.
137. Isometsä E, Aro S, Aro H. Depression in Finland: A computer assisted telephone interview study. Acta Psychiatr Scand 1997; 96:122–128.
138. Lindeman S, Hämäläinen J, Isometsä E, et al. The 12-month prevalence and risk factors for major depressive episode in Finland: Representative sample of 5993 adults. Acta Psychiatr Scand 2000; 102:178–184.
139. Madianos MG, Gournas G, Stefanis CN. Depressive symptoms and depression among elderly people in Athens. Acta Psychiatr Scand 1992; 86:320–326.
140. Carta MG, Carpiniello B, Morosini PL, et al. Prevalence of mental disorders in Sardinia: A community study in an inland mining district. Psychol Med 1991; 21:1061–1071.
141. Beekman AT, Deeg DJ, van Tilburg T, et al. Major and minor depression in later life: A study of prevalence and risk factors. J Affect Disord 1995; 36:65–75.
142. Wells JE, Browne MA, Scott KM, et al. New Zealand Mental Health Survey Research Team. Prevalence, interference with life and severity of 12 month DSM-IV disorders in Te Rau Hinengaro: The New Zealand Mental Health Survey. Aust N Z J Psychiatry 2006; 40:845–854.
143. Singleton N, Bumpstead R, O'Brien M, et al. Psychiatric morbidity among adults living in private households,2000: The report of a survey carried out by Social Survey Division of the Office for National Statistics on behalf of the Department of Health, the Scottish Executive and the National Assembly for Wales. London, UK: Stationary Office, 2001.
144. Ohayon MM, Priest RG, Guileminault C, et al. The prevalence of depressive disorders in the United Kingdom. Biol Psychiatry 1999; 45:300–307.
145. Alonso J, Angermeyer MC, Bernert S, et al. ESEMeD/MHEDEA 2000 Investigators, European Study of the Epidemiology of Mental Disorders (ESEMeD) Project. Prevalence of mental disorders in Europe: Results from the European Study of the Epidemiology of Mental Disorders (ESEMeD) project. Acta Psychiatr Scand Suppl 2004; 420:21–27.
146. Shen YC, Zhang MY, Huang YQ, et al. Twelve-month prevalence, severity, and unmet need for treatment of mental disorders in metropolitan China. Psychol Med 2006; 36:257–267.
147. Kawakami N, Takeshima T, Ono Y, et al. Twelve-month prevalence, severity, and treatment of common mental disorders in communities in Japan: Preliminary finding from the World Mental Health Japan Survey 2002–2003. Psychiatry Clin Neurosci 2005; 59:441–452.
148. Karam EG, Mneimneh ZN, Karam AN, et al. Prevalence and treatment of mental disorders in Lebanon: A national epidemiological survey. Lancet 2006; 367:1000–1006.
149. Levinson D, Zilber N, Lerner Y, et al. Prevalence of mood and anxiety disorders in the community: Results from the Israel national health survey. Isr J Psychiatry Relat Sci 2007; 44:94–103.
150. Streiner DL, Cairney J, Veldhuizen S. The epidemiology of psychological problems in the elderly. Can J Psychiatry 2006; 51:185–191.
151. Kramer M, German PS, Anthony JC, et al. Patterns of mental disorders among the elderly residents of eastern Baltimore. J Am Geriatr Soc 1985; 33:236–245.
152. Kawamura T, Shioiri T, Takahashi K, et al. Survival rate and causes of mortality in the elderly with depression: A 15-year prospective study of a Japanese community sample, the matsunoyama-niigata suicide prevention project. J Investig Med 2007; 55:106–114.
153. Ben-Ezra M, Shmotkin D. Predictors of mortality in the old-old in Israel: The cross-sectional and longitudinal aging study. J Am Geriatr Soc 2006; 54:906–911.

154. Kamphuis MH, Kalmijn S, Tijhuis MA, et al. Depressive symptoms as risk factor of cardiovascular mortality in older European men: The Finland, Italy and Netherlands Elderly (FINE) study. Eur J Cardiovasc Prev Rehabil 2006; 13:199–206.
155. Bergdahl E, Gustavsson JM, Kallin K, et al. Depression among the oldest old: The Umeå 85+ study. Int Psychogeriatr 2005; 17:557–575.
156. Adamson JA, Price GM, Breeze E, et al. Are older people dying of depression? Findings from the Medical Research Council trial of the assessment and management of older people in the community. J Am Geriatr Soc 2005; 53:1128–1132.
157. Blazer DG, Hybels CF. What symptoms of depression predict mortality in community-dwelling elders? J Am Geriatr Soc 2004; 52:2052–2056.
158. Vinkers DJ, Stek ML, Gussekloo J, et al. Does depression in old age increase only cardiovascular mortality? The leiden 85-plus study. Int J Geriatr Psychiatry 2004; 19:852–857.
159. Fröjdh K, Håkansson A, Karlsson I, et al. Deceased, disabled or depressed–a population-based 6-year follow-up study of elderly people with depression. Soc Psychiatry Psychiatr Epidemiol 2003; 38:557–562.
160. Schoevers RA, Geerlings MI, Beekman AT, et al. Association of depression and gender with mortality in old age. Results from the Amsterdam Study of the Elderly (AMSTEL). Br J Psychiatry 2000; 177:336–342.
161. Saz P, Launer LJ, Día JL, et al. Mortality and mental disorders in a Spanish elderly population. Int J Geriatr Psychiatry 1999; 14:1031–1038.
162. Pulska T, Pahkala K, Laippalla P, et al. Major depression as a predictor of premature deaths in elderly people in Finland: A community study. Acta Psychiatr Scand 1998; 97:408–411.
163. Engedal K. Mortality in the elderly: A 3-year follow-up of an elderly community sample. Int J Geriatr Psychiatry 1996; 11:467–471.
164. Kay DW, Henderson AS, Scott R, et al. Dementia and depression among the elderly living in the Hobart community: The effect of the diagnostic criteria on the prevalence rates. Psychol Med 1985; 15:771–788.
165. Newman SC, Bland RC, Orn HT. The prevalence of mental disorders in the elderly in Edmonton: A community survey using GMS-AGECAT. Geriatric mental state-automated geriatric examination for computer assisted taxonomy. Can J Psychiatry 1998; 43:910–914.
166. Chen R, Copeland JR, Wei L. A meta-analysis of epidemiological studies in depression of older people in the People's Republic of China. Int J Geriatr Psychiatry 1999; 14:821–830.
167. Chen R, Hu Z, Qin X, et al. A community-based study of depression in older people in Hefei, China—The GMS-AGECAT prevalence, case validation and socio-economic correlates. Int J Geriatr Psychiatry 2004; 19:407–413.
168. Schaub RT, Linden M, Copeland AJR. comparison of GMS-A/AGECAT, DSM-III-R for dementia and depression, including subthreshold depression (SD)—Results from the Berlin Aging Study (BASE). Int J Geriatr Psychiatry 2003; 18:109–117.
169. Meller I, Fichter M, Schröppel H, et al. Mental and somatic health and need for care in octo- and nonagenerians. An epidemiological community study. Eur Arch Psychiatry Clin Neurosci 1993; 242:286–292.
170. Kim JM, Stewart R, Shin IS, et al. Lifetime urban/rural residence, social support and late-life depression in Korea. Int J Geriatr Psychiatry 2004; 19:843–851.
171. van Ojen R, Hooijer C, Bezemer D, et al. Late-life depressive disorder in the community. I. The relationship between MMSE score and depression in subjects with and without psychiatric history. Br J Psychiatry 1995; 166:311–315
172. Uwakwe R. The pattern of psychiatric disorders among the aged in a selected community in Nigeria. Int J Geriatr Psychiatry 2000; 15:355–362.
173. Kua EH. A community study of mental disorders in elderly Singaporean Chinese using the GMS-AGECAT package. Aust N Z J Psychiatry 1992; 26:502–506.
174. Chuan SK, Kumar R, Matthew N, et al. Subsyndromal depression in old age: Clinical significance and impact in a multi-ethnic community sample of elderly Singaporeans. Int Psychogeriatr 2008; 20:188–200.

175. Chong MY, Tsang HY, Chen CS, et al. Community study of depression in old age in Taiwan: Prevalence, life events and socio-demographic correlates. Br J Psychiatry 2001; 178:29–35.
176. Ghubash R, El-Rufaie O, Zoubeidi T, et al. Profile of mental disorders among the elderly United Arab Emirates population: Sociodemographic correlates. Int J Geriatr Psychiatry 2004; 19:344–351.
177. Bhatnagar K, Frank J. Psychiatric disorders in elderly from the Indian sub-continent living in Bradford. Int J Geriatr Psychiatry 1997; 12:907–912.
178. Saunders PA, Copeland JR, Dewey ME, et al. The prevalence of dementia, depression and neurosis in later life: The Liverpool MRC-ALPHA study. Int J Epidemiol 1993; 22:838–847.
179. Copeland JR, Dewey ME, Wood N, et al. Range of mental illness among the elderly in the community. Prevalence in Liverpool using the GMS-AGECAT package. Br J Psychiatry 1987; 150:815–823.
180. Copeland JR, Gurland BJ, Dewey ME, et al. Is there more dementia, depression and neurosis in New York? A comparative study of the elderly in New York and London using the computer diagnosis AGECAT. Br J Psychiatry 1987; 151:466–473.
181. McDougall FA, Kvaal K, Matthews FE, et al. Medical Research Council Cognitive Function and Ageing Study. Prevalence of depression in older people in England and Wales: The MRC CFA study. Psychol Med 2007; 37:1787–1795.
182. Lobo A, Dewey M, Copeland J, et al. The prevalence of dementia among elderly people living in Zaragoza and Liverpool. Psychol Med 1992; 22:239–243.
183. Copeland JR, Beekman AT, Braam AW, et al. Depression among older people in Europe: The EURODEP studies. World Psychiatry 2004; 3:45–49.

4 Bipolar Disorder in Later Life

Brent P. Forester

Geriatric Psychiatry Program, McLean Hospital, Belmont, and Department of Psychiatry, Harvard Medical School, Boston, Massachusetts, U.S.A.

Brittany Jordan

Geriatric Psychiatry Program, McLean Hospital, Belmont, Massachusetts, U.S.A.

INTRODUCTION

Bipolar disorder in older adults is a complex neuropsychiatric syndrome that presents clinicians with both diagnostic and therapeutic challenges. Mania in later life can represent the recurrence of an illness first manifested in adolescence or early adulthood; alternately, it can represent the new onset of a state arising in later life from medical or neurologic causes. In either case, the presentation and treatment of bipolar disorder in later life are frequently complicated by medical comorbidity, especially cardiovascular and cerebrovascular illness (1). Despite clinical lore that bipolar disorder "burns out" with aging, cross-sectional analyses have reported that older adults with bipolar disorder continue to use health services at high rates (2). Unfortunately, there has been little longitudinal study to date on the effects of aging on the course of bipolar disorder.

Many clinical challenges arise during the evaluation and management of the geriatric bipolar patient (3). What are the effects of lithium treatment acutely and chronically on an aging brain? How do older adults with acute mania respond to treatments, including lithium, divalproex or the atypical antipsychotic agents that carry an FDA indication for treatment of acute mania or mixed states? What is the appropriate pharmacologic management of bipolar depression in the elderly, a condition that overshadows mania in its frequency yet has been less thoroughly investigated? What is the natural history of early-onset bipolar disorder through the life cycle? How does a clinician differentiate between the syndromes of mania, delirium, and dementia in a patient with a history of bipolar disorder presenting with mood instability, anxiety, and increased confusion? Finally, what are the long-term effects of bipolar disorder on cognitive functioning and, specifically, are patients with bipolar disorder at an increased later risk of developing degenerative dementias?

Many of these questions remain unanswered given the paucity of prospective, controlled clinical research in any phase of bipolar disorder in a geriatric population. Rather, the current approach to treatment for older adults with bipolar disorder relies predominantly on a careful psychiatric, medical, and neurologic evaluation and the judicious use of pharmacologic treatments that do have evidence-based support from studies of younger adults with bipolar disorder. In this chapter, we will present a case vignette highlighting some of the critical clinical issues that arise in the management of an older adult with bipolar disorder. We will then discuss epidemiologic data, differential diagnosis, and evidence-based pharmacotherapeutic and psychosocial interventions for the treatment of bipolar disorder in older adults.

CASE VIGNETTE ADAPTED FROM

Mrs. Smith, a 74-year-old widow with a 30-year history of bipolar disorder, was referred because of concerns about increasing depression (4). She had remained stable on lithium carbonate since 1979, most recently at a dose of 900 mg/day. Over the past few months, her family had noted increasing apathy, lack of motivation, and a decline in her functional capacity, although she had denied feeling depressed. The dosage of a diuretic medication, furosemide, had been recently increased in order to treat her hypertension. On examination, Mrs. Smith had an intention tremor of both hands, a Mini-Mental Status Examination (MMSE) score of 28 out of 30, clinically apparent deficits in concentration, and a lithium level of 0.9 mEq/L. Because lithium neurotoxicity was suspected, her lithium dosage was decreased to 450 mg/day, with a follow-up serum lithium level of 0.5 mEq/L. Within 2 weeks, Mrs. Smith's daughter called to report that her mom was "no longer depressed," with improved motivation, energy, and concentration, and a return to independent functioning.

Two years later, a routine check of Mrs. Smith's renal function revealed a creatinine level of 1.4 mg/dL and a 24-hour creatinine clearance that indicated significant renal insufficiency. A nephrology consultation recommended gradually discontinuing her lithium. This recommendation caused the patient severe anxiety and sleeplessness, leading to a brief hospitalization for a mixed episode with racing thoughts, irritable mood, and pressured speech.

Still on lithium carbonate, Mrs. Smith was discharged with the addition of olanzapine 5 mg/day at bedtime. As an outpatient, she was started on lamotrigine, which was titrated to 100 mg/day over a 2-month period. Lithium was then tapered and discontinued, and olanzapine was maintained at 2.5 mg/day at bedtime. Over the next six months, Mrs. Smith's condition remained stable with no further mood episodes. Repeat neuropsychological testing after two years indicated a stable impairment in memory retrieval and executive functioning.

This case highlights a number of important clinical issues when treating older adults with bipolar disorder, including age-related pharmacokinetic and pharmacodynamic changes that impact the efficacy and tolerability of lithium in older adults (e.g., the increasingly narrow therapeutic index of lithium), an understanding of cognitive changes that can be related to the underlying illness, the complication of a superimposed delirium or adverse medication effect, the risk of renal insufficiency with long-term use of lithium, the challenges in switching from lithium to alternative mood-stabilizing therapies, and the use of combination pharmacotherapy. Furthermore, the psychosocial adversities related to bipolar illness continue to be a major complication of bipolar disorder in later life.

EPIDEMIOLOGY

Geriatric bipolar disorder is a grossly understudied area with large gaps in the literature. Today, much of what we know about the epidemiology of geriatric bipolar disorder derives from data collected from mixed-age adult populations. Bipolar disorder is a highly recurrent disorder that can significantly impact the function of an individual. Approximately 85% to 100% of patients experience a recurrence of symptoms after their initial episode (5). Of all disabilities that originate from a medical disorder, bipolar disorder ranks as the sixth leading cause of disability in developed countries (6).

Lifetime prevalence rates of bipolar disorder appear uniform across cultures and are similar between men and women in adult samples (7). However, gender differences change within the bipolar population when stratified by age with a 2:1 ratio, woman to men respectively, in an older bipolar cohort (8). The 1-year prevalence of bipolar disorder among adults 65 years and older is 0.4%, significantly lower than that in younger adults (1.4%) (9).

Bipolar disorder is often considered to be a heterogeneous diagnosis comprised primarily of two groups, those with early-onset illness who are aging and those who develop the first episode of mania after the age of 50 years (later onset). In as many as 10% of all patients with bipolar disorder, the illness develops after the age of 50 years (10). Later-onset bipolar disorder is associated with a lower rate of familial illness than early-onset cases, a higher rate of medical and neurologic comorbidity, and an increased vulnerability to relapse (11). Later-onset bipolar disorder that has developed after a history of unipolar depression is poorly understood but could be linked to medication, vascular-related factors, or other brain mechanisms (12). In patients with a history of unipolar depression, mania may not develop until later life (11), and so misdiagnosis is common, especially in type II bipolar disorder. In a recent study, a majority of the 54% of misdiagnosed geriatric bipolar patients was originally believed to have had unipolar depression (13).

Finally, older patients with bipolar disorder have a lower incidence of substance abuse, but a higher severity of cognitive and functional impairment, than their younger counterparts (8). Data from a U.S. Veterans' Bipolar Disorder Database reports an 8.9% co-occurrence of substance misuse, a 9.7% co-occurrence of anxiety disorders, and a 4.5% co-occurrence of dementia (14).

Little is known about utilization of mental health services by geriatric bipolar patients (8).While 10% to 20% of geriatric outpatients with mood disorders have bipolar disorder (15), bipolar patients represent 5% to 12% of all geriatric psychiatry inpatient admissions in the course of a year (16). A study of health care expenditures associated with the treatment of bipolar disorder examined 13,471 mixed-age bipolar patients in the Medicaid system. Researchers reported that 30% of the total cost was related to the treatment of bipolar disorder and 70% was attributed to the treatment of comorbid conditions (17). The same authors also found high costs attributed to hospitalizations, antipsychotic medication use, and personal care (17).

DIFFERENTIAL DIAGNOSIS

The DSM-IV TR diagnostic classification system is used for the diagnosis of bipolar disorder in the elderly (18). This includes the diagnosis of bipolar disorder, Type I (recurring episodes of mania with or without depression); bipolar disorder, Type II (hypomania and recurrent major depression); and cyclothymic disorder (hypomanic symptoms alternating with subthreshold depression). DSM-IV TR also identifies bipolar, mixed state and bipolar disorder, rapid cycling subtypes as important considerations. Please see Table 1 for an adapted list of DSM-IV TR criteria for bipolar disorder (18).

Although these criteria are clear, the presenting symptoms of these disorders are often less easy to discern and distinguish in the geriatric patient. The diagnostic picture of bipolar disorder in the elderly is often confounded by the presence of delirium, dementia, and medical or neurologic conditions. Another factor often overlooked when diagnosing the geriatric bipolar patient is comorbid substance use, the presence of which can have acute and long-term effects that can impact a patient's mood state, cognition, and level of independent functioning.

TABLE 1 DSM-IV TR Criteria for Bipolar Disorder

Bipolar I disorder requires the presence of at least one manic episode in patient's lifetime

Manic episode

1. A distinct period of abnormally and persistently elevated, expansive, or irritable mood lasting at least 1 week.
2. During the period of mood disturbance, three or more of the following symptoms persisted and have been present to a significant degree.
   (a). inflated self-esteem or grandiosity
   (b). decreased need for sleep
   (c). more talkative than usual or pressured speech
   (d). flight of ideas or racing thoughts
   (e). distractibility
   (f). increase in goal-directed activity or psychomotor agitation
   (g). excessive involvement in pleasurable activities that have a high consequence for painful consequences (e.g., buying sprees, sexual indiscretion)
3. The mood disturbance is sufficient to cause marked impairment in occupational or social functioning or to necessitate hospitalization, or if there are psychotic features.
4. The symptoms are not due to the direct physiological effects of a substance or a general medical condition.

Hypomanic episode

1. A distinct period of abnormally and persistently elevated, expansive, or irritable mood, lasting at least 4 days, that is clearly different from the usual nondepressed mood.
2. The episode is associated with an unequivocal change in functioning that is uncharacteristic of the person, when not symptomatic.
3. Remainder of manic episode criteria, except that the episode is not severe enough to cause a marked impairment in social or occupational functioning, or to necessitate hospitalization, and there are no psychotic features.

Mixed episode

1. The criteria are met for both a manic and a major depressive episode (except for duration) nearly everyday during at least a 1-week period.
2. The mood disturbance is sufficient to cause marked impairment in occupational or social functioning or to necessitate hospitalization, or if there are psychotic features.
3. The symptoms are not due to the direct physiological effects of a substance or a general medical condition.

Bipolar disorder criteria sets include:

Bipolar I disorder, Single manic episode
Bipolar I disorder, Most recent episode hypomanic
Bipolar I disorder, Most recent episode manic
Bipolar I disorder, Most recent episode depressed
Bipolar I disorder, Most recent episode unspecified

For all bipolar disorder criteria sets, the following specifiers may apply:

Severity/Psychotic/Remission specifiers
With catatonic features
With postpartum onset
Longitudinal course specifiers (with and without interepisode recovery)
With seasonal pattern
With rapid cycling (at least 4 episodes of a mood disturbance in the last 12 months that meet criteria for either a major depressive, manic, mixed, or hypomanic episode)

Bipolar II Disorder (Recurrent Major Depressive Episodes with Hypomanic Episodes)

Source: Adapted from Ref. 18.

Because of these confounding issues an evaluation of manic symptoms in an older adult requires a thorough differential diagnosis. The clinical history is key to determining the accurate diagnosis and developing a proper treatment plan.

Geriatric Mania

Although the DSM-IV TR criteria for mania focus on the presence of abnormal and persistent elevation of mood, expansiveness, or irritability (18), older manic adults often present with a confusing combination of depressed and manic symptoms described as a mixed presentation (19). The presence of mixed symptoms, along with differing symptomatology from that of bipolar disorder in younger populations, can decrease the sensitivity of the DSM-IV TR criteria when being used as a guide for diagnosing bipolar disorder in a geriatric individual. Although mood congruent delusions often occur in both young and older adult populations, instances of mood incongruent delusions increase in the geriatric patient (19). The hyperactivity and flight of ideas often seen in younger adult populations more often present as irritability in the older adult manic patient (10). Older adult manic patients are also less likely to present with increases in activity, sexual interest, religiosity, and initiating and making plans than their younger counterparts (20). The incidence of cognitive impairment is higher in older adult manic patients than younger ones, which may be due to medical and neurologic issues discussed in greater detail later in this chapter (21).

Despite all these differences, there are still similarities among the younger and older populations of manic bipolar patients. Sleep difficulties are still present in both populations along with thought disorders such as incoherence, loose associations, derailment, illogical thinking, and neologism (22). The severity of these thought disorders can be as severe as in schizophrenia in both the younger and older adult populations (22).

Secondary Mania

As previously mentioned, the presence of delirium, dementia, and medical or neurologic conditions often clouds the diagnosis of mania in older bipolar patients. When mania presents purely in the context of medical or neurologic factors, it is described as "secondary mania" and is diagnosed in DSM-IV TR as a mood disorder due to a general medical condition, with manic features (293.83) (18). Sorting out the differences between mania in the context of bipolar disorder and these medical factors can be difficult. Neuropsychiatric symptoms of patients with secondary mania can present very similarly to those of a patient with new onset or even recurrent primary mania. Secondary mania is most often seen with a late onset and secondary to the presence of a medical or neurologic illness or an adverse reaction to a pharmacologic treatment (23). Secondary mania is less frequently correlated with a family history of mood disorder, as it is rooted in medical and neurologic origins (23). Table 2 lists some of the conditions that have been reported to present as secondary mania.

To highlight the prevalence of neurologic disorders and their effects on secondary mania, a retrospective study conducted by Tohen demonstrated the high frequency of medical etiologies in late-life mania. Tohen assessed 50 manic subjects older than 65 years of age and found that within that cohort, neurologic disorders were reported in 74% of the manic patients with late onset and 28% of those with early onset (24).

TABLE 2 Causes of Secondary Mania

Neurologic disorders (10,20,23,60,94–97)	**Especially right orbitofrontal & right basotemporal localities** Space-occupying lesions or other head injuries Epilepsy, especially right temporal focus Alzheimer disease Vascular dementia Parkinson disease Pick disease (Frontotemporal Dementia) Tourette Syndrome Wilson disease Encephalitis
Lesions (10,20,60)	Chronic alcoholism Multiple sclerosis Endocrine disorders Right hemisphere cerebrovascular disease
Infections (20,23,60,98)	Viral: influenza, AIDS Rickettsial: Q fever Spirochetes: neurosyphilis
Pharmacologic agents or ECT (10,23,60)	Antidepressants Benzodiazepines Corticosteroids Estrogen Thyroid replacement Amphetamines/cocaine Levodopa Captopril Isoniazid Enalapril Procarbazine Lithium Decongestants ECT Bronchodilators Metoclopromide Calcium Procyclidine Stimulant appetite suppressants Phencyclidine
Toxins (10,23)	Bromide
Metabolic disturbances (10,23,60)	End-stage renal disease Hemodialysis-related metabolic changes Postoperative metabolic disturbances Anemia Hyperthyroidism B12 deficiency Niacin deficiency

Source: Reference for Table 2 is reprinted from Ref. 19.

Differentiating Among Mania, Dementia, and Delirium

Dementia and delirium can present with manic symptoms such as irritable mood, emotional lability, sleep disturbance, and impaired social judgment. Further evaluation, once manic symptoms have subsided, may reveal the early stages of dementia. The co-occurrence of significant signs of confusion, fluctuation of alertness, or evidence of autonomic dysfunction can indicate the presence of delirium and requires a thorough medical and neurologic evaluation (3). For any patient with a history of bipolar disorder, any change in baseline mood symptoms or functioning suggesting a decompensation, warrants a workup for a concurrent medical condition (3).

In the presence of dementia, the diagnosis of mania is particularly problematic. McDonald and Nemeroff (25) highlight the difficulties in distinguishing mania from dementia, delirium, or agitated depression among patients older than 70 years with MMSE scores below 15 on the 30-point scale. The following "clinical pearls" (19) may assist in the differential diagnosis in patients who present with a combination of manic and cognitive symptoms.

1. A rapid decline in cognitive functioning in a demented patient, along with fluctuations in mood, energy, and sleep, can indicate the onset of a manic episode.
2. Mixed manic and depressive symptoms are common in older manic patients.
3. Focal neurologic findings such as aphasia, apraxia, or impaired visuospatial functioning are typically associated with dementia rather than with mania.
4. Nighttime agitation and confusion (sundowning) are more typically associated with dementia or delirium than with mania.
5. A negative family history for bipolar disorder may be unreliable, because an older patient's siblings and ancestors may have been diagnosed (or misdiagnosed) prior to the modern diagnostic classification. Prior to the widespread availability of mood stabilizing agents, clinicians were less sensitive to the presence of bipolar disorder (26).

Table 3 lists characteristic features of mania as contrasted with delirium and dementia.

Bipolar Depression

Unfortunately, there has been little in the literature concerning the differences between the clinical presentation of geriatric bipolar depression in the older adult population as compared to the younger bipolar depressed population (11). In addition, the question of whether the common clinical perception that symptoms such as hypersomnia, hyperphagia, and psychomotor retardation occur more often in adult bipolar depression as opposed to unipolar depression, remains unresolved in an elderly cohort (3).

Substance Abuse

The long-term and acute effects of substance abuse can contribute to the difficulty in making an accurate diagnosis of bipolar disorder. Recognizing comorbid substance use is a critical part of treating an older adult patient with bipolar disorder. Today's cohort of older adults appears to more commonly misuse or abuse alcohol, benzodiazepines, prescription pain medications, or over-the-counter medications that have anticholinergic side effects than the drugs abused in younger bipolar patients, such as heroin or cocaine (3). It is important to thoroughly assess all substances a patient is taking, whether over-the-counter, prescribed, or used as dietary supplements

TABLE 3 Diagnostic Considerations in Geriatric Bipolar Disorder

Data source	Mania	Dementia	Delirium	Secondary mania
History	At least 1-week duration of elevated, expansive, or irritable mood and distractibility	Gradual onset	Rapid onset, with fluctuation during course of day	There is a close temporal relationship between a manic episode and a primary medical disorder in 20% of patients (a latent period of months to years may be observed)
Physical examination	Not attributable to a medical condition; neurologic signs such as ataxia and frontal release signs may be present	Identifiable functional decline; movement disorders are common	Evidence of physical illness (e.g., urinary tract infection, upper respiratory tract infection)	Evidence of accompanying neurologic or nonneurologic disorders
Family history	Mood disorders	Dementia	No association	No association with family history of bipolar disorder
Mental status examination	Alert Symptoms (2 or more): Grandiosity Pressured speech Psychomotor agitation Flight of ideas Increased goal-directed activity Excessive behaviors	Alert Aphasia, apraxia, agnosia Impaired executive functioning Usually absent: Mood elevation and expansiveness, inflated self-esteem, flight of ideas, and excessive involvement in pleasurable activities	Disturbance of consciousness, orientation, and sleep/wake cycle	Irritable mood, persecutory delusions of mood incongruent type, grandiose delusions not as common as with mania

Attention and concentration	Tangential; flight of ideas, with grandiosity; easily distracted	Decreased ability to register new data, but may respond well to prompting	Easily distracted; ability to maintain and shift focus is impaired	May or may not be relevant, depending on primary condition
Speech	Pressured	Aphasia	Varies	May be pressured but disorganized because of primary condition
Sleep	Decreased need; common	No direct association, but sleep/wake cycle reversal	Sleep/wake cycle disturbances common; daytime sleepiness/nighttime agitation	Sleep/wake cycle disturbance due to agitation and irritability
Laboratory and other associated findings			Lab abnormalities common; associated with underlying medical condition	Lab abnormalities associated with primary condition, but mostly nondiagnostic
Neuroimaging and EEG	Increased perfusion in orbital and supragenual medial frontal cortex	Neuroimaging may reveal cerebral atrophy, but mostly no uniform findings	EEG abnormal; frequently generalized slowing	Neuroimaging supporting neurologic disorders or head trauma, right-sided lesions of frontal projection pathways are more common

Abbreviation: EEG, electroencephalogram.
Source: Adapted from Ref. 19.

(including nutritional agents and herbal therapies), when evaluating an older bipolar individual (3).

DIAGNOSTIC ASSESSMENTS

Cognitive Functioning

Recent years have seen an increased number of publications that address the cognitive function of bipolar patients. Researchers have recognized that cognitive impairment can be present even during periods of euthymic mood. For bipolar adults, in general, neurocognitive impairment can be a trait rather than a state variable, or even a slowly evolving process (3). Cavanaugh and colleagues reviewed controlled studies and concluded that significant deficits in verbal memory, as assessed by the California Verbal Learning Test, are present among euthymic bipolar adults (27). Other researchers have replicated this finding and have added evidence of impaired executive function and sustained attention in euthymic bipolar patients. These include a controlled study of 18 euthymic bipolar patients aged 60 years and above that found executive dysfunction on the Mattis Dementia Rating Scale and the executive interview (28). There was no association among age of first episode, duration of illness, or use of specific mood stabilizers and cognitive dysfunction. Kessing and Nilsson report an increased risk of hospitalization for dementia in patients that have been hospitalized previously for mania (29). Kessing and Anderson report that with every episode that leads to hospitalization for a bipolar patient, the risk of dementia increases by 6% (30).

A recent comprehensive study compared the performance of middle-aged and older bipolar patients to age-matched controls and schizophrenic patients on a battery of neuropsychological tests assessing vocabulary, attention/working memory, verbal learning memory, visual learning memory, information processing speed, and reasoning/problem solving. (31) The bipolar group was designated as stable but not uniformly euthymic. Based on an overall mean score of "global cognitive functioning," 56% of the bipolar patients were designated as cognitively impaired compared with 65% of schizophrenic patients and 12% of normal controls. The bipolar group differed significantly from the control group on all but three specific measures: WAIS-R vocabulary, Story Memory Learning, and the Boston Naming Test. Although patients taking lithium or antipsychotic medications had significantly worse scores than patients who were not, the scores of the bipolar group not taking lithium or antipsychotics were still significantly lower than the normal controls. Depp and colleagues found these results to be independent of symptom severity or duration of illness (31).

There is some evidence in the literature of a positive correlation between the degree of impairment in verbal learning and memory and the number and cumulative duration of manic episodes in a given patient, a finding that would seem to have implications for geriatric patients with early-onset bipolar disorder (27). However, in a recent study by Schouws, geriatric bipolar patients with early-onset bipolar disorder (before age 50) were found to have cognitive deficits consistent with those found in younger adults, suggesting a trait-related dysregulation that is independent of age (32).

A recent study by Nunes examined 66 elderly euthymic bipolar patients on chronic lithium therapy compared with 48 without recent lithium treatment (33). The mean duration of bipolar disorder for this sample was greater than 25 years.

The prevalence of Alzheimer dementia was 5% for those on lithium compared with 33% not on lithium, suggesting a neuroprotective effect in patients treated chronically with lithium. Biologically, lithium inhibits the enzyme glycogen synthase kinase 3 (GSK 3), a key enzyme in the metabolism of amyloid precursor protein and the phosphorylation of tau protein, implicated in the pathophysiology of Alzheimer disease.

Many hypotheses regarding the causes of cognitive impairment in geriatric bipolar disorder have been offered including neurodevelopmental abnormalities, "toxicity" of recurrent mood episodes, cerebrovascular disease, substance abuse comorbidity, and medication side effects (28). Whatever the cause, the phenomenon of cognitive impairment in elderly patients with bipolar disorder demands wider acknowledgment and attention, as evidenced in a sobering study by Gildingers et al. reporting a significant correlation between cognitive deficits in euthymic elderly bipolar patients and poor performance on measures of independent activities of daily living (28).

Neuroimaging

Neuroimaging studies of bipolar disorder have primarily focused on cerebral volume loss and cerebrovascular changes. SPECT scans have demonstrated a relative decrease in cerebral blood flow in the right basal temporal cortex of bipolar patients (34). Structural imaging studies have shown significantly larger amygdala volumes and larger lateral and third ventricles in bipolar patients (26), suggesting a reduction in the volume of the thalamus or hypothalamus (35). Others have discovered a significant reduction of gray matter in the left subgenual area of the prefontal cortex (36). A neuroimaging study of first episode bipolar patients reported smaller volumes of total corpus callossom, total body, and isthmus in bipolar patients compared with healthy controls, as well as a negative correlation between these volumetric measures and scores on the Young Mania Rating Scale (37).

Recent advances in neuroimaging technology have permitted a greater focus on cerebrovascular correlates of bipolar disorder. McDonald et al. in one of the earliest of such studies, reported increased subcortical hyperintensities in elderly manic patients, in the inferior half of the frontal lobe (38). Later, Steffens and Krishnan coined the term "vascular mania" referring to manic episodes associated with cortical cerebrovascular lesions and white matter intensities.(39). Zanetti et al. reported an interesting case study of a 72-year-old woman with a 14-year history of depression who presented with a manic episode at the age of 61 followed by rapid cycling(12). An MRI revealed significant white matter hyperintensities. The authors speculate that "vascular white matter intensities can provoke late-onset bipolar disorder by damaging frontolimbic circuits implicated in the pathophysiology of mania" (12). Although white matter hyperintensities (WMHs) have also been observed in children and adolescents with bipolar disorder, the authors speculate that WMHs associated with late-onset bipolar disorder may be more ischemic in origin, as is the case for WMHs in late-life depression.

The study of the neurophysiologic correlates of bipolar disorder in later life is in its infancy and there is still much to be discovered regarding the differences between older adults with late-onset bipolar disorder, those with longstanding bipolar disorder, and younger bipolar patients. Future findings that also measure brain metabolites with magnetic resonance spectroscopy will hopefully shed further light not only on treatment strategies, but possibly preventive measures as well (40).

TREATMENT STRATEGIES FOR GERIATRIC BIPOLAR DISORDER

Psychopharmacology

Most of what we know about the treatment of bipolar disorder comes from randomized, controlled clinical trials in adult or mixed-age populations. There are no double-blind, placebo-controlled studies in geriatric bipolar disorder. There are a number of plausible explanations for this lack of controlled clinical data. Diagnostic overlap between geriatric mania, delirium, and dementia, as well as other clinical syndromes such as secondary mania, not only confound diagnosis but also make assessment of efficacy and tolerability of pharmacologic interventions more challenging. Furthermore, Young and colleagues (41) note that the large numbers of patients with geriatric bipolar disorder necessary for prospective clinical trials are not available at single-site academic centers, suggesting the utility of multicenter collaborative studies.

Despite limited data available on best treatment practices in elderly, bipolar patients, a recent naturalistic study assessed patterns of psychopharmacologic treatment and treatment response in 138 acutely ill, bipolar patients older than the age of 60 years (42). Standard mood stabilizers (lithium, valproate, carbamazepine, and lamotrigine) were the most prescribed medications (68%), followed by antipsychotics (54%) and antidepressants (34%). Combination therapy was more common than monotherapy (57% vs. 38%) and remission was achieved in 35% of subjects, while 32% showed no significant improvement. The authors point out that these findings are consistent with current clinical guidelines for mixed-age bipolar patients (42).

As with younger adults, the pharmacologic approach to the treatment of geriatric bipolar disorder can be broken down into three clinical scenarios (Table 4).

1. Treatment of acute geriatric mania (including subtypes of mixed states and rapid cycling).
2. Treatment of geriatric bipolar depression.
3. Maintenance, treatment/prevention of recurrent mania and bipolar depression.

The pharmacologic treatment section of this chapter will consider each one of these scenarios, reviewing the evidence-based literature in geriatric bipolar disorder, commenting on controlled data in younger adults and then making recommendations about clinical choice of medication and suggested dosing.

Geriatric Mania

Although there are currently no published double-blind, placebo-controlled treatment studies of geriatric mania, the first double-blind, prospective, controlled trial in geriatric bipolar disorder, funded by NIMH, is now underway and is evaluating the efficacy and tolerability of lithium and divalproex in individuals aged 60 years and older with mania, hypomania, or mixed states (43). This study may help inform clinical practice, but for now, the appropriate management of geriatric mania begins with the identification of comorbid medical and neurologic disorders and includes the elimination of other unnecessary psychotropic medications. In younger patients, polypharmacy is often used from the outset for rapid symptom control. In contrast, monotherapy is usually the first step of treatment in geriatric mania to reduce the potential for the additional side-effect burden of combined treatment. As we

TABLE 4 Pharmacotherapeutic approaches to Geriatric Bipolar Disorder

I. GERIATRIC MANIA

A. Acute Mania (treat for minimum of 3–4 weeks)

MEDICATION	DOSAGE	ADVERSE EFECTS	COMMENTS
(1) Lithium Carbonate	300 to 900 mg/d in divided doses	Impaired cognition, tremor, renal compromise, hypothyroidism, increased appetite/weight gain, others	Target blood level: 0.4 and 0.8 mEq/l Higher levels (0.8–1.0 mEq/l) needed in some cases
(2) Divalproex Sodium (Depakote)	500 to 1000 mg/d	Sedation, gait disturbance, thrombocytopenia, impaired cognition, increased appetite/weight gain, others; Rare: hepatotoxicity, pancreatitis	Target blood level: 50 and 100 mcg/ml Higher levels associated with significant increase in adverse effects
(3) Atypical antipsychotic		Class effects: sedation, postural hypotension, constipation, impaired cognition, extrapyramidal symptoms including tardive dyskinesia, increased appetite/weight gain, metabolic syndrome, possible increased mortality, others	Class recommendations: Cerebrovascular adverse events and increased mortality in patients with dementia related psychosis. Pre-treatment and periodic monitoring suggested for weight, waist circumference, serum glucose, lipid profile.
(a) Olanzapine (Zyprexa)	5–15 mg/d		
(b) Risperidone (Risperdal and others)	2–6 mg/d		
(c) Quetiapine (Seroquel)	100–200 mg/d		
(d) Aripiprazole (Ability)	5–30 mg/d		
(e) Ziprasidone (Geodon)	80–160 mg/d		
(4) Carbamazepine (Tegretol, Equetro, and others)	100–800 mg/d	Cardiovascular effects, gait disturbance, sedation, impaired cognition, hematological effects, increased appetite/weight gain, others	Second-line choice. Work–up should include EKG, liver function tests and hematology. Serum level = 6-12 mcg/L. Induction of 3A4 hepatic enzymes may result in drug interactions or lower carbamazepine level over time.
(5) Combination therapy: lithium or divalproex plus atypical antipsychotic	Monotherapy range doses may be required for each medication	Adverse effects may be additive or synergistic	Monitoring of adverse effects for both agents is necessary.
(6) Electroconvulsive therapy (ECT)	See Chapter 16 for detailed discussion	See Chapter 16 for detailed discussion	Consider in patients: ∗Refractory to pharmacotherapy ∗Rapid cycling ∗With severe acute suicidality ∗With dangerously poor nutritional status Note that no systematic data compare ECT to pharamacotherapy in elderly bipolar patients

TABLE 4 Pharmacotherapeutic approaches to Geriatric Bipolar Disorder (*Continued*)

MEDICATION	DOSAGE	ADVERSE EFFECTS	COMMENTS
I. GERIATRIC MANIA			
B. Refractory Mania/Mixed Symptoms			
(1) Lithium plus atypical antipsychotic	Monotherapy doses may be needed for both agents.	Adverse effects may be additive or synergistic	
(2) Lithium plus divalproex	As above	Adverse effects may be additive or synergistic. As above	
(3) Clozapine (Clozaril and others)	50–400 mg/d	Sedation, postural hypotension, hematologic effects, cardiovascular effects, endocrine effects, impaired cognition, increased appetite/weight gain, metabolic syndrome	Follow WBC weekly for 6 months, then every other week
(4) Electroconvulsive therapy (ECT)	See above	See above	See above
C. Bipolar Depression			
(1) Lithium carbonate	See above	See above	
(2) Quetiapine	See above	See above	
(3) Olanzapine/fluoxetine (Symbiax)	3/25–12/50 (1st number is mg of olanzapine, 2nd is mg of fluoxetine)	Sedation, edema, increased appetite/weight gain, metabolic syndrome, impaired cognition, tremor	
(4) Lamotrigine (Lamictal and others)	50–200 mg/d	Rash/hematologic effects, impaired cognition, dizziness, ataxia, sedation	Starting at 12.5 mg every day, titrate upwards every two weeks to target dosage
(5) Lithium or atypical antipsychotic or anticonvulsant plus antidepressant			Antidepressant selection based on treatment history and adverse effects. SSRIs have been safe for the treatment of older adults with major depression.
(6) Electroconvulsive therapy (ECT)	See above	See above	See above
D. Maintenance Pharmacotherapy			
(1) Lithium or DVP with or without atypical antipsychotic	Monotherapy doses may be needed for both agents.	Adverse effects may be additive or synergistic	Pharmacotherapy that has proven effective for acute treatment of mania or bipolar depression should be continued 6–12 months. Mood stabilizer continuation is essential; monitored tapering of antidepressants, antipsychotics or antianxiety agents can be attempted.
(2) Lamotrigine with or without atypical antipsychotic	As above	As above	
(3) Quetiapine alone	As above	As above	

consider the treatment of geriatric mania, it is important to define not only adequate treatment dose, but also duration (41).

Antipsychotic Medications

In treating manic older adults, conventional antipsychotic medications historically have been used in treating the acute phase of the disorder, when a patient's safety or health might be endangered by awaiting the therapeutic effects of less rapidly acting approaches. To minimize side-effect burden, McDonald and Nemeroff (25) recommend low dosages of haloperidol 0.25 mg to 0.5 mg intramuscularly or orally, followed one hour later by lorazepam 0.5 mg intramuscularly or orally. Repeated alternating doses can be given on an hourly basis until the patient is calm but not oversedated. In addition to sedation, other side effects to monitor include orthostatic hypotension, extrapyramidal symptoms, and neuroleptic malignant syndrome. The risk of tardive dyskinesia (TD) is heightened with long-term use and is increased in older adults, females, and mood disorder patients. A review by Jeste and colleagues (44) found the cumulative incidence of TD in older adults prescribed conventional antipsychotics to approximate 29% after one year, 50% after two years, and 63% after three years. The concurrent administration of lorazepam, though useful in limiting the maximum necessary antipsychotic dose, is not without its own complications. These can include unwanted sedation, ataxia, falls, cognitive impairment, withdrawal symptoms (if lorazepam is used regularly for more than 2–3 weeks), and disinhibition (45).

Largely due to the adverse effects associated with conventional antipsychotic medications, atypical antipsychotic agents have generally supplanted conventional antipsychotic medications as first line treatments in geriatric clinical practice (46). In the elderly, atypical antipsychotic agents can be used alone or in combination with mood stabilizers (47). Clozapine, risperidone, olanzapine, quetiapine, ziprasidone, and aripiprazole have each been shown beneficial in younger manic patients in controlled or uncontrolled trials, but no controlled trials yet attest to their safety and efficacy in older adults (48). All the atypical antipsychotics, except for clozapine and paliperidone, have been FDA approved for the treatment of acute mania in adults.

Overall, the atypical antipsychotics are associated with less severe extrapyramidal effects but many of them can produce adverse effects including weight gain, glucose intolerance, hyperprolactinemia, orthostatic hypotension, gait disturbance, and sedation. Furthermore, a 2003 FDA warning of cerebrovascular adverse events and a 2005 FDA boxed warning of increased mortality (49) has limited the use of atypical antipsychotic medications in older adults with dementia-related psychosis. These warnings did not include older adults with bipolar disorder, although due to the lack of controlled trials in geriatric mania thus far and the relative dearth of subjects in uncontrolled reports, little is known about the potential risk of cerebrovascular adverse events and increased mortality when prescribing atypical antipsychotic in geriatric bipolar individuals.

Dosing of atypical antipsychotics in the elderly is typically half to one-third the daily dose recommended for younger patients, although effective dosing varies with such factors as comorbid medical illness and age (50). McDonald and Nemeroff recommend risperidone 0.5 mg/day or olanzapine 5.0 mg/day as acceptable alternatives to haloperidol in the regimen described above (51). Mixed-age patients may benefit from using adjunctive risperidone with divalproex or lithium, (52,53).

Uncontrolled data give some support to the use of atypical antipsychotic medications in geriatric mania. A secondary analysis of olanzapine and divalproex monotherapy treatment in acute mania demonstrated superior efficacy of both medications compared with placebo for the treatment of mania in mixed-age patients (Total $N = 97$, mean age = 57) (47). Quetiapine has also demonstrated efficacy in acute mania in a secondary analysis of a subgroup of older adults (quetiapine $N = 28$, mean age = 63; placebo $N = 31$, mean age = 61) studied in two double-blind controlled trials for bipolar mania (54). Manic symptoms in these older adults improved by day 4 at a mean dose of 550 mg/day. Side effects included dry mouth, postural hypotension, somnolence, weight gain, and dizziness. Although not supported by prospective controlled trials, the relatively high dose and rapid dose escalation of quetiapine may have contributed to the tolerability findings. In clinical practice, a lower dose of around 300 mg/day, in divided doses, may be better tolerated. Furthermore, aripriprazole has demonstrated significant reductions in scores on the Hamilton Depression Rating Scale (HAM-D), Young Mania Rating Scale (YMRS), and Clinical Global Impression scale (CGI) after 12 weeks of open label prospective treatment in 20 older bipolar patients (mean age = 59.6) minimally responsive to previous treatment with mood stabilizing medications (55). These individuals were predominantly bipolar depressed at study entry. The mean dose of aripriprazole was 10.3 mg/day with a low frequency of side effects including sedation, restlessness, weight gain, drooling, and loose stools. Finally, for the management of refractory geriatric bipolar mania, Shulman reported the use of clozapine in doses ranging from 25 to 112.5 mg/day (56). Despite apparent efficacy and an improved side-effect profile compared with the conventional antipsychotic agents, there is a need for further controlled data on the use of atypical antipsychotic agents in older adults with mania (57).

Lithium

While many clinicians have come to rely on atypical antipsychotic medications during the acute treatment of geriatric mania, some authorities still include lithium salts among the first-line agents for both acute and longer term treatment. Available as lithium carbonate or as the liquid lithium citrate, lithium salts have not been studied in the elderly under double-blind conditions but have been reported effective as acute or prophylactic treatments in several open trials (48). Lithium pharmacokinetics is altered in the aging body. Age-associated decreases in volume of distribution and renal clearance, for example, increases the elimination half-life of lithium in the elderly, from the 24 hours typical for younger adults to about 28 to 36 hours (57). Perhaps even more than in younger patients, lithium treatment of older patients can be associated with troublesome side effects such as polyuria, tremor, mental slowing and memory difficulties, sinus node dysfunction, peripheral edema, hypothyroidism or nontoxic goiter, nausea, diarrhea and a worsening of arthritis, acne, and psoriasis (3). These effects can become intolerable even at serum levels often well below those regarded as toxic in younger adults. The presence of cognitive impairment or preexisting tremor can increase the likelihood of side effects (58).

An ongoing and active review of concomitant medications while prescribing lithium is essential. Lithium's serum level can be raised by many nonsteroidal anti-inflammatory agents (NSAIDs), cyclooxygenase 2 (COX-2) inhibitors, furosemide, thiazide diuretics, angiotensin converting enzyme inhibitors and dehydration (59). Other treatments can decrease serum lithium levels including acetazolamide, caffeine, aminophylline, mannitol, and theophylline (59). For these reasons, the pretreatment workup should include a thorough list of current medications as well as an electrocardiogram, electrolytes, BUN, creatinine, and TSH (3). Serum creatinine levels can be imprecise in an elderly individual due to decreased skeletal muscle mass along with a concomitant decrease in glomerular filtration rate, so a 24-hour creatinine clearance is useful for establishing an accurate baseline measure of renal function (21). Despite this recommendation, serum creatinine is the most widely used measure of renal function over time. If the serum creatinine rises, or if there is concern about the risk of lithium-induced renal insufficiency, a 24-hour creatinine clearance can inform further treatment decisions regarding the use of lithium salts.

Lithium treatment can be initiated at a dosage of 150 to 300 mg at bedtime (3). Lithium citrate, the liquid form of lithium, provides a simple means for dose titration or for using lower dosages. If nausea is present, lithobid or Eskalith CR, the slow release preparations of lithium, may be better tolerated. For patients with diarrhea, the sustained release preparations can exacerbate the problem. Administration of the entire lithium dose at bedtime sometimes reduces daytime sedation. The dose range of lithium typically used is 300 to 900 mg/d, with serum levels between 0.6 and 1.0 mEq/L (60), although lower levels such as 0.4 to 0.8 mEq/L have also been advocated as effective (61). Lithium levels and other laboratory parameters should be monitored at regular intervals as well as in response to such events as dosage changes, changes in sodium or water intake, or coadministration of medications that affect lithium metabolism (3).

Interestingly, serum lithium levels may not correlate with brain lithium levels in older adults with bipolar disorder based on preliminary findings from MR spectroscopy studies (64). Studies have demonstrated an increased brain-to-peripheral lithium concentration ratio with increased age potentially increasing vulnerability to neurocognitive toxicity (62,63). These findings may have clinical implications for an older patient on lithium and support the decreased serum levels needed to maintain therapeutic effect and avoid excess toxicity.

Divalproex

Divalproex sodium (DVP), a mood-stabilizing anticonvulsant, is effective for the acute treatment of mania in younger adults. In the geriatric population, it is modestly effective and fairly well tolerated although no double-blind, placebo-controlled trials are yet available (65). There have been five retrospective and open studies of DVP in geriatric bipolar patients ($N = 137$) with evidence of antimanic efficacy with serum divalproex levels between 25 and 125 μg/mL (41). A mixed-age population of lithium refractory patients and those with neurologic abnormalities appears to be particularly responsive to DVP (66), suggesting possible efficacy in treating mania comorbid with neurologic disorders. Additional support for the use of DVP in older manic patients comes from the observation that younger patients with mixed states respond better to divalproex than to lithium (67). While DVP use appears to have become more prevalent than lithium among older bipolar patients in recent years (68), lithium remains superior to DVP in preventing suicide attempts (69).

Treatment with DVP can be accompanied by side effects including nausea, tremor, ataxia, asymptomatic serum hepatic transaminase elevations, alopecia, increased appetite, weight gain, and sedation (70). Initial treatment of acute geriatric mania often requires higher doses and serum levels of DVP. However, after stabilizing, clinicians should beware of the subsequent development of toxic side effects, including sedation, gait disturbance and cognitive side effects (3). Hepatic and pancreatic toxicity is infrequent among the elderly, although baseline liver functions should be obtained (3). DVP is highly protein bound, and thus capable of interacting with other highly protein bound medications such as warfarin (21). In addition, DVP strongly inhibits certain glucuronidation enzymes leading to a clinically significant increase in the levels of lamotrigine when coprescribed (3).

DVP is available as capsules, sprinkles, an extended release version (Depakote ER) and Depakene syrup, accommodating patients who have difficulty swallowing. The starting dose of DVP in older adults is 125 to 250 mg at bedtime, with a recommended increase over several days to 250 mg bid and eventual increase from 500 to 1000 mg/day (Brent chapter). Blood levels between 60 and 100 mcg/mL are usually optimal (8), although clinical efficacy in the elderly may sometimes be achieved with lower levels.

Other Mood Stabilizing Anticonvulsants

Other anticonvulsants have also been used in the elderly for acute mania, despite limited support from controlled studies. Carbamazepine, problematic because of its neurologic side effects, has largely been superseded by DVP (3) (3,71). Oxcarbazepine is often better tolerated than carbamazepine; however, efficacy data for oxcarbazepine in geriatric bipolar disorder is lacking. Gabapentin, topiramate, levetiracetam, and zonisamide, all require further study in elderly bipolar patients before a recommendation for use can be made (3).

ECT

For treatment-resistant patients, or for those who require rapid symptomatic resolution, ECT is an appropriate option in the acute treatment of late-life mania. Most responders can then be switched to pharmacotherapeutic maintenance, with or without continued ECT maintenance (40). There has been one small positive case series of three geriatric patients with mania and comorbid dementia who responded well to acute ECT with improvement in symptoms of mania, agitation, and mental status scores (72). Coadministration of lithium and ECT should be avoided, due to an association with increased risk of delirium (11).

Geriatric Bipolar Depression

Bipolar depression in older adults is a complex condition that is both insufficiently studied and difficult to treat. The goal of treatment for any patient with bipolar depression is to relieve depressive symptoms without inducing a switch into mania or an acceleration of cycle frequency. While antidepressants can increase the risk of mania and rapid cycling over the long-term, mood-elevating mood stabilizers are associated with a lower risk of switching (19). The diagnosis of bipolar depression is often overlooked due to overlapping symptoms in common with unipolar depression, and to the frequent difficulty in identifying past hypomanic and manic episodes. Compared to lamotrigine and certain atypical antipsychotic agents, the traditional mood stabilizers—lithium and DVP—have limited efficacy in bipolar depression, notwithstanding their strong antimanic effects (3). Despite the potential risk of a switch into hypomania or mania, the addition of an antidepressant drug to ongoing mood stabilizer treatment is often the chosen treatment (73). Although more comparative data are needed, preliminary studies support the notion that bupropion or an SSRI are associated with less risk of switch into mania than a tricyclic or MAO inhibitor.

Lamotrigine has been shown to have acute and prophylactic antidepressant effects both in younger adults and in the elderly (74). In addition, its generally benign side-effect profile makes lamotrigine an attractive treatment option for the elderly. In an 8-week, double-blind, placebo-controlled, mixed-age bipolar cohort, Calabrese and colleagues observed that either 50 mg ($N = 66$) or 200 mg ($N = 63$) per day of lamotrigine were superior to placebo ($N = 63$) by week 3 onward in treating acute bipolar depression (75). Lamotrigine's FDA-indicated use as a maintenance treatment for prevention of bipolar depression is supported by two large, double-blind, placebo-controlled maintenance trials of 18 months duration in which lamotrigine monotherapy ($N = 59$) was compared to either lithium monotherapy ($N = 46$) or placebo ($N = 70$) in patients with bipolar disorder, type I, who were recently manic or hypomanic (76,77). Lamotrigine and lithium were equivalent to each other and both were superior to placebo in delaying the time to a mood episode. In particular, lamotrigine strongly delayed the onset of bipolar depression, while lithium and placebo did not. In contrast, lithium was superior to both lamotrigine and placebo in delaying the recurrence of mania or hypomania. In a secondary analysis of these data including 86 patients older than 55 years, the time to relapse for any mood episode was prolonged for lamotrigine treated patients (median 202 days) compared with placebo (median 99 days) or lithium (median 139) (74). The mean lamotrigine dose in the older patients (median age—63 years) was 220 mg/day. No cases of serious rash were reported in this sample and adverse effects of lamotrigine were similar to those of placebo.

Lamotrigine therapy should be initiated at 12.5 to 25 mg/day, increasing no more than 12.5 to 25 mg/day every 2 weeks, with a target dosage of 200 mg/day in younger adult patients (3). Target dosages of lamotrigine for a geriatric population are not known. "Starting low and going slow" will minimize the risk of benign skin rash and greatly reduce the likelihood of Stevens-Johnson syndrome. The most significant known drug interaction for lamotrigine is with divalproex sodium (DVP) (3). Conjugation via glucuronidation is the major route of lamotrigine metabolism. DVP can double the serum level and half-life of lamotrigine via inhibition of the UDP-glucuronosyltransferase enzyme mediating lamotrigine glucuronidation (3). If lamotrigine is started in a patient already receiving divalproex sodium, it is important to reduce the rate of lamotrigine dosage titration by approximately 50%, minimizing the risk of a severe rash. This same pharmacokinetic interaction will lead to a marked drop in lamotrigine serum levels if DVP is discontinued.

Adverse effects from lamotrigine include the occurrence of benign skin rashes and the rare presentation of more serious and life-threatening dermatologic reactions, notably Stevens-Johnson syndrome (SJS) (78,79). Early detection and treatment of the SJS reduces its mortality rate greatly (80). The majority of skin rashes are benign and improve spontaneously even with continued lamotrigine therapy (3). If a lamotrigine-associated rash develops, many clinicians hold the dose constant or lower the dose, until the rash subsides. Once the rash is gone, the dose titration should resume, but at a slower pace (3). This gradual titration reduces the risk of SJS to that of most other drugs, but unfortunately precludes the rapid use of lamotrigine for acute bipolar depression or mixed states.

Limited data suggest that carbamazepine can also be an effective treatment agent in bipolar depression, although its effects can diminish over the long term (81). Lithium is a long-standing treatment agent for bipolar depression, and was recently shown to have definite prophylactic efficacy in bipolar depression for older adults (82). Although lithium is the only mood stabilizer with demonstrated antisuicide effects, it can be neurotoxic or deadly in overdose. The optimal serum lithium level for bipolar depression remains unclear, but the usual therapeutic range is 0.6 to 1.0 mEq/L with lower doses and serum levels (0.4–0.8 mEq/L) generally being adequate for older patients.

In 2005, the atypical antipsychotic medication olanzapine, in combination with the antidepressant fluoxetine (marketed under the brand name Symbyax™), became the first FDA-indicated medication for treatment of bipolar depression (83). However, there are no clinical data published for the fluoxetine/olanzapine combination in the geriatric bipolar population, and clinical experience is limited. More recently, quetiapine was indicated by the FDA for the treatment of adult-aged bipolar depression (84). A small post hoc analysis found quetiapine to be as efficacious in treating bipolar depressive episodes in older adults as in younger adults (74). Preliminary studies have also shown adjunctive aripiprazole to improve depressive symptoms in bipolar older adults (age 55–65 years) who are suboptimally responsive to traditional mood stabilizers (74). Controlled studies with older and larger patient cohorts are needed to confirm the efficacy of quetiapine and aripiprazole in treating geriatric bipolar depression. Finally, there are no known controlled studies of Omega 3 fatty acids, inositol, St. John's Wort (Hypericum perforatum), and S-adenosyl-L-methionine (SAMe) in geriatric bipolar patients (3).

For patients with severe or treatment-refractory bipolar depression, more aggressive pharmacotherapy or ECT is indicated (40). Aggressive pharmacotherapy generally involves the use of a mood stabilizer with an antidepressant, with or without an augmentation agent.

Maintenance Therapy

Little information is available regarding maintenance treatment and prevention of recurrent episodes of mania and depression in older adults with bipolar disorder. DVP and lithium are widely used maintenance medications in younger adults, and a recent double-blind, placebo-controlled study confirmed the prophylactic efficacy of lithium in the geriatric population (85). Lamotrigine, olanzapine, aripriprazole, and lithium are all FDA-indicated for the maintenance treatment of bipolar disorder. Of these drugs, only lamotrigine has been shown to delay mood and depressive episode recurrences in the elderly under double-blind conditions (74). For patients who show poor response to maintenance medication regimens, maintenance ECT is an option.

Although pharmacotherapy may have much to offer even in the absence of a thorough evidence base, poor medication adherence complicates the treatment course at all stages (3). A recent assessment of medication adherence among veterans receiving lithium and anticonvulsant medications from the Department of Veterans Affairs found that only 54.1% of patients were fully adherent while 21.4% were nonadherent (74). Younger age, diagnosis of a substance abuse disorder, and fewer outpatient psychiatric visits were found to be associated with poorer medication adherence. Sajatovic and colleagues also found that bipolar patients placed substantial emphasis on the interactional component within the patient–provider relationship in promoting treatment adherence, highlighting the significance of the patient–provider relationship in treatment outcome (86).

Psychotherapeutic Interventions with Geriatric Bipolar Patients

There are no controlled studies to date on the efficacy of psychotherapy for bipolar geriatric patients (3). A large scale study of the efficacy of psychotherapy for bipolar patients as an adjunctive therapy has been funded by the National Institute for Mental Health as part of their STEP-BD program (87). The potential value of psychotherapeutic treatment of a geriatric cycling mood disorder is suggested by findings of psychotherapeutic efficacy in geriatric unipolar depression (3). Researchers stress the efficacy of combined psychosocial and pharmacologic treatments for older depressed adults when compared to either form of treatment alone (88). In some preliminary studies, interventions that teach bipolar patients to monitor and manage stress have been effective in reducing rates of recurrence (89–91). Perhaps the most frequently cited "psychosocial trigger" of relapse in the bipolar patient is poor medication adherence. A number of studies, importantly, have demonstrated the efficacy of psychotherapy in improving medication adherence (92–94).

While many clinicians would agree that individual psychotherapy with an unstabilized manic patient may not be an effective intervention, psychosocial interventions can be accomplished with a program designed for the patient's family (3). For the manic patient, the therapist maintains a delicate balance between setting limits and validating the bipolar patient as the patient attempts to return to baseline modes of effective communication. For the bipolar patient in a depressed state, the initial goal in group therapy becomes gradual encouragement of the patient to participate with other group members in more advanced stages of stabilization serving as models for productive self-expression (40). Clearly more research is needed to generate psychotherapeutic approaches that can be standardized for the treatment of geriatric bipolar disorder.

CONCLUSION

Bipolar disorder continues to be an under-recognized mood disorder in later life encompassing individuals who have lived for years with recurrent mood episodes, and a smaller minority who develop an index episode of mania in later life. Distinguishing among syndromes of delirium, dementia, and mania often presents clinicians with difficulties when standard DSM-IV TR criteria for mania are used. The occurrence of manic symptoms in an older adult must prompt a careful clinical evaluation to identify treatable medical conditions. Somatic and psychosocial approaches can be helpful in acute and maintenance treatment of late-life mania as well as bipolar depression. Unfortunately, prospective randomized controlled trials in geriatric bipolar disorder of all phases are currently lacking. Psychotherapy is critical to enhance treatment adherence, educate patients and family members about relapse risk and help patients cope with the realities of a chronic mental disorder (3). A systematic approach to controlled clinical research along with collaborations in the fields of genetics, molecular biology, and functional neuroimaging, will help improve our understanding of the neurobiologic causes of geriatric bipolar disorder and eventually lead to the development of more specific and effective treatment strategies (3) for these patients.

REFERENCES

1. Subramaniam H, Dennis MS, Byrne EJ. The role of vascular risk factors in late onset bipolar disorder. Int J Geriatr Psychiatry 2007; 22(8):733–737.
2. Bartels SJ, Forester B, Miles KM, et al. Mental health service use by elderly patients with bipolar disorder and unipolar major depression. Am J Geriatr Psychiatry 2000; 8(2):160–166.
3. Forester B, Stoll AL, Antognini F. Geriatric bipolar disorder. In: Agronin ME, Maletta GJ, eds. Principles and Practice of Geriatric Psychiatry. Baltimore, MD: Lippincott Williams & Wilkins, 2006.
4. Trinh N, Forester B. Bipolar disorder in the elderly: Differential diagnosis and treatment. Psychiatric Times 2007; 24(14):38–43.
5. Angst J, Sellaro R. Historical perspectives and natural history of bipolar disorder. Biol Psychiatry 2000; 48(6):445–457.
6. Murray CJ, Lopez AD. Evidence-based health policy: Lessons from the Global Burden of Disease Study. Science 1996; 274(5288):740–743.
7. Weissman MM, Bland RC, Canino GJ, et al. Cross-national epidemiology of major depression and bipolar disorder. JAMA 1996; 276(4):293–299.
8. Depp CA, Lindamer LA, Folsom DP, et al. Differences in clinical features and mental health service use in bipolar disorder across the lifespan. Am J Geriatr Psychiatry 2005; 13(4):290–298.
9. Weissman MM, Leaf PJ, Tischler GL, et al. Affective disorders in five United States communities. Psychol Med 1988; 18(1):141–153.
10. Yassa R, Nair NP, Iskandar H. Late-onset bipolar disorder. Psychiatr Clin North Am 1988; 11(1):117–131.
11. Young RC. Bipolar mood disorders in the elderly. Psychiatr Clin North Am 1997; 20(1):121–136.
12. Zanetti MV, Cordeiro Q, Busatto GF. Late onset bipolar disorder associated with white matter hyperintensities: A pathophysiological hypothesis. Prog Neuropsychopharmacol Biol Psychiatry 2007; 31(2):551–556.
13. Sobow T, Kisiela E, Luczak O, et al. Depression in the course of bipolar disorder and recurrent depressive disorder in the elderly: Diagnostic difficulties. Psychiatr Pol 2005; 39(5):963–975.
14. Sajatovic M, Blow FC, Ignacio RV. Psychiatric comorbidity in older adults with bipolar disorder. Int J Geriatr Psychiatry 2006; 21(6):582–587.
15. Aziz R, Lorberg B, Tampi RR. Treatments for late-life bipolar disorder. Am J Geriatr Pharmacother 2006; 4(4):347–364.
16. Sajatovic M, Blow FC, Ignacio RV, et al. New-onset bipolar disorder in later life. Am J Geriatr Psychiatry 2005; 13(4):282–289.
17. Guo JJ, Keck PE, Li H, et al. Treatment costs related to bipolar disorder and comorbid conditions among Medicaid patients with bipolar disorder. Psychiatr Serv 2007; 58(8):1073–1078.
18. American Psychiatric Association. Diagnostic and Statistical Manual of Mental Disorders, 4th ed. Text Revision. Washington, D. C.: American Psychiatric Association, 2000.
19. Forester BP, Antognini F, Sivrioglu EY, et al. Geriatric mania. Dir Psychiatry 2004; 24(1):43–55.
20. Shulman KI, Herrmann N. The nature and management of mania in old age. Psychiatr Clin North Am 1999; 22(3):649–665.
21. Satlin A, Liptzin B. Diagnosis and treatment of mania. In: Salzman C, ed. Clinical Geriatric Psychopharmacology. Baltimore, MD: Lippincott Williams & Wilkins, 1998:310–330.
22. Harrow M, Grossman LS, Silverstein ML, et al. Thought pathology in manic and schizophrenic patients. Its occurrence at hospital admission and seven weeks later. Arch Gen Psychiatry 1982; 39(6):665–671.
23. Krauthammer C, Klerman GL. Secondary mania: Manic syndromes associated with antecedent physical illness or drugs. Arch Gen Psychiatry 1978; 35(11):1333–1339.
24. Tohen M, Castillo J, Pope HG Jr, et al. Concomitant use of valproate and carbamazepine in bipolar and schizoaffective disorders. J Clin Psychopharmacol 1994; 14(1):67–70.

25. McDonald W, Nemeroff CB. Practical Guidelines for Diagnosing and Treating Mania and Bipolar Disorder in the Elderly. Medscape Psychiatry Mental Health eJournal [serial online] 1998; 3(2):1–6. http://www.medscape.com/viewarticle/430757
26. Stoll AL, Tohen M, Baldessarini RJ, et al. Shifts in diagnostic frequencies of schizophrenia and major affective disorders at six North American psychiatric hospitals,1972–1988. Am J Psychiatry 1993; 150(11):1668–1673.
27. Cavanagh JT, Van Beck M, Muir W, et al. Case-control study of neurocognitive function in euthymic patients with bipolar disorder: An association with mania. Br J Psychiatry 2002; 180:320–326.
28. Gildengers AG, Butters MA, Seligman K, et al. Cognitive functioning in late-life bipolar disorder. Am J Psychiatry 2004; 161(4):736–738.
29. Kessing LV, Nilssonb FM. Increased risk of developing dementia in patients with major affective disorders compared to patients with other medical illnesses. J Affect Disord 2003; 73(3):261–269.
30. Kessing LV, Andersen PK. Does the risk of developing dementia increase with the number of episodes in patients with depressive disorder and in patients with bipolar disorder? J Neurol Neurosurg Psychiatry 2004; 75:1662–1666.
31. Depp CA, Moore DJ, Sitzer D, et al. Neurocognitive impairment in middle-aged and older adults with bipolar disorder: Comparison to schizophrenia and normal comparison subjects. J Affect Disord 2007; 101(1–3):201–209.
32. Schouws SN, Zoeteman JB, Comijs HC, et al. Cognitive functioning in elderly patients with early onset bipolar disorder. Int J Geriatr Psychiatry 2007; 22(9):856–861.
33. Nunes PV, Forlenza OV, Gattaz WF. Lithium and risk for Alzheimer's disease in elderly patients with bipolar disorder. Br J Psychiatry 2007; 190:359–360.
34. Migliorelli R, Starkstein SE, Teson A, et al. SPECT findings in patients with primary mania. J Neuropsychiatry Clin Neurosci 1993; 5(4):379–383.
35. Videbech P. MRI findings in patients with affective disorder: A meta-analysis. Acta Psychiatr Scand 1997; 96(3):157–168.
36. Drevets WC, Price JL, Simpson JR Jr, et al. Subgenual prefrontal cortex abnormalities in mood disorders. Nature 1997; 386(6627):824–827.
37. Atmaca M, Ozdemir H, Yildirim H. Corpus callosum areas in first-episode patients with bipolar disorder. Psychol Med 2007; 37(5):699–704.
38. McDonald WM, Krishnan KR, Doraiswamy PM, et al. Occurrence of subcortical hyperintensities in elderly subjects with mania. Psychiatry Res 1991; 40(4):211–220.
39. Steffens DC, Krishnan KR. Structural neuroimaging and mood disorders: Recent findings, implications for classification, and future directions. Biol Psychiatry 1998; 43(10):705–712.
40. Forester BP, Antognini FC, Jordan B, et al. Geriatric bipolar disorder: A review of diagnostic and therapeutic challenges. Dir Psychiatry 2008; 28(1):1–15.
41. Young RC, Gyulai L, Mulsant BH, et al. Pharmacotherapy of bipolar disorder in old age: Review and recommendations. Am J Geriatr Psychiatry 2004; 12(4):342–357.
42. Beyer JL, Burchitt B, Gersing K, et al. Patterns of pharmacotherapy and treatment response in elderly adults with bipolar disorder. Psychopharmacol Bull 2008; 41(1):102–114.
43. Young RC. Evidenced based approach to treatment of geriatric bipolar disorder in AAGP Meeting. Orlando, Florida, 2008.
44. Jeste DV, Caligiuri MP, Paulsen JS, et al. Risk of tardive dyskinesia in older patients. A prospective longitudinal study of 266 outpatients. Arch Gen Psychiatry 1995; 52(9):756–765.
45. Young RC. Use of lithium in bipolar disorder. In: Nelson JC, ed. Geriatric Psychopharmacology. New York, NY: Marcel Dekker, Inc., 1998:259–272.
46. Jeste DV, Rockwell E, Harris MJ, et al. Conventional vs. newer antipsychotics in elderly patients. Am J Geriatr Psychiatry 1999; 7(1):70–76.
47. Beyer J, Siegal A, Kennedy J, et al. Olanzapine, divalproex, and placebo treatment non-head-to-head comparisons of older-adult acute mania, in 10th Congress of the International Psychogeriatric Association. Nice, France, 2001.

48. Umapathy C, Mulsant BH, Pollock BG. Bipolar disorder in the elderly. Psychiatric Annals 2000; 30:473–480.
49. FDA Public Health Advisory: Deaths with Antipsychotics in Elderly Patients with Behavioral Disturbances [on-line]. Available at www.fda.gov/cder/drug/advisory/antipsychotics.htm.
50. Fuller MA, Sajatovic M. Drug Information for Mental Health. Cleveland, OH: Lexi-Comp, Inc., 2001.
51. McDonald WM, Nemeroff CB. The diagnosis and treatment of mania in the elderly. Bull Menninger Clin 1996; 60(2):174–196.
52. Niedermier JA, Nasrallah HA. Clinical correlates of response to valproate in geriatric inpatients. Ann Clin Psychiatry 1998; 10(4):165–168.
53. Regenold WT, Prasad M. Uses of intravenous valproate in geriatric psychiatry. Am J Geriatr Psychiatry 2001; 9(3):306–308.
54. Sajatovic. Quetiapine for the treatment of mania in older adults, in American Psychiatric Association Annual Meeting. Atlanta, GA: 2005.
55. Sajatovic M, Coconcea N, Ignacio RV, Blow FC, Hays RW, Cassidy KA, Meyer WJ. Aripiprazole therapy in 20 older adults with bipolar disorder: a 12-week, open-label trial. J Clin Psychiatry. 2008 Jan; 69(1):41–6.
56. Shulman RW, Singh A, Shulman KI. Treatment of elderly institutionalized bipolar patients with clozapine. Psychopharmacol Bull 1997; 33(1):113–118.
57. Sajatovic M. Treatment of bipolar disorder in older adults. Int J Geriatr Psychiatry 2002; 17(9):865–873.
58. Nambudiri DE, Meyers BS, Young RC. Delayed recovery from lithium neurotoxicity. J Geriatr Psychiatry Neurol 1991; 4(1):40–43.
59. Dunner DL. Drug injections of lithium and other antimanic/mood-stablizing medications. J Cin Psychiatry 2003; 64(suppl 5):38–43.
60. McDonald WM. Epidemiology, etiology, and treatment of geriatric mania. J Clin Psychiatry 2000; 61(supp 13):3–11.
61. Schaffer CB, Garvey MJ. Use of lithium in acutely manic elderly patients. Clin Gerontol 1984; 3:58–60.
62. Gonzalez RG, Guimaraes AR, Sachs GS, et al. Measurement of human brain lithium in vivo by MR spectroscopy. AJNR Am J Neuroradiol 1993; 14(5):1027–1037.
63. Moore CM, Demopulos CM, Henry ME, et al. Brain-to-serum lithium ratio and age: An in vivo magnetic resonance spectroscopy study. Am J Psychiatry 2002; 159(7):1240–1242.
64. Forester BP, Streeter CC, Berlow YA, Tian H, Wardrop M, Finn CT, Harper D, F. RP, Moore CM. Brain lithium levels and effects on cognition and mood in geriatric bipolar disorder. American Journal of Geriatric Psychiatry. Expedited E-published. 2008; July 14, 2008.
65. Risinger RC, Risby ED, Risch SC. Safety and efficacy of divalproex sodium in elderly bipolar patients. J Clin Psychiatry 1994; 55(5):215.
66. Stoll AL, Banov M, Kolbrener M, et al. Neurologic factors predict a favorable valproate response in bipolar and schizoaffective disorders. J Clin Psychopharmacol 1994; 14(5):311–313.
67. Bowden CL. Anticonvulsants in bipolar elderly. In: Nelson J, ed. Geriatric Psychopharmacology. New York, NY: Marcel Dekker, Inc., 1998:285–299.
68. Shulman KI, Rochon P, Sykora K, et al. Changing prescription patterns for lithium and valproic acid in old age: Shifting practice without evidence. Bmj 2003; 326(7396): 960–961.
69. Goodwin FK, Fireman B, Simon GE,et al . Suicide risk in bipolar disorder during treatment with lithium and divalproex. JAMA 2003; 290(11):1467–1473.
70. Bowden CL. Valproate. Bipolar Disorder 2003; 5(3):189–202.
71. Goldberg JF, Harrow M, Whiteside JE. Risk for bipolar illness in patients initially hospitalized for unipolar depression. Am J Psychiatry 2001; 158(8):1265–1270.
72. McDonald WM, Thompson TR. Treatment of mania in dementia with electroconvulsive therapy. Psychopharmacol Bull 2001; 35(2):72–82.

73. American Psychiatric Association. Practice guideline for the treatment of patients with bipolar disorder. Am J Psychiatry 1994; 151(12 suppl):1–36.
74. Sajatovic M, Ramsay E, Nanry K, et al. Lamotrigine therapy in elderly patients with epilepsy, bipolar disorder or dementia. Int J Geriatr Psychiatry 2007; 22(10):945–950.
75. Calabrese JR, Bowden CL, Sachs GS, et al. A double-blind placebo-controlled study of lamotrigine monotherapy in outpatients with bipolar I depression. Lamictal 602 Study Group. J Clin Psychiatry 1999; 60(2):79–88.
76. Bowden CL, Calabrese JR, Sachs G, et al. A placebo-controlled 18-month trial of lamotrigine and lithium maintenance treatment in recently manic or hypomanic patients with bipolar I disorder. Arch Gen Psychiatry 2003; 60(4):392–400.
77. Calabrese JR, Bowden CL, Sachs G, et al . A placebo-controlled 18-month trial of lamotrigine and lithium maintenance treatment in recently depressed patients with bipolar I disorder. J Clin Psychiatry 2003; 64(9):1013–1024.
78. Matsuo F. Lamotrigine. Epilepsia 1999; 40(suppl 5):S30–S36.
79. Messenheimer J, Mullens EL, Giorgi L, et al. Safety review of adult clinical trial experience with lamotrigine. Drug Saf 1998; 18(4):281–296.
80. Rzany B, Correia O, Kelly JP, et al. Risk of Stevens-Johnson syndrome and toxic epidermal necrolysis during first weeks of antiepileptic therapy: A case-control study. Study Group of the International Case Control Study on Severe Cutaneous Adverse Reactions. Lancet 1999; 353(9171):2190–2194.
81. Greil W, Kleindienst N. The comparative prophylactic efficacy of lithium and carbamazepine in patients with bipolar I disorder. Int Clin Psychopharmacol 1999; 14(5):277–281.
82. Lepkifker E, Iancu I, Horesh N, et al. Lithium therapy for unipolar and bipolar depression among the middle-aged and older adult patient subpopulation. Depress Anxiety 2006; 24:571–576.
83. Tohen M, Vieta E, Calabrese J, et al. Efficacy of olanzapine and olanzapine-fluoxetine combination in the treatment of bipolar I depression. Arch Gen Psychiatry 2003; 60(11):1079–1088.
84. Calabrese JR, Keck PE Jr, Macfadden W, et al. A randomized, double-blind, placebo-controlled trial of quetiapine in the treatment of bipolar I or II depression. Am J Psychiatry 2005; 162(7):1351–1360.
85. Sajatovic M, Gyulai L, Calabrese JR, et al. Maintenance treatment outcomes in older patients with bipolar I disorder. Am J Geriatr Psychiatry 2005; 13(4):305–311.
86. Sajatovic M. Bipolar disorder: Disease burden. Am J Manag Care 2005; 11(3 suppl):S80–S84.
87. Miklowitz DJ, et al. Psychosocial treatments for bipolar depression: a 1year randomized trial from the Systematic Treatment Enhancement Program. Arch Gen Psychiatry 2007; 64(4):419–26.
88. Cerbone M, Mayo JA, Cuthbertson BA, et al. Group therapy as an adjunct to medications in the management of bipolar affective disorder. 1992(16):174–187.
89. Frank E, Hlastala S, Ritenour A, et al. Inducing lifestyle regularity in recovering bipolar disorder patients: Results from the maintenance therapies in bipolar disorder protocol. Biol Psychiatry 1997; 41(12):1165–1173.
90. Frank E, Swartz HA, Mallinger AG, et al. Adjunctive psychotherapy for bipolar disorder: Effects of changing treatment modality. J Abnorm Psychol 1999; 108(4):579–587.
91. Satterfield JM. Adjunctive cognitive-behavioral therapy for rapid-cycling bipolar disorder: An empirical case study. Psychiatry 1999; 62(4):357–369.
92. Peet M, Harvey N. NIMH workshop report on treatment of bipolar disorder. Psychopharmacology Bulletin 1991; 26:409–427.
93. Shakir SA, Volkmar FR, Bacon S, et al. Group psychotherapy as an adjunct to lithium maintenance. Am J Psychiatry 1979; 136(4 A):455–456.
94. Volkmar FR, Bacon S, Shakir SA, et al. Group therapy in the management of manic-depressive illness. Am J Psychother 1981; 35(2):226–234.

95. Starkstein SE, Manes F. Mania and manic-like disorders. In: Bogousslavsky J, Cummings JL, eds. Behavior and Mood Disorders in Focal Brain Lesions. Cambridge, UK: Cambridge University Press, 2000:202–216.
96. Cummings JL. Frontal-subcortical circuits and human behavior. Arch Neurol 1993; 50(8):873–880.
97. Starkstein SE, Robinson RG. Mechanism of disinhibition after brain lesions. J Nerv Ment Dis 1997; 185(2):108–114.
98. Jorge RE, Robinson RG, Starkstein SE, et al. Secondary mania following traumatic brain injury. Am J Psychiatry 1993; 150(6):916–921.
99. Lyketsos CG, Hanson AL, Fishman M, et al. Manic syndrome early and late in the course of HIV. Am J Psychiatry 1993; 150(2):326–327.

5 Barriers to the Safe and Effective Treatment of Late-Life Mood Disorders

Helen H. Kyomen

McLean Hospital, Belmont, and Department of Psychiatry, Harvard Medical School, Boston, Massachusetts, U.S.A.

Gary L. Gottlieb

Department of Psychiatry, Harvard Medical School, and Brigham and Women's Hospital, Boston, Massachusetts, U.S.A.

INTRODUCTION

Mood disorders are common in the elderly and include depressive and manic conditions. Major depression has been reported to occur in 1% to 3% of the general elderly population (1–5). Estimates of the prevalence of geriatric mania in treatment populations range from 5% to 19%, but reliable community-based rates are not known (6).

Despite the substantial prevalence of mood disorders in the elderly, many elderly with diagnosable mood symptoms are not reliably identified (6,7). Diagnosis is often complicated by comorbid medical illness, cognitive impairment, and adverse life events. Only about 30% to 40% of the elderly with identified depressive signs and symptoms receive appropriate treatment for these problems (8,9). Even fewer elderly with mania are apt to receive treatment. As many as 70% to 80% of elderly with depression and likely, even more with mania, do not receive needed intervention. In addition, among elderly persons treated for mood disorders, compliance with treatment frequently is incomplete (10,11).

Taken together, these circumstances—common occurrence of mood disorders among elderly persons, obscured identification of these signs and symptoms, insufficient provision of indicated interventions for these conditions, and inadequate compliance with treatment among treated patients—suggest that there are important operative barriers to care among elderly persons with mood disorders. Identifying these barriers to care may be a useful early step in their attenuation.

This chapter will discuss barriers to care for mood disorders in the elderly. The salient barriers to care are multiform and related to patient, provider, as well as organizational/financial, interventional, and societal issues. Suggestions for an action and research agenda to improve the care of elderly with mood disorders will close the discussion.

PATIENT-RELATED BARRIERS TO RECOGNITION AND CARE

Patient-related barriers to care range from emotional and physiologic changes occurring in the elderly patient due to the affective condition, through problems of exacerbation of co-occurring medical illnesses, to difficulties based in the psychosocial network, economic status, and ethnocultural background of the patient.

Mood disorders in elderly patients, just as in younger adults, can range from mild symptom combinations suggesting a subsyndromal state to full-scale illness with psychotic features. Available data indicate that older adults use considerably fewer than expected mental health services relative to their prevalence of mood disorders (12,13).

Many individuals have a gradual, insidious onset of illness that progressively impairs their ability to retain insight into their condition. In contrast to depression or mania experienced by many younger adults, many elderly persons do not endorse symptoms of sadness (14,15) or euphoria, and may experience the illness differently from younger adults (see Chapter 1 of this book). Thus, the elderly patient may be unaware of the mood disorder–related changes that are occurring and may not recognize the need to seek evaluation for a consequential illness.

Those elderly who do recognize that affective symptoms are having a significant impact on their lives may not acknowledge that these symptoms may need to be assessed and treated by appropriate clinicians. If somatic concerns predominate, the affective symptoms may be experienced as stemming from physical illness, perhaps leading to assessment by the family doctor. Indeed, this approach may be favored by many elderly patients, especially where there are concurrent medical conditions (16,17). Alternatively, and very commonly, the affective condition may be considered as something that the patient can take care of on her/his own or that will go away with time (17).

Even when the affective condition is recognized, and the need for mental health evaluation is acknowledged, impaired motivation and insight may deter the patient from seeking help. The depressed patient may feel hopeless and believe that no assistance is available, or, if sought, that the aid will be ineffective. The patient, due to thought disturbances from the depressive illness or lack of knowledge about health benefits, may feel that she or he does not have adequate financial resources or health insurance to pay for physician visits, medications, or other treatments (18,19). The manic patient may insist that she or he is fine and see no reason to seek assistance or treatment. The tasks of identifying appropriate sources of care and of obtaining this assistance can feel overwhelming for an elderly person experiencing disabling depressive symptoms. Obtaining transportation to a treatment site may be perceived as eminently problematic, especially for elderly living in regions where mental health care services are limited (20,21).

Many elderly persons perceive a stigma associated with depression (22), mania, or other mental illnesses, and attach a negative connotation to mental illness or the need for mental health treatment. These stigmatization issues, often linked with ageism, can become accentuated in the depressed state, to the extent that self-esteem plummets and feelings of guilt about having a mental illness or being "too old to be worth helping" supervene, further dissuading the patient from seeking treatment. The manic patient may resort to extreme denial of illness and thus, may see no reason to seek or follow through with treatment.

Isolation and inadequate social supports, common among the elderly, present additional obstacles to receiving care (23). Isolated older adults are at risk of deterioration emotionally and physically. Those with depression may have such severe anhedonia and even anorexia, and those with acute mania may have such problems with focusing and organizing their thoughts, that they may not buy food or ask others to help them with food shopping. The resulting inadequate food or fluid intake may lead to dehydration, metabolic derangement, and nutritional deficits (24).

These conditions, in turn, may result in confusion, weakness, and frailty, diminishing motivation and undermining ability to seek help.

Even when the potential patient manages to seek out treatment, she/he may de-emphasize mood symptoms because other problems, in particular somatic symptoms in depressed patients (25) or external issues in manic patients, are more easily discussed. Few older adults with depressive symptoms, and most likely few with manic symptoms, discuss their complaints with their primary care providers. The majority of these individuals refuse psychiatric referral when it is offered (26). When a patient's wish for rapid relief of a somatic complaint takes center stage, a thorough assessment of mood and behavioral concerns may be averted and a mood disorder diagnosis missed.

Limited adherence to an appropriate treatment plan constitutes a further obstacle to treatment. This lack of adherence may reflect a limited understanding of the need for acute and ongoing treatment or of medication directions (27,28), reluctance to follow through with recommendations due to illness-related symptoms such as decreased motivation or nihilistic thinking in the depressed patient, or disbelief of illness in the manic patient. Suicidal ideation may develop (29), and suicide increasingly may be seen as a reasonable, inevitable, or even impulsive choice, prevailing over any thoughts of recovery through treatment. For a substantial fraction of elderly patients, this is a mortal risk, if the means for completion of a suicidal act are available and the likelihood of rescue is low (30). The rates of active suicide rise and are greatest for elderly Caucasian men, compared to Caucasian women and black men and women. "Passive suicide," commonly seen in geriatric settings, occurs when individuals stop eating and taking fluids or needed medications. To our knowledge, there are no controlled studies of this phenomenon.

Increasingly, language and communication barriers due to failing sensorial and cognitive abilities and, for ethnic minority elderly, the inability to convey information adequately due to language and cultural differences, are important impediments to care for elderly persons with affective symptoms.

In summary, patient-related barriers to care for elderly persons with affective symptoms include multiple complex psychiatric and medical problems, patient–provider communication issues, stigmatization and other attitudinal concerns, compliance difficulties, and ethnocultural differences.

PROVIDER-RELATED BARRIERS TO RECOGNITION AND CARE

Providers in this context are health care professionals in direct treatment roles, providing care to elderly patients. Provider-related barriers to care stem from a number of issues, including nonrecognition or misdiagnosis of an affective condition in an elderly patient, initiation of suboptimal or even inappropriate evaluation and treatment, and lack of patient referral for additional expert geropsychiatric evaluation and management when these are indicated.

The subtlety of some affective symptoms in many elderly patients, and the similarity of these symptoms to effects of primary medical disorders that are highly prevalent in this population, may limit the ability of even the most adept clinician to diagnose and treat affective disorders effectively. Indeed, affective conditions in the elderly are often unrecognized by health care professionals (31–33). Nonrecognition of depression may occur when the older patient asserts anxiety or various somatic concerns such as pain, fatigue, or insomnia, without explicitly endorsing a depressed mood. Manic behavior may be mistaken as ebullience, irritability, a driven personality style, or eccentricity. Various factors, including inherent differences in how elderly experience affective illness compared to younger patients, the coexistence of additional medical illness, or the patient's reluctance to acknowledge symptoms of a mental illness that can be perceived as stigmatizing, may contribute to this presentation (14,15,25).

There is further diagnostic complication when the depressed patient is also experiencing psychotic features, alterations of consciousness, or significant cognitive impairment, all common in elderly patients (34–37). Cognitive disturbances, labile or altered mood, irritability, sleep problems, and changes in energy level or motivation are all nonspecific symptoms that may accompany not only depression or mania but also delirium or dementia. In these contexts, a diagnosis of a possible affective illness may not receive priority consideration. Frequently, there is limited history from both the patient and collateral historians. Elderly with affective symptoms may underreport the severity of their symptoms (38). Respondents may not agree on key history issues (39,40). Screening instruments used to identify depression may yield both high false-positive and high false-negative results (41), a shortcoming also of instruments used to screen for mania. Unless the clinician has substantial experience with elderly patients enduring depression or mania with and without psychotic features, delirium, and/or dementia, co-occurring conditions may go partially unrecognized and receive inadequate management.

Between one-half and two-thirds of all psychiatric care delivered to older adults is provided by primary care providers in the general health care sector (42–44). Primary care providers are a diverse group, comprised largely of general practitioners, family practitioners, internists, and gynecologists. The majority of these providers have limited training in the special needs of older adults with affective illness. Yet, elderly patients with mood disturbances are most often evaluated and treated in primary care settings and are less likely than younger patients to see a mental health specialist (45,46).

With some clinicians, the presenting signs and symptoms of affective illness may be unintentionally subjected to stigmatization (47) and ageist-based misinterpretations, so that the provider assesses the patient to be eating less or sleeping poorly due to a normal aging process. The frequent result is failure to evaluate for affective illness.

The time constraints and economic incentives inherent in primary care practice settings limit the availability of adequate time to perform extensive diagnostic assessments and to distinguish disorders of mood from concomitant medical illness. Systematic screening for mental disorders in primary care practices confirm a substantial prevalence of untreated psychiatric symptoms and disorders in these settings (48–51). Primary care providers identify, and then appropriately treat and/or refer, only a small proportion of the older patients with affective illness in their practices. One study reported that primary care providers are more than 50% less likely to record a diagnosis of depression in elderly patients compared to younger adult patients (50). Older patients in academic medical center primary care and Medicare Health Maintenance Organization (HMO) settings have been found to have low rates of treatment for depression, ranging from 4% to 7% in all persons studied, to 12% to 25% among patients with probable depression (Centers for Epidemiologic Studies Depression Scale [DES-D] score ≥ 21) (51).

Nearly 80% of elderly patients with psychiatric diagnoses receive pharmacotherapy without psychosocial interventions for their psychiatric diagnoses (43). Most of this treatment is provided by primary care practitioners. Nearly 85% of all older adults see a primary care physician at least once per year and most have multiple visits (43). Approximately 10% of medical visits by older adults are associated with prescription of a psychotropic medication (52,53).

Primary care providers are also responsible for the overwhelming majority of psychiatric care and prescription of psychotropics in institutional settings. Approximately 50% to 60% of nursing home patients are prescribed some kind of psychotropic medication in any given year (54,55). The rates of depression in the elderly are higher for nursing home patients than for noninstitutionalized, non–medically ill elderly (56). It has been estimated that more than 9 out of 10 nursing home residents who would benefit from treatment for psychiatric disorders, including depression and mania, receive no treatment whatsoever (57,58). This estimate may be conservative, as other data indicate that a substantial proportion of nursing home residents who receive psychiatric treatment are not treated for the correct disorder or are not treated with the appropriate intervention (57–59). But not all of the assessment difficulties associated with affective conditions in elderly persons relate to under-recognition. In some elderly patients, affective conditions may be overdiagnosed, perhaps due to misinterpretation of the symptoms of other medical or psychiatric problems, and patients may be prescribed inappropriate treatment. One study suggests that, in an acute hospital setting, approximately 40% of specialty referrals for depression involved problems other than depression, including delirium, dementia, and anxiety (60). Delirium and anxiety may be mistaken for mania in many older adults. Overdiagnosis can be significant if the presumption of affective illness delays assessment for other medical, neurologic, or psychiatric conditions.

If an affective illness is considered and diagnosed, the severity of the illness may be misjudged so that appropriate referrals to experts in geropsychiatry are not considered. As a result, adequate evaluation for suicide risk, mood-congruent delusions, or other psychiatric illness may not occur, averting treatment initiation or resulting in suboptimal/inappropriate interventions.

Treatments for mood disorders in the elderly include pharmacologic agents; psychotherapy, including individual, couples, family, and group therapies; psychosocial treatments including behavioral and milieu interventions; electroconvulsive therapy (ECT), and in some centers, transcranial magnetic stimulation (TMS). Some providers may not consider this range of possible treatments. The plan of treatment for an elderly patient is frequently much more complicated than in a younger patient due to medical and social comorbidities, requiring expert multidisciplinary care.

In summary, provider-related barriers to care affecting elderly patients with mood disorders extend from affective illness-identification problems with older patients to provider difficulties in selection and application of appropriate treatments.

ORGANIZATIONAL AND FINANCIAL BARRIERS TO RECOGNITION AND CARE

Barriers to care related to organizational and financial factors include organization-specific mission and philosophy issues, unavailability of a sufficiently wide range of different modalities of psychiatric care to older adults with affective illness, financial incentives/disincentives, and transportation issues.

The diverse group of professionals and paraprofessionals who provide mental health services to older adults work in a fragmented system. They have limited commonality in training, philosophy, therapeutic approach, and the objectives of care. These providers deliver care to elders with affective symptoms under conditions of extraordinary uncertainty. Even in severe cases, definitions of illness remain controversial and triage and clinical decision making are not well standardized.

The mental health specialty sector, providing care to older adults, comprises a large and growing group of diversely trained professionals and paraprofessionals from several major disciplines: nursing, social work, counseling, psychology, and psychiatry. Unquantified amounts of nonspecialty services are provided to elders with affective symptoms by social workers and caseworkers in social agencies and by clergy in religious settings. Training in diagnosis and management among these providers is highly variable. Considering the complexity and subtlety of geriatric affective illness, it is highly likely that case identification among these providers is incomplete, and appropriate referral almost surely is limited to settings that are relatively well connected to the mental health specialty sector or where innovative training programs have been initiated.

The availability of specialty training for the care of older adults in each of the clinical disciplines is limited, although growing in recent years. Virtually all of the disciplines have developed minimum criteria for specialty psychiatric training and for subspecialty training in geriatrics. Nursing, social work, psychology, and psychiatry have all undertaken extensive efforts to increase subspecialty geriatric training (61–65) and to provide incentives for trainees to pursue careers focused on the care of elderly patients (64,65).

Even with improvement in standardization of training, there remains considerable variability in the skills and objectives of providers from each of the disciplines. Each of the provider disciplines involved in mental health care for older adults has a unique ethos. Standards for training have been linked traditionally to the philosophy and the identified tasks associated with each provider group. Additionally, the dominance of private practice by mental health providers in an environment of limited economic resources has led to vigorous competition among disciplines (44). The equivocal nature of criteria for treatment of affective illness in elderly patients has permitted providers from different disciplines to treat patients in accordance with their training, but in ways that do not necessarily reflect current knowledge-based practice.

Mental health specialty care is provided in a large variety of settings, few of which are designed specifically for the care of older adults. Private practice continues to dominate psychiatric service delivery (66), although this is steadily changing with the continued growth of managed care plans. Many private practitioners maintain that late-life psychiatric disorders do not fit with their chosen style of practice. They also question the appropriateness of traditional psychiatric treatments for problems associated with aging. For example, some psychiatrists in private practice attribute their avoidance of geriatric patients to the complex nature of the care of elderly patients who commonly have co-occurring medical problems. They claim that the resource requirements of this population are matched poorly with the structural limitations of solo and group private psychiatric practice (67,68).

Because of similar limitations, community mental health centers (CMHCs), which are designed primarily to serve younger, chronically mentally ill patients, often have limited programs for and expertise in the care of older adults with affective illness, particularly in the presence of medical comorbidity (69). CMHCs are commonly inadequately integrated with the social service agencies and the network of primary care providers in the community from which referrals are likely to originate (53). Several innovative programs have improved access to care for older adults with mental disorders. These programs have been successful largely because of their ability to recruit specialty-trained geriatric clinicians and because of innovative programs linking them to social agencies that provide services for older adults (70–73).

In recent years, mental health specialty providers in general and private psychiatric hospital settings have become more actively involved in providing geriatric mental health services. However, the nature of traditional general hospital and private psychiatric inpatient facilities, steeped in milieu therapies for behavioral control and functional improvement for younger populations, limits access to appropriate care for older adults who have concomitant medical disorders requiring acute attention. The advent of medical psychiatric units and geropsychiatric inpatient units (42,74–76) has provided a new resource for the treatment of frail, elderly psychiatric patients in acute-care settings.

Clinical uncertainty is said to emanate from three key factors: (*i*) the ability of the clinician to classify the existence of illness; (*ii*) the ability of the clinician to understand the probability of a successful outcome given a specific treatment; and (*iii*) the correspondence of the clinician's desires and benefits with those of the patient's (77). Providers of mental health services to older adults have substantial variability in training, treatment philosophy, economic incentives, and perceived available treatment options. In a well-organized delivery system, this diversity could provide a richness of service delivery alternatives to meet the complex needs of older adults. However, given the fragmentation of the service delivery system and the substantial barriers to access, this diversity has the effect of increasing the level of uncertainty that individual providers face in clinical decision making. The somewhat paradoxical result is that the appropriate matching of services to needs is less likely to occur for elderly patients.

Some health services organizations may choose to de-emphasize care of the older, mentally ill patient because of a perception that provision of such services will project a negative public image. For example, some clinics may wish to project a health and wellness image, and accordingly, emphasize treatment putatively focused on maintaining health among those who are relatively young, healthy, and with "intact" minds. Providing care to the elderly with mental illness may not accord well with this image.

In most health services organizations, there is vigorous competition for limited financial resources, and in this context, provision of care for mental illness may not be considered to be adequately profitable. Certainly, compared to many inpatient surgical procedures, the revenue generated in outpatient psychiatric care to elderly patients may not be substantial. This revenue-generation focus can have a profound effect on the way some health services organizations view and provide care to elderly patients with affective symptoms.

Even in organizations (or organizational components) with a strong commitment to providing health care to the aged with mental illness, there can be important, sometimes unrecognized, barriers to care. There may be limited availability of psychiatric and/or mental health expertise, limited access to some care modalities (such as ECT), and a restrained pharmacy formulary so that options for pharmacologic care are significantly reduced. The latter situation can be especially problematic if a patient needs a nonformulary drug to continue ongoing maintenance treatment or because of adverse reactions to drugs on formulary.

The growth of managed care in the general health care sector is likely to affect access to appropriate psychiatric care for older adults. As health maintenance organizations (HMOs) have gained increased market penetration throughout the country and while federal regulations have provided incentives for the inclusion of Medicare populations, older adult participation in HMOs has grown steadily. Of more than 44 million Americans enrolled in Medicare in 2007, more than 19% participated in the Medicare Advantage (previously known as "Medicare + Choice") plans authorized under the 1997 Balanced Budget Act (78). Enrollment was encouraged following new and expanded plans in 2005 by the Centers for Medicare and Medicaid Services. The Medicare Advantage plans resemble a traditional HMO plan, in that members are permitted to obtain services only from providers who participate in the plan or on referral from the plan, with monthly payment by Medicare of a fixed capitated amount to the insurer or HMO that the Medicare beneficiary chooses. Medicare-eligible persons choosing Part B coverage pay a modest premium for this coverage, and many choose to supplement this coverage with "Medigap insurance" purchased from private insurers. Some Medicare benefits under part B supplemental (non-inpatient) coverage are subject to 20% copayment, with some services also subject to an annual deductible. Prior to the enactment of the Mental Health Parity Act of 1996, included in the Health Insurance Portability and Accountability Act (HIPAA) of 1996 (Public Law 104–191, 1996) (79), mental health services were treated in a discriminatory manner by Medicare, with a 50% copayment required instead of the 20% to which other medical services were subject. The Mental Health Parity Act of 1996 established parity for mental health benefits provided by large group insurance plans, changing copayment requirements from the previously discriminatory 50% Medicare and 50% beneficiary formula for outpatient mental health services to the 80% to 20% formula applied for all other medical services. Enactment of the Paul Wellstone and Pete Domenici Mental Health Parity and Addiction Equity Act of 2008, included in the Emergency Economic Stabilization Act of 2008, H.R. 1424, amends the Mental Health Parity Act of 1996 to ensure that all financial requirements and treatment limitations for mental health care are no more restrictive than those placed on medical/surgical benefits for health plans of groups with more than 50 employees. Provisions of this law are planned to be phased in over six years and fully in place by 2014.

Medicare part A (inpatient services) is provided to all Medicare beneficiaries at no premium cost. Part A covers inpatient hospital services, skilled nursing facility (SNF) benefits following a 3-day hospital visit, home health visits following a hospital or SNF stay, and certain other services. A copayment is required of Medicare beneficiaries for hospital stay days 61 to 90; the amount increases for days 91to 150, and then to 100% of all costs after day 150. SNF care costs nothing during the first 20 days, then a copayment is required until day 100, after which the beneficiary pays all costs (80). Nothing in these Medicare provisions affects patients with affective symptoms any differently from the way that patients with other medical problems are affected. But because of the chronicity of affective illness, these financial constraints impact much more heavily on Medicare beneficiaries with affective illness or other chronic medical problems than on Medicare enrollees whose medical problems are more episodic and less persistent over time. In this sense, these Medicare coverage rules differentially affect elderly persons with affective illness and other chronic problems.

Yet, in practical terms, these Medicare part A requirements for beneficiary participation in the payment for acute inpatient and SNF care probably do not have a significant deterrent effect on care seeking. In these situations, the need for care is so strong that, for the beneficiary, viable alternatives are not available. For Medicare part B, the situation is quite different. Here, the need to pay a copayment, either out-of-pocket or through one of the Medigap insurance coverages (for which the insurance premium costs are paid out-of-pocket), may have a substantial deterrent effect among elderly Medicare beneficiaries with affective illness.

Since the advent of Medicare part D, insurance coverage for medications has become possible for more elderly. Yet, the premium for and cost-sharing nature of Medicare part D may cause many participants to stop or ration the use of needed psychotropic medication, jeopardizing optimal care. For elderly persons in managed care plans, an additional mechanism intended to control health care expenditures is the mental health "carve-out" (81). This mechanism provides for a separate preapproval and service limitation system, administered by a third-party contractor, for treatment of mood disorders, substance abuse, and other mental health conditions. These carve-out contractors are most commonly large, for-profit companies or group practices specializing in managed mental health care. Psychiatric carve-outs may focus on utilization control, without prioritizing patient care and outcomes, and this may disproportionately impact certain covered subgroups that are primarily elderly (82). To our knowledge, no data quantifying, whether these carve-out programs significantly affect the quality of care, providing Medicare/Medicaid beneficiaries with affective symptoms are yet available. However, these programs have been put into operation to attempt to control putative overutilization, so that it seems likely that their net effect is to reduce the volume of services that provided elders with problems with affective illness.

Transportation issues can be problematic for elderly persons seeking to access mental health services. Available data, while limited in scope, clearly indicate that utilization and accessibility vary closely together among elderly persons needing health services (83). Some health organizations invest in community outreach activities, providing transportation between patients' homes and the health care facilities at which services are delivered. However, these programs can be costly and are not common. Obviously, to the extent that unavailability of appropriate transportation inhibits the delivery of needed health services, this can be an important barrier to care for elderly persons with affective illness.

In summary, organizational and financial barriers to care include fragmentation of care issues, insurance copayment, and deductible provisions that obstruct access to services, especially pharmaceutical services, and transportation issues.

TREATMENT-/INTERVENTION-RELATED BARRIERS TO RECOGNITION AND CARE

By intervention-related barriers, we mean issues embedded in the pathophysiology of the illness and related to somatic and psychotherapeutic treatments for affective illness.

There is a growing but still relatively underdeveloped understanding of the pathophysiology of depression and mania in elderly. The dynamics leading to affective illness are complex in any circumstance, and especially so in elderly patients, who may also be affected by various aging-related changes, as well as a wide spectrum of medical problems. Mechanisms of action of various interventions used in the treatment of affective illness, including psychotropic medications, ECT, and various psychotherapeutic treatments, are still incompletely understood. Knowledge about the tolerability and effectiveness of the psychotropic medications among elderly patients varies widely by the type and dose of treatment (84–86).

Very active research initiatives are examining the risk factors, pathophysiology, diagnostic specificity, and progression over time of affective illness in the elderly. However, despite the vigor with which this research is being pursued, current knowledge remains relatively limited. Compared to other medical conditions that affect the elderly significantly, such as hypertension or myocardial infarction, current levels of scientific understanding of affective illness in the elderly are at nascent levels.

Diagnostic assignments are affected by the limited scientific knowledge about the etiology, risk factors, and longitudinal pathophysiology of late-life affective illness. This has resulted in the routine use among elderly patients of nosologic diagnostic categories mostly devised for a younger population. A consequence of this practice has been a widespread willingness to consider that the treatment indications and prognostic circumstances associated with these nosologic categories apply equally well to elderly as to the younger patients who were the clinical trial subjects upon which they were based. As well, and perhaps ominously, various pharmacologic and nonpharmacologic intervention strategies originally developed for younger patients have been extended for use with elderly patients, sometimes without the benefit of adequate safety, tolerability, and efficacy research. For example, more than a dozen antidepressants are currently marketed; many of these are widely used among elderly depressed patients, even though efficacy research specific to elderly patients has been carried out less frequently and has yielded conflicting results (84,85).

Available data suggest that the unconstrained use, among older patients, of treatments for affective illness that were developed within nonelderly cohorts may result in suboptimal results. Data on adverse drug reactions (ADRs) indicate that these events are a leading cause of morbidity and mortality, with the highest incidence occurring in patients aged 60 and older. A meta-analysis concluded that ADRs were among the leading causes of death, ranking 4th to 6th, depending on study inclusion rules (ahead of diabetes and pneumonia), and that approximately three-fourths of ADRs were dose dependent (87). Another study found that risk factors associated with ADRs among hospitalized elderly included inappropriate medications (IMs), number of prior diagnoses, and number of prescribed medications (88). It was reported that anticholinergic antidepressants, cerebral vasodilators, long-acting benzodiazepines, and concurrent use of multiple psychotropic drugs from the same treatment class were the most frequent IMs (89).

Some authorities recommend that physicians give older patients lower initial doses than are prescribed for younger patients. The reasons for this recommendation include (*i*) older patients have reduced rates of drug metabolism and elimination compared with younger adults; (*ii*) chronic or multiple disease processes, which are common in older patients, may alter drug response; and (*iii*) drug–drug interactions are a particular concern among older patients because of the high likelihood that they are taking more than one medication. Most practicing physicians rely on the Physicians' Desk Reference (PDR) for medication dosing information

(90). Yet, the PDR does not provide recommendations for reduced initial dosing of many medications for older patients.

Polypharmacy in the elderly possibly could be reduced if there were regular reviews of therapy already prescribed. This would enable the identification of those medicines that are no longer required, those without clear indication, those prescribed for side effects that could be avoided by therapy changes, and those that duplicate similar medicines. All of these actions would reduce the frequency of polypharmacy and thereby reduce the likelihood of life-threatening ADRs.

In addition to pharmaceutical treatments for geriatric affective illness, various nonpharmacologic interventions are also widely used. Psychotherapeutic interventions include interpersonal psychotherapy, behavioral therapy, cognitive behavioral therapy, and psychodynamic therapy. Counseling/social interventions of various types have been used to treat affective illness in elderly patients (91). Scientific knowledge about the outcomes of such treatments in the elderly is very limited.

Efficacy research on other nonpharmacologic interventions in elderly cohorts is equally sparse. For example, efficacy research on ECT in the elderly is limited (92, and see Chapter 16 of this book). The limited data that are available suggest that ECT therapy results in favorable outcomes in elderly with affective illness, who are less able to tolerate the prolonged response times common with pharmaceutical therapies. Transcranial Magnetic stimulation (TMS), recently indicated by the FDA for treatment of depression in adults, has shown potential as an ECT alternative and merits further exploration as a treatment for depressed elders (93–95).

The association of affective illness in elderly patients with physical-illness risk factors could result in a weakening of some barriers to care. Although there are numerous reports of linkages of depression or mania with elevated mortality risk for patients with cardiovascular and other illnesses (96–98), as yet, no credible scientific data have been published that indicate that effective treatment can result in mortality reduction. If it is found that treatment of affective illness can result in reduced mortality risk in patients with cardiovascular and other illnesses, this could lead to dramatic improvements in the evaluation and management of affective illness in the elderly.

If the risk factors for affective illness in elderly could be established more clearly, targeted prevention strategies might be more effectively instituted, to decrease the incidence and eventually the prevalence of late-life mood disorders. Were the etiology and pathophysiology of affective illness in the elderly understood more clearly, more specific therapies with greater effectiveness and fewer side effects might be developed. Many elderly have a number of co-occurring psychiatric or medical conditions that likely need treatment with various medications from different classes. This increases the risk for illness–drug and drug–drug interactions so that the development of effective, safe psychotropic treatments is a very high priority goal. The availability of medications with improved tolerability and efficacy for use with the elderly will likely ameliorate some patients' reluctance to accept treatment and will improve compliance with acute and relapse prevention treatment, resulting in improved long-term treatment effectiveness.

In summary, intervention-related barriers to safe and effective care for mood disorders in the elderly include limitations in the understanding of pathophysiologic and ethologic issues in this age group, limited efficacy data, significant risks associated with polypharmacy, and vulnerability to adverse drug reactions and treatment intolerance.

SOCIETAL BARRIERS TO RECOGNITION AND CARE

Sociodemographic characteristics have been shown to influence patient demand and the use of mental health services in general populations. Sex, age, race, education, marital status, residence location, and attitudes toward mental health services exert independent effects on the likelihood of pursuing mental health care (99–102). Socioeconomic status may determine access both to primary care and to mental health specialty providers who are specially trained to provide services for older adults. Similarly, geographic location may be an important factor in determining access to appropriate care for affective illness in elderly persons (20,21).

The stigma associated with psychiatric disorder and the pursuit of mental health services by older adults has its roots in a culture and tradition that have discouraged the recognition and the importance of psychiatric syndromes. The controversial nature of psychiatric treatments makes them especially vulnerable to public scrutiny and potential regulation. Social and legal pressures from local communities controlling the use of psychotropic medications and electroconvulsive therapy may limit the availability of safe and effective treatments for geriatric mood disorders (103). Societal denial of the importance of psychiatric disorders and discrimination against individuals with mental disorders continues to exert an influence over public policy governing payment for health services.

Although recent reforms in the Medicare program have eliminated the discriminatory regulation of mental health services in comparison to services for other medical problems, these discriminatory policies continue in force in numerous ways within the Medicaid program. For example, federal participation in Medicaid has been disallowed for young adults in institutions for mental disease (IMD). An IMD has been defined as a facility with more than 16 beds that specializes in psychiatric care. This exclusion had its roots in the 1950 amendments to the Social Security Act. There has been a debate over whether nursing homes can be considered IMDs; according to a 1995 Supreme Court ruling, nursing homes can be designated as IMDs if they meet the criteria. When this happens, the nursing home may no longer be eligible for any Medicaid funding (104–106). Limitations in Medicaid reimbursement levels provide additional disincentives for some hospitals and many private providers to deliver psychiatric care to older adults.

Data on ethnicity differences in rates of identification of, and treatment for, affective symptoms in elderly patients are limited. One study, using data from the 1997 to 1998 National Ambulatory Medical Care Surveys, determined that primary care physicians were 37% less likely to record a diagnosis of depression during visits by African-Americans compared to Caucasians, and 35% less likely to do so during visits by Medicaid patients compared to patients with private insurance coverage (50). In making these comparisons, the investigators controlled for symptom presentation. It is possible, although unlikely given the magnitude of these differences, that the African-American and Medicaid patients were 37% and 35%, respectively, less likely to present with significant depressive symptoms, and that the diagnostic assignments thus were validly made. Another interpretation is that these differential rates reflect discriminatory societal attitudes. It is unknown if these differential diagnostic rates for African-Americans and Medicaid recipients obtain in geriatric populations. Perhaps, future research of this kind can help to determine whether these rate differentials are due to actual differences in illness prevalence or are attributable to discriminatory attitudes.

In summary, societal barriers to care include discriminatory health policy factors that treat mental health services in ways that are substantively different from, and inferior to, other medical services.

IMPROVING ACCESS TO CARE: AN ACTION AND RESEARCH AGENDA

Prevention

Identifying risk factors for affective illness in later life through longitudinal epidemiologic studies would be invaluable for instituting preventive strategies. Providing informative bulletins through different media to familiarize the public with affective signs and symptoms in the elderly and identifying mood disorders with well-known figures or celebrities may help to destigmatize such illness, raise the population's consciousness regarding affective illness, and encourage patients with depressive or manic symptoms to seek help. Routine screening of at-risk individuals, followed by appropriate evaluation and management over time, may improve patients' access to care and delay the incidence, prevalence, and progression of late-life mood disorders (107,108).

Translational Research

Translational research suggests a bridging of knowledge, gained through basic and clinical scientific work, to application in the clinical realm. Inherent in applying these concepts to the elderly is the focus on change as a person becomes older. Important are (*i*) identifying and harnessing molecular mechanisms regarding the etiology and pathophysiology of affective illness over time and as a person ages; (*ii*) unveiling longitudinal genotypic and phenotypic markers for affective illness that are practicable, sensitive and specific, and can be identified cost effectively; (*iii*) developing longitudinal dimensional and categorical models of affective illness; (*iv*) shaping diagnostic criteria applicable to affective illness in the elderly; and (*v*) emphasizing pathways out of illness and into health in later life. Translational research can impact the diagnostic and interventional capabilities in medical and scientific realms.

Interventional Studies

Changes in pharmacokinetics and pharmacodynamics in aging individuals, and uncertainties around medical comorbidities, polypharmacy, and adverse effects in the elderly make it imperative to conduct drug-intervention trials with elderly subjects. Food and Drug Administration (FDA) approval for drug use in older patients may be made contingent on clinical trials in the elderly. In addition to safety, efficacy, and tolerability of the interventions, additional measures to assess impact on compliance, functional ability, cognitive capabilities, well-being, and comorbid physical illnesses such as cardiovascular disease, endocrinologic illness, or rheumatologic conditions may be especially relevant in the elderly.

Investigations of nonpharmacologic interventions are just as important and include ECT, TMS, psychotherapeutic, psychosocial, behavioral, and milieu interventions as well as case management. Alternative interventions such as exercise and nutritional supplements, and ethnic minority/cultural group and gender issues also warrant scientific appraisal. Ethnocultural factors influence presentations of mental disorders, description of psychiatric symptoms, and diagnoses and treatments received. Ethnic and gender differences in pharmacokinetics and pharmacodynamics contributing to differential drug responsiveness deserve investigation as well. Efficacy of pharmacologic versus nonpharmacologic interventions in the elderly, alone or in combination, needs further exploration.

Because geriatric affective illness is chronic and recurrent, it is necessary to study the course of the illness longitudinally, over extended time periods of at least 18 to 24 months. Most of the existing outcomes research in geriatric mood disorders has been limited to studies a few weeks or months in length.

Health Services Research

Managed care and long-term care have greatly influenced the delivery of health care to the elderly. Although interventional studies may help to uncover efficacious treatments, health services research may be better suited to determine if, in "real world" situations, the treatments are effective. Health services research should consider whether treatments are truly effective, with the financial and other constraints placed on treatments due to managed care and other considerations. Interventional clinical trials typically utilize stringent inclusion and exclusion criteria so that the population studied may not be representative of the many patients who are frail, have multiple comorbid illnesses such as delirium, dementia, cardiovascular disease, or diabetes, and are taking multiple medications. Population-based studies could also establish study samples more representative of the general, ill elderly population, and may be able to identify morbidity risks associated with affective illness in such an ill population. Also needed are the data that identify the morbidity risks associated with the use of antidepressant and mood-stabilization medication in combination with other commonly used treatments for medical problems in frail elderly. The role of specialty mental health services, development and implementation of practice guidelines, and evaluation of outcomes are important to explore. Systematic research designed to assess the impact among elderly of affective illness on functioning, mortality, and quality of life is needed.

Training

Training in geriatric mental health needs to be improved at all levels, including patients, clinicians of various backgrounds, public workers who may come in contact with elderly living alone, the public at large, and policy makers. Patients who know more about affective illness and how it interacts with medical conditions may be more willing to seek and continue with treatment, and volunteer for studies on affective illness. Training collaborations among existing mental health services and centers with expertise on geriatric psychiatry and gerontology may help to improve and extend services for the elderly. Patients and service organizations may be more active in letting their needs be known to government officials to influence mental health policy and insurance groups to achieve greater mental health parity, improve insurance coverage for prescription drugs with the lifting of arbitrary drug-benefit caps, pay for clinical trials, and contribute data for research.

REFERENCES

1. Mojtabai R, Olfson M. Major depression in community-dwelling middle-aged and older adults: Prevalence and 2-and 4-year follow-up symptoms. Psychol Med 2004; 34:623–634.

2. Steffens DC, Skoog I, Norton MC, et al. Prevalence of depression and its treatment in an elderly population. Arch Gen Psychiatry 2000; 57:601–607.
3. Beekman ATF, Copeland JRM, Prince MJ. Review of community prevalence of depression in later life. Br J Psychiatry 1999; 174:307–311.
4. Cole MG, Bellavance F, Mansour A. Prognosis of depression in elderly community and primary care populations: A systematic review and meta-analysis. Am J Psychiatry 1999; 156:1182–1189.
5. Regier DA, Myers JK, Kramer M, et al. The NIMH Epidemiologic Catchment Area Program: Historical context, major objectives, and study population characteristics. Arch Gen Psychiatry 1984; 41:934–941.
6. Depp CA, Jeste DV. Bipolar disorder in older adults: A critical review. Bipolar Disord 2004; 6:343–367.
7. Mulsant BH, Ganguli M. Epidemiology and diagnosis of depression in late life. J Clin Psychiatry 1999; 60(suppl 20):9–15.
8. Unutzer J, Katon W, Callahan CM, et al. Depression treatment in a sample of 1801 depressed older adults in primary care. J Am Geriatr Soc 2003; 51:505–514.
9. Gottlieb GL. Barriers to care for older adults with depression. In: Schneider LS, Reynolds CF III, Lebowitz BD, et al. eds. Diagnosis and Treatment of Depression in Late Life. Washington D. C.: American Psychiatric Press, 1994:377–396.
10. Copeland LA, Zeber JE, Salloum IM, et al. Treatment adherence and illness insight in veterans with bipolar disorder. J Nerv Ment Dis 2008; 196:16–21.
11. McDonald HP, Garg AX, Haynes RB. Interventions to enhance patient adherence to medication prescriptions: Scientific review. JAMA 2002; 288:2868–2879.
12. Klap R, Tschantz K, Unützer J. Caring for mental disorders in the United States: A focus on older adults. Am J Geriatr Psychiatry 2003; 11:517–524.
13. Older Adults and Mental Health: Issues and Opportunities. Rockville, MD, Administration on Aging, 2001.
14. Gallo JJ, Rabins PV. Depression without sadness: Alternative presentations of depression in late life. Am Fam Physician 1999; 60:820–826.
15. Gottfries CG. Is there a difference between elderly and younger patients with regard to the symptomatology and aetiology of depression? Int Clin Psychopharmacol 1998; 13(suppl 5):S13–S18.
16. Katona C, Livingston G, Manela M, et al. The symptomatology of depression in the elderly. Int Clin Psychopharmacol 1997; 12(suppl 7):S19–S23.
17. Sherrill JT, Frank E, Geary M, et al. Psychoeducational workshops for elderly patients with recurrent major depression and their families. Psychiatr Serv 1997; 48:76–81.
18. Raccio-Robak N, McErlean MA, Fabacher DA, et al. Socioeconomic and health status differences between depressed and nondepressed ED elders. Am J Emerg Med 2002; 20:71–73.
19. Mickus M, Colenda CC, Hogan AJ. Knowledge of mental health benefits and preferences for type of mental health providers among the general public. Psychiatr Serv 2000; 51:199–202.
20. McCarthy JF, Blow FC. Older patients with serious mental illness: Sensitivity to distance barriers for outpatient care. Med Care 2004; 42:1073–1080.
21. Fortney J, Rost K, Zhang M, et al. The impact of geographic accessibility on the intensity and quality of depression treatment. Med Care 1999; 37:884–893.
22. Sirey JA, Bruce ML, Alexopoulos GS, et al. Perceived stigma as a predictor of treatment discontinuation in young and older outpatients with depression. Am J Psychiatry 2001; 158:479–481.
23. Mistry R, Rosansky J, McGuire J, et al. UPBEAT Collaborative Group. Social isolation predicts re-hospitalization in a group of older American veterans enrolled in the UPBEAT program. Int J Geriatr Psychiatry 2001; 16:950–959.
24. Pisani MA, Murphy TE, Van Ness PH, et al. Characteristics associated with delirium in older patients in a medical intensive care unit. Arch Intern Med 2007; 167:1629–1634.
25. O'Connor DW, Rosewarne R, Bruce A. Depression in primary care 1: Elderly patients' disclosure of depressive symptoms to their doctors. Int Psychogeriatr 2001; 13:359–365.

26. Waxman HM, Carner EA. Physicians' recognition, diagnosis and treatment of mental disorders in elderly medical patients. Gerontologist 1984; 24:23–30.
27. Kairuz T, Bye L, Birdsall R, et al. Identifying compliance issues with prescription medicines among older people: A pilot study. Drugs Aging 2008; 25:153–162.
28. Lauber C, Nordt C, Falcato L, et al. Lay recommendations on how to treat mental disorders. Soc Psychiatry Psychiatr Epidemiol 2001; 36:553–556.
29. Alexopoulos GS, Bruce ML, Hull J, et al. Clinical determinants of suicidal ideation and behavior in geriatric depression. Arch Gen Psychiatry 1999; 56:1048–1053.
30. Szanto K, Gildengers A, Mulsant BH, et al. Identification of suicidal ideation and prevention of suicidal behaviour in the elderly. Drugs & Aging 2002; 19:11–24.
31. Depp CA, Lindamer LA, Folsom DP, et al. Differences in clinical features and mental health service use in bipolar disorder across the lifespan. Am J Geriatr Psychiatry 2005; 13:290–298.
32. Pouget R, Yersin B, Wietlisbach V, et al. Depressed mood in a cohort of elderly medical inpatients: Prevalence, clinical correlates and recognition rate. Agin Clin Exp Re 2000; 12:301–307.
33. Garrard J, Rolnick SJ, Nitz NM, et al. Clinical detection of depression among community-based elderly people with self-reported symptoms of depression. J Gerontol (Series A) 1998; 53:92–101.
34. Cepoiu M, McCusker J, Cole MG, et al. Recognition of depression in older medical inpatients. J Gen Intern Med 2007; 22:559–564.
35. Khousam HR, Emes R. Late life psychosis: Assessment and general treatment strategies. Compr Ther 2007; 33:127–143.
36. Brooks JO III, Hoblyn JC. Secondary mania in older adults. Am J Psychiatry 2005; 162:2033–2038.
37. Hoblyn J. Bipolar disorder in later life. Older adults presenting with new onset manic symptoms usually have underlying medical or neurologic disorder. Geriatrics 2004; 59:41–44.
38. Lyness JM, Cox C, Curry J, et al. Older age and the underreporting of depressive symptoms. J Am Geriatr Soc 1995; 43:216–221.
39. Heun R, Muller H. Interinformant reliability of family history information on psychiatric disorders in relatives. Eur Arch Psychiatry Clin Neurosc 1998; 248:104–109.
40. Long K, Sudha S, Mutran EJ. Elder-proxy agreement concerning the functional status and medical history of the older person: The impact of caregiver burden and depressive symptomatology. J Am Geriatr Soc 1998; 46:1103–1111.
41. Papassotinopoulos A, Heun R. Screening for depression in the elderly: A study on misclassification by screening instruments and improvement of scale performance. Prog Neuropsychopharmacol Biol Psychiatry 1999; 23:431–446.
42. Ettner SL, Hermann RC. Provider specialty choice among Medicare beneficiaries treated for psychiatric disorders. Health Care Financ Rev 1997; 18:43–59.
43. Burns BJ, Taube CA. Mental health services in general medical care and in nursing homes. In: Fogel BS, Furino A, Gottlieb GL, eds. Mental Health Policy for Older Americans: Protecting Minds at Risk. Washington, D. C.: American Psychiatric Press, 1990:53–83.
44. Gottlieb GL. Market segmentation. In: Fogel BS, Furino A, Gottlieb GL, eds. Mental Health Policy for Older Americans: Protecting Minds at Risk. Washington, D. C.: American Psychiatric Press, 1990:135–155.
45. Pingitore D, Snowden L, Sansone RA, et al. Persons with depressive symptoms and the treatments they receive: A comparison of primary care physicians and psychiatrists. Int J Psychiatry Med 2001; 31:41–60.
46. Olfson M, Shea S, Feder A, et al. Prevalence of anxiety, depression, and substance use disorders in an urban general medicine practice. Arch Fam Med 2000; 9:876–883.
47. Raue PJ, Meyers BS. An overview of mental health services for the elderly. New Dir Ment Health Serv 1997; 76:3–12.

48. Sajatovic M, Kales HC. Diagnosis and management of bipolar disorder with comorbid anxiety in the elderly. J Clin Psychiatry 2006; 67(suppl 1):21–27.
49. Edlund MJ, Unutzer J, Wells KB. Clinician screening and treatment of alcohol, drug, and mental problems in primary care: Results from healthcare for communities. Med Care 2004; 42:1158–1166.
50. Harman JS, Schulberg HC, Mulsant BH, et al. The effect of patient and visit characteristics on diagnosis of depression in primary care. J Fam Pract 2001; 50:1068.
51. Unutzer J, Simon G, Belin TR, et al. Care for depression in HMO patients aged 65 and older. J Am Geriatr Soc 2000; 48:1011–1013.
52. Schneider LS. Pharmacological considerations in the treatment of late life depression. Am J Geriatr Psychiatry 1996; 4(suppl 1):S51–S65.
53. Lebowitz BD, Niederehe G. Concepts and issues in mental health and aging. In: Birren JE, Sloane RB, Cohen GD, eds. Handbook of Mental Health and Aging, 2nd ed. San Diego, CA: Academic Press, 1992:3–26.
54. Grossberg GT, Grossberg JA. Epidemiology of psychotherapeutic drug use in older adults. Clin Geriatr Med 1998; 14:1–5.
55. Beardsley RS, Larson DB, Burns BJ, et al. Prescribing of psychotropics in nursing home patients. J Am Geriatr Soc 1989; 37:327–330.
56. Nelson JC. Diagnosing and treating depression in the elderly. J Clin Psychiatry 2001; 62(suppl 24):18–22.
57. Teresi J, Abrams R, Holmes D, et al. Prevalence of depression and depression recognition in nursing homes. Soc Psychiatry Psychiatr Epidemiol 2001; 36:613–620.
58. Burns BJ, Kamerow DB. Psychotropic drug prescriptions for nursing home residents. J Fam Pract 1988; 26:155–160.
59. Mort JR, Aparasu RR. Prescribing of psychotropics in the elderly – Why is it so often inappropriate? CNS Drugs 2002; 16:99–109.
60. Boland RJ, Diaz S, Lamdan RM, et al. Overdiagnosis of depression in the general hospital. Gen Hosp Psychiatry 1996; 18:28–35.
61. Fichtner CG, Hardy D, Patel M, et al. A selfassessment program for multidisciplinary mental health teams. Psychiatr Serv 2001; 52:1352–1357.
62. Howe JL, Hyer K, Mellor DJ, et al. Educational approaches for preparing social work students for interdisciplinary teamwork on geriatric health care teams. Soc Work Health Care 2001; 32:19–42.
63. Belza B, Baker MW. Maintaining health in well older adults: Initiative for schools of nursing and The John A. Hartford Foundation for the 21st century. J Gerontolog Nurs 2000; 26:8–17.
64. Cohen GD. The future of mental health and aging. In: Birren JE, Sloane RB, Cohen GD, eds. Handbook of Mental Health and Aging, 2nd ed. San Diego, CA: Academic Press, 1992:894–914.
65. Mezey MD, Lynaugh JE. The teaching nursing home program: Outcomes of care. Nurs Clin North Am 1989; 24:769–780.
66. Zarin DA, Pincus HA, Peterson BD, et al. Characterizing psychiatry with findings from the 1996 National Survey of Psychiatric Practice. Am J Psychiatry 1998; 155:397–404.
67. Mitchell JB, Cromwell J, Schurman R, et al. Psychiatric office practice study: Final Report submitted to the National Institute of Mean Health. Needham, MA: Health Economics Research, 1989.
68. Mitchell JB, Schurman J. Practice patterns and earnings of private psychiatrists: Report submitted to National Institute of Mental Health. Needham, MA: Health Economics Research, 1986.
69. Shear MK, Greeno C, Kang J, et al. Diagnosis of nonpsychotic patients in community clinics. Am J Psychiatry 2000; 157:581–587.
70. Moak G, Borson S. Mental health services in long-term care—Still an unmet need. Am J Geriatr Psychiatry 2000; 8:96–100.
71. Rosenheck R. Primary care satellite clinics and improved access to general and mental health services. Health Serv Res 2000; 35:777–790.

72. Lebowitz BD, Light E, Bailey F. Mental health center services for the elderly: The impact of coordination with area agencies on aging. Gerontologist 1987; 27:699–702.
73. Light E, Lebowitz BD, Bailey F. CMHCs and elderly services: An analysis of direct and indirect services and service delivery sites. Community Ment Health J 1986; 22: 294–302.
74. Kominski G, Andersen R, Bastani R, et al. UPBEAT: The impact of a psychogeriatric intervention in VA medical centers. Unified Psychogeriatric Biopsychosocial Evaluation and Treatment. Med Care 2001; 39:500–512.
75. Weintraub D, Mazour I. Clinical and demographic changes over ten years on a psychogeriatric inpatient unit. Ann Clin Psychiatry 2000; 12:227–231.
76. Fogel BS, Kroessler D. Treating late-life depression on a medical-psychiatric unit. Hosp Community Psychiatry 1987; 38:89–831.
77. Wennberg JE, Barnes BA, Zubkoff M. Professional uncertainty and the problem of supplier-induced demand. Soc Sci Med 1982; 16:811–824.
78. http://www.statehealthfacts.org/comparetable.jsp?ind=327&cat=6. (Accessed May 30, 2008).
79. Public Law No. 104–191, 110 Stat. 2023 (1996), 42 U.S.C. 1320(d)-3. The Health Insurance Portability and Accountability Act of 1996.
80. http://questions.medicare.gov/ (Accessed May 30, 2008).
81. Frank RG, Huskamp HA, McGuire TG, et al. Some economics of mental health 'carve-outs'. Arch Gen Psychiatry 1996; 53:933–937.
82. Kihlstrom LC. Managed care and medication compliance: Implications for chronic depression. J Behav Health Serv Res 1998; 25:367–376.
83. Field KS, Briggs DJ. Socio-economic and locational determinants of accessibility and utilization of primary health-care. Health Social Care Community 2001; 9:294–308.
84. Mottram P, Wilson K, Strobl J. Antidepressants for depressed elderly. Cochrane Database of Syst Rev 2006; (1). Art. No.: CD003491. doi: 10.1002/14651858.CD003491.pub2.
85. Volz HP, Gleiter CH. Monoamine oxidase inhibitors. A perspective on their use in the elderly. Drugs Aging 1998; 13:341–355.
86. Aziz R, Lorberg B, Tampi RR. Treatments for late-life bipolar disorder. Am J Geriatr Pharmacother 2006; 4:347–364.
87. Lazarou J, Pomeranz BH, Corey PN. Incidence of adverse drug reactions in hospitalized patients: A metaanalysis of prospective studies. JAMA 1998; 279:1200–1205.
88. Passarelli MCG, Jacob-Filho W, Figueras A. Adverse drug reactions in an elderly hospitalised population: Inappropriate prescription is a leading cause. Drugs Aging 2005; 22:767–777.
89. Laroche ML, Charmes JP, Nouaille Y, et al. Is inappropriate medication use a major cause of adverse drug reactions in the elderly? Br J Clin Pharmacol 2006; 63:177–186.
90. Physicians' Desk Reference, 62nd ed. Montvale, NJ: Thomson Healthcare. 2007.
91. Freudenstein U, Jagger C, Arthur A, et al. Treatments for late life depression in primary care—A systematic review. Fam Pract 2001; 18:321–327.
92. Stek M, Van der Wurff FB, Hoogendijk W, et al. Electroconvulsive therapy for the depressed elderly. Cochrane Database Syst Rev 2003; (2): Art. No.: CD003593. doi: 10.1002/14651858.CD003593.
93. Holtzheimer P. Treatment refractory depression in the elderly: A possible role for repetitive transcranial magnetic stimulation. Curr Psychosis Ther Rep 2006; 4: 74–78.
94. Hasey G. Transcranial magnetic stimulation in the treatment of mood disorder: A review and comparison with electroconvulsive therapy. Can J Psychiatry 2001; 46:720–727.
95. McNamara B, Ray JL, Arthurs J, et al. Transcranial magnetic stimulation for depression and other psychiatric disorders. Psychol Med 2001; 31:1141–1146.
96. Blazer DG, Hybels CF, Pieper CF. The association of depression and mortality in elderly persons: A case for multiple, independent pathways. J Gerontol A Biol Sci Med Sci 2001; 56:M505–M509.

97. Ariyo AA, Haan M, Tangen CM, et al. Depressive symptoms and risks of coronary heart disease and mortality in elderly Americans. Circulation 2000; 102:1773–1779.
98. Schulz R, Beach SR, Ives DG, et al. Association between depression and mortality in older adults: The Cardiovascular Health Study. Arch Intern Med 2000; 160:1731–1732.
99. Husaini BA, Sherkat DE, Levine R, et al. Race, gender, and health care service utilization and costs among Medicare elderly with psychiatric diagnoses. J Aging Health 2002; 14:79–95.
100. Wells KB, Manning WG, Duan N, et al. Sociodemographic factors and the use of outpatient mental health services. Med Care 1986; 24:75–85.
101. Gallo JJ, Cooperpatrick L, Lesikar S. Depressive symptoms of whites and African Americans aged 60 years and older. J Gerontol (Series B) 1998; o53:277–286.
102. Leaf PJ, Livingston MM, Tischler GL, et al. Contact with health professionals for the treatment of psychiatric and emotional problems. Med Care 1985; 23:1322–1337.
103. Curlik S, Frazier D, Katz I. Psychiatric aspects of long-term care. In: Sadavoy J, Lazarus LW, Jarvik LF, eds. Comprehensive Review of Geriatric Psychiatry. Washington, D. C.: American Psychiatric Press, 1991:547–564.
104. http://mentalhealth.samhsa.gov/publications/allpubs/sma03-3830/. (Accessed May 30, 2008).
105. U.S. Department of Health and Human Services (USDHHS). State Medicaid manual. HCFA Pub. Washington, D.C.: USDHHS, 1994:45–4.
106. U.S. Department of Health and Human Services (USDHHS). Medicaid and institutions for mental diseases. HCFA Pub 03339. Washington, D.C.: USDHHS, 1992.
107. Gottlieb GL. Financial issues. In: Sadavoy J, Lazarus LW, Jarvik LF, eds. Comprehensive Review of Geriatric Psychiatry. Washington, D.C.: American Psychiatric Press, 1991:667–686.
108. Gottlieb GL. Cost implications of depression in older adults. Int J Geriatr Psychiatry 1988; 3:191–200.

6 Economic Burden of Late-Life Depression: Cost of Illness, Cost of Treatment, and Cost Control Policies

Kiran Verma

Department of Accounting and Finance, University of Massachusetts Boston, Boston, Massachusetts, U.S.A.

Benjamin C. Silverman

MGH/McLean Adult Psychiatry Residency Training Program, Clinical Fellow in Psychiatry, Harvard University, Cambridge, Massachusetts, U.S.A.

INTRODUCTION

Depressive symptoms are highly prevalent among the elderly. Prevalence estimates for clinically significant depressive symptoms in the elderly range from about 10% for persons living independently in the community to about 25% for those with comorbid lung disease, arthritis, or Alzheimer disease (1). This rate is likely to be even higher among the elderly residing in long-term care facilities. More alarmingly, rates of major depressive disorder in younger cohorts have risen markedly over the past decade indicating that in the future with increases in the numbers of elderly in the population, prevalence of this disease in the elderly is also likely to rise significantly. It is predicted that by 2020 depression will be second only to heart disease in its contribution to the global burden of illness as measured by disability-adjusted life years (2).

The adverse effects of depression include reduced function, increased pain and suffering, and accelerated mortality from both suicide and exacerbation of morbidity associated with medical illness. It is estimated that although the elderly comprise only 12.4% of the U.S. population, people older than 65 years account for 16% of the suicides in the United States, with the rate among elderly white males (aged 85 years and older) more than 5.5 times the national rate of about 11 per 100,000. It has been noted in a number of studies that suicide among elderly persons is strongly associated with the presence of diagnosable depression (3–5). In this chapter we examine elements of the cost of depression in the elderly, research on evidence-based cost-effective treatments, impact of nonadherence to treatment regimens, and the potentially adverse effects of third party payers' policies on delivery of effective treatments.

COSTS OF DEPRESSION IN THE ELDERLY

Health care expenditures in the United States are highest among the elderly, and health care spending is projected to continue growing at a rate exceeding the annual growth rate of the overall economy (6.7%) through 2017. By that time, U. S. health care costs are estimated to reach $4.3 trillion per year, approximately 19.5% of the gross domestic product (6). In 2004, annual per person spending for individuals 65 years and older was $14,797, slightly higher than five times the amount spent on children (0–18 years) and more than three times the amount spent on working-age adults (19–64 years) (7). In this time frame, the elderly composed approximately 12% of the U.S. population and accounted for 34% of personal health care spending ($531.5 billion). The large costs of caring for the elderly pose challenges to both medical and mental health providers, who must balance quality health care with available resources.

Depression in the elderly results in considerable economic burden, both in terms of direct as well as indirect costs. Direct costs include the costs of diagnosis and treatment including medication, outpatient therapy, and hospitalization for the index admission and subsequent admissions. Indirect costs include costs of failed interventions resulting in impaired health status and suicide, exacerbation of comorbid medical conditions, and caregiver burden resulting from lost wages and/or increased health care costs for the caregiver. Although these indirect costs are more difficult to measure, as discussed below, there is evidence that they are considerable.

INCREASED UTILIZATION OF HEALTH SERVICES

A review by the Geriatric Psychiatric Alliance concludes that depression is linked to increased utilization of health care services (8). Other studies in primary care show that even after controlling for effects of medical comorbidity, the presence of depression and anxiety disorders increased health care costs (9,10). In a study by Unutzer et al., outpatient visits by depressed primary care patients increased in direct proportion to the severity of the depression, and the total median annual health care costs were twice as high for patients with severe depression as compared to nondepressed control subjects (11). Similarly, Katon et al. reported that depressed older adults incurred costs that were higher in every category examined (primary care visits with or without a mental health diagnosis, diagnostic tests, specialty medical visits, emergency department visits, pharmacy costs [including antidepressant and nonantidepressant], and other outpatient costs) (12). In another study focusing on veterans, costs of index admissions were 77% higher for patients with more severe depressive symptoms than for patients in the least symptomatic group. These costs were almost completely attributable to inpatient expenditures based on increased inpatient medical days. In this study the authors also noted that the actual mental health costs for the more severely depressed patients were only 1.8% of total medical costs. The authors concluded that for older patients, higher levels of depressive symptoms are a strong predictor of increased medical expenditures (13).

In 2008, Luppa et al. published a report on the direct costs of geriatric depression in Germany. In their study, 451 primary care patients aged 75 years and older participated in clinician interviews to assess depressive symptoms and complete a cost diary. The authors noted a statistically significant difference in the extrapolated yearly costs (by approximately one-third) of treating depressed elderly persons compared to nondepressed elderly persons ($5241 vs. $3648). Differences persisted despite controlling for chronic medical illnesses. Examined direct costs included outpatient physician and nonphysician provider visits, inpatient stays, medications, medical supplies and dentures, home care services (e.g., household services and meal delivery), assisted living days, and transportation. Depressed individuals accounted for statistically significant higher costs in three areas—medications, medical supplies and dentures, and home care services (14).

In a cross-sectional study examining the relative association of depression severity and comorbid conditions among primary care patients, Noel et al. found that although study participants had an average of 3.8 chronic medical illnesses, after controlling for sociodemographic differences and the presence of 11 chronic medical conditions, severity of depression made a larger independent contribution to three of the four general health indicators (mental function, disability, and quality of life). They concluded that as depression has the potential of being one of the more treatable chronic illnesses among the elderly, effective treatment for depression could lead to greater improvements in functional status, disability, and quality of life than interventions for other chronic illnesses in this age group (15).

CAREGIVER BURDEN

Depressive symptoms can impair initiative, energy, and executive function in older individuals making it more difficult for them to live independently. In turn, this increases the need for caregiving from family members or paid professionals. It is clear that informal care giving contributes to the burden of depression on the elderly in a variety of ways. In 1997, an estimated 25.8 million persons provided informal care to the elderly, equating to a cost of $196 billion (16). This value far exceeded the costs for formal home health care ($32 billion) and nursing home costs ($83 billion) and accounted for approximately 18% of total national health spending. As the population ages, it is likely that these costs will continue to rise. In 2006, an estimated 34 million persons provided informal care, with an estimated value of $354 billion (17).

A large part of these informal care costs are attributable to depression in the elderly. In a study of 82 elderly outpatients receiving care for depression and their related caregivers in Sao Paulo, Brazil, caretaker burden assessed by a Burden Interview scale was positively associated with severity and duration of depression, caregivers perception of patients' mood and behavioral problems, and need for assistance with activities of daily living (18). The authors note that overall levels of burden were similar to those reported for caretakers of elderly patients with dementia in a number of other studies. Studies directly comparing caretakers of patients with depression and/or dementia have found both sets of caretakers to experience significant burden and stress, though results on the relative impact of each condition have been mixed (19–23).

Informal care giving leads to emotional and physical strain on caretakers, often leading them to increase their own use of health care resources. Notably, a significant portion of caretakers for older persons are elderly themselves. A recent study by Thompson et al. found elderly patients with depression who provided care to others experienced 30 more days of depression over a 2-year period than those without a caregiving role (24). In a sample of 97 elderly, cognitively intact, medical inpatients in Montreal, McCusker et al. examined the impact of depression on informal caretakers after six months of follow-up (25). They found caregivers of patients with a diagnosis of major depression to have lower mental health scores after six months than those caring for individuals without depression. In another study of 392 caregivers and 427 noncaregivers aged between 66 and 96 years, estimated risks for mortality were 63% higher based on self-reported emotional or physical strain related to caregiving for participants who were providing care to their live-in spouses than for noncaregiving controls (26). In addition to increased health care costs, caregivers may experience loss of income and other benefits, such as social security and health insurance by giving up work or reducing work hours (27–29).

Although it is difficult to accurately assess the exact financial cost of caregiving related to depression in the elderly, a study based on prevalence estimates of depressive symptoms from the nationally representative sample of the AHEAD study estimated that among the U.S. population approximately 8.3 million older individuals had one to three depressive symptoms and 3.1 million had four to eight depressive symptoms. They further estimated that elderly individuals with no depressive symptoms received, on an average, 2.9 hrs/wk of informal care, while those with one to three symptoms received 4.3 hrs/wk, and those with four to eight symptoms received 6.0 hrs/wk. Using a median home health aide wage of $8.23 per hour, they calculated that the additional caregiving cost for persons with one to three depressive symptoms is $5.0 billion per year and for persons with four to eight symptoms, it is $9.1 billion. They also noted in their study that this estimate is probably low, as the care provided by a committed spouse or child is likely to be of higher quality and effective, and thus of value greater than the $8.23 rate cited above. In addition, the authors pointed out that the costs for informal caregiving, which are difficult to measure, are often overlooked in cost-effectiveness analyses. This omission could unfavorably bias conclusions about the cost-effectiveness of other health care interventions in the depressed elderly population (30).

UNDERTREATMENT FOR DEPRESSION IN THE ELDERLY

In spite of the awareness of the importance of early diagnosis and aggressive treatment of depressive disorders in the elderly, the actual number of individuals who receive appropriate treatment is small. Reasons for this include the perceived stigma attached with mental illness, presence of comorbid conditions that make diagnosis more difficult, cost of medications, and a lack of adequate awareness among the primary care physicians who are usually the first-line health care providers for this population. The complexity of detecting depressive disorders in frail older adults imposes an additional obstacle, because mood symptoms may be obscured by complaints about somatic or cognitive concerns or simply attributed to the aging process (31).

Ideally, to achieve long-term remission or recovery from this disease, not only early diagnosis and effective treatment but also adequately attentive follow-up are needed. Many studies have sought to identify appropriate interventions that could improve outcomes. Such interventions include preventive measures to help identify those at risk, early recognition of symptoms that can be addressed in order to prevent the development of a full depressive syndrome, and employment of treatment plants that incorporate and integrate the use of pharmacotherapy, other somatic therapies, psychosocial therapies and other nonmedical treatments (32–37). In a meta-analysis of randomized controlled trials of psychological treatments for late-life depression, Cuijpers et al. concluded that although the quality of the studies varied, evidence supports the effectiveness of psychological treatments of depression in older adults. Furthermore, they reported similar efficacy of psychological and pharmacological treatments, though no clear differences emerged among the specific psychological treatments studies (38).

Cost-Effective Treatments

In the current cost-conscious health care environment, in which treatments for the elderly are most often paid for by third party payers such as Medicare or Medicaid, it is very important that the recommended treatment protocols be both efficacious and cost effective for successful implementation and reimbursement. As discussed below, several recent studies have examined the issue of cost-effectiveness of treatments for depression in the elderly. There are two streams of research examining this issue, one examining preventive interventions targeting at-risk individuals in the early stages of depression, and the other examining treatment interventions targeting clinically depressed individuals in later stages of the disease.

Depression is costly to treat and treatment effectiveness is limited; therefore, preventive treatment may be a more cost-effective alternative from the public health perspective. A number of studies have shown that by targeting appropriate preventative measures at subjects identified as possessing known risk factors for major depression such as subsyndromal depression, disability, living alone, or bereavement, the burden of this illness can be reduced (39,40). A targeted intervention to reduce even three or four selected risk indicators could potentially avoid enough new onsets of depression to save at least $1.9 million for every one million elderly people in the population, provided that the cost of the preventive interventions does not exceed the estimated total cost savings from avoided onsets of depression (41).

To examine the cost-effectiveness of treatment regimens for depressed elderly primary care patients, an Australian study used epidemiological data to measure the impact of optimal care versus usual or current care. In this study Andrews et al., calculated the cost of the disability-adjusted life years (DALYs) averted through implementing recommended treatments. A measure of the years of healthy life lost due to premature death or disability is expressed as DALYs lost. This measure of burden of illness can be lessened via appropriate interventions and treatments thereby reducing or "averting" the number of DALYs lost. The cost-effective benefit from treatment can then be measured in terms of DALYs averted. From their analysis, using this metric, the authors concluded that optimal care was more cost effective because it led to an estimated 28,632 DALYs averted at a cost of AU $295 million as compared with 19,297 DALYs averted at a cost of AU $720 million for patients under current care (42).

In a randomized controlled trial labeled IMPACT (Improving Mood: Promoting Access to Collaborative Treatment), the cost-effectiveness of collaborative care was studied from a payer's perspective. The IMPACT intervention was a 1-year stepped collaborative care program in which a nurse or a psychologist care manager augmented the patient's regular primary care physician's role by providing education about depression, antidepressant medication and psychotherapy treatment options. Depression care managers used behavioral activation with all patients and offered a choice of treatment with antidepressant medication or problem-solving treatment in primary care via a 6- to 8-session program designed for primary care patients (43). The trial was carried out in 18 primary care clinics from 8 health care organizations in 5 states. A total of 1801 patients, 60 years or older, with major depression (17%) dysthymic disorder (30%), or both (53%) participated in the study. Data from the trial showed that over a 2-year follow-up period, relative to usual care, intervention patients experienced 107 more depression free days. This benefit increased total health care costs slightly (by $295) over the 2-year study period (44).

In a subsequent study encompassing a longer term (4 years) IMPACT trial from two health maintenance organizations for which 4-year cost data for 551 enrollees in the trial were available, it was found that over this longer follow-up period, intervention patients had lower average health care cost, i.e., $29,422 as compared to $32,785 for usual care patients. In addition it was found that the intervention patients had lower health care costs than usual care patients in every cost category observed (outpatient and inpatient mental health specialty costs, outpatient and inpatient medical and surgical costs, pharmacy costs, and other outpatient costs). These research studies suggest that investments in better depression care may be initially more costly, but are ultimately more cost effective over a longer term (45).

Despite identification of efficacious and cost-effective antidepressant and psychosocial treatments in late-life depression, much remains to be accomplished. Detection of depression is suboptimal in many settings, and clinicians may fail to provide an appropriate treatment. Nonadherence to an optimal regimen accounts for additional depressive burden. In a study examining the relationship of medication nonadherence to changes in depression scores during 12 months of treatment of a sample of older adults, nearly 28% of patients reported being nonadherent with their antidepressant medication. Nonadherence, along with other psychosocial variables, was related to increased 12-month depression scores (46).

Cost-Related Treatment Nonadherence

For any intervention for a chronic disease to be effective, patients need to adhere to the prescribed treatment regimen including the right doses of medications, therapy, and other indicated protocols. Many times that does not happen because of cost and reimbursement reasons. For example, for IMPACT-like interventions, although evidence shows that nurses or nurse practitioners who are not health care specialists can function as care managers, third party insurance providers including Medicare and Medicaid, do not reimburse for care-management services. Similarly, Medicare and Medicaid do not pay for supervision by a psychiatrist, even though many states make this a prerequisite for a nurse clinical specialist's work (47).

There is considerable evidence that economic reasons contribute significantly to elderly depressed patients' nonadherence with a recommended treatment plan. Treatments costs can be quite expensive for many older people living on fixed incomes. Cost-related medication nonadherence (CRN) occurs when patients attempt to save money by reducing or omitting medication doses. In a study examining how the chronically ill elderly make choices to underuse one or more of their prescription drugs based on costs, it was found that patients are more likely to underuse symptom-relief medications such as for arthritis or depression than preventive medications such as for diabetes or hypertension (48).

Risk factors for CRN include high total medication costs, limited or no drug coverage, and increases in copayments. For the elderly who depend on Medicare or Medicaid for their health coverage, there are many restrictions on inpatient as well as outpatient interventions. Disincentives for prolonged hospital stays, limits on the availability of certain medications, and restrictions on the provision of psychosocial therapies including psychotherapy may interfere with a patient's ability to follow the clinician's intended treatment plan. The techniques used to restrict care take the form of caps on coverage, deductibles, copayments, formulary limitations and utilization reviews, each of which can increase out-of-pocket expenditures for the recommended treatment, thereby increasing nonadherence (49–51). The primary goal of the newly enacted Medicare Prescription Drug, Improvement and Modernization Act (MMA) of 2003 that created the voluntary drug benefit, Medicare Part D, was to increase access to medications for seniors and other Medicare enrollees. By providing more affordable drug coverage to the elderly, Medicare Part D aimed to reduce CRN for this population. Many embedded incentives in the design of the Medicare Part D benefit, however, have made it difficult to achieve this goal.

MEDICARE PART D AND ACCESS TO PRESCRIPTION DRUGS

The elderly must join a Medicare part D drug plan to get prescription drug coverage under Medicare. Private insurance companies approved by Medicare run these plans. Medicare drug plans vary in cost and formulary coverage (52). Although this benefit has increased the number of seniors who have prescription coverage, many are required to pay a substantial percentage of the prescription drug costs. Projections of the average Part D cost sharing under standard benefit are $1095 in 2006, $1325 in 2007, and $1357 in 2008. These numbers are likely to be much higher when comorbid medical conditions are present. In addition, these out-of-pocket costs can vary based on elements of the selected plan such as the plan's deductible, coverage gap (donut-hole), and catastrophic threshold (53). To put these costs in perspective, the median income of households headed by someone aged 65 or older was $24,509 in 2004 (54).

Medicare Part D plans also vary in terms of premiums, deductibles, copays, and coverage of popular drugs. On average, plans compensate for lower deductibles by charging both a higher premium and higher copayments. As plans are at some financial risk for drug costs, they have the incentive to structure their benefit in such a way as to discourage high-use enrollees and to encourage low-use enrollees. Plans can achieve this through their formulary design and associated utilization management programs that make it more difficult to access certain medications. Formularies are lists of medications available to enrollees and tiered formularies provide financial incentives for the enrollees to use cheaper drugs on the list. Although through thoughtful formulary design it is possible to achieve cost savings without negatively impacting enrollees' health, adoption of three tiered formulary and/or increased cost sharing for prescription drugs has been associated with discontinuation of medications in the United States (55,56). One element of formulary design that impacts on access to medications is the definition of therapeutic categories and classes. By defining a class of covered drugs broadly, for example, a formulary can exclude more medications for certain conditions. For example, "antidepressants" can be defined as a category and "reuptake inhibitors" as a class, with the latter including SSRIs, SNRIs, and the TCAs, an older class of antidepressants with more problematic side-effect profiles for many patients. Then with a formulary policy that requires coverage of at least two drugs from each class, it is possible for the plan to cover only two TCAs and none of the newer, albeit more expensive SSRIs or SNRIs. In a study examining the availability and cost sharing for 12 of the most popular brand-name drugs among the elderly in 15 representative Medicare part D plans, brand-name Celexa was found to be the least likely to be covered, and when it was covered, it had the highest copay (55).

Another way to limit access to more expensive drugs is through formulary drug selection and tier assignment. For example, under a 3-tier drug plan, the cheapest, typically generic drugs are associated with the lowest copayments (e.g.,

5%), the second tier includes some brand-name drugs with higher cost sharing (e.g., 20%), and the third tier includes nonpreferred drugs with the highest cost sharing (e.g., 40–100%). Then if the plan's formulary includes older but cheaper drugs with lower efficacy or problematic side effects on tiers 1 and 2, patients for whom the more expensive drug would be more efficacious are discouraged from obtaining the more expensive drug by the higher required copayment. Similarly, patients who need their medications in a timely manner will be deterred by a time-consuming reconsideration process to get approval for drugs that are not in the formulary or are categorized in a formulary tier that requires high copayments.

Finally, plans can discourage medication use through implementing utilization management programs such as fail-first policies that mandate that patients have to fail at a certain number of medication regimens using cheaper drugs before a more costly drug can be prescribed. When specific properties of a more costly drug suggest that it would increase a particular patient's chance for improvement, a fail-first policy may require the patient to undergo potentially demoralizing trials of other medications first in order to gain access to the one that a clinician would have wished available from the start (56,57).

Financial viability of insurance plans requires that the enrolled population includes participants who are likely to be low users of plan services, to offset costs from others who are likely to be high users. This phenomenon in economics is known as "adverse selection" and to guard against it, the incentives embedded in most insurance plans including Medicare Part D plans are designed to discourage participants with potentially high drug costs. These users can include many depressed elders with coexisting comorbid conditions that require many medications and higher costs, thus potentially leaving them without adequate coverage for their prescription drug needs. These kinds of understandable but ultimately perverse incentives lead many elders to play what is akin to "Russian Roulette" with their prescribed medicines, by either not taking them consistently or by taking them in less than prescribed doses. All this is counterproductive as it can lead to relapses, recurrences, and ultimately to poorer health outcomes and higher costs.

CONCLUSION

In conclusion, we can say that the economic burden of late-life depression is considerable and that research has helped identify cost-effective interventions that have the potential of decreasing this burden. Access to the specific treatment options, however, is based not solely on efficacy research but also on health care payers' coverage policies. Recent enactment of the prescription drug benefit, Medicare Part D, has the potential to help alleviate some of the burden of depression in the elderly by making psychopharmacological treatments more available to many who previously were not able to afford them. At the same time, however, many of the policies enacted by the insurance companies that offer these Medicare approved drug plans can also hinder effective implementation of the prescribed interventions. This trend is likely to get worse as Congress may phase out many of the initial subsidies it gave these plans to get them to take on the financial risk of paying for prescription drug treatments of the elderly. Because the loss of these subsidies is likely to diminish profitability of these plans, the effect of this squeeze on policies, such as copayments, restrictive formularies, and utilization management that are employed by these plans, needs to be monitored so prevent insurers from further restricting access and thereby increasing the burden of this debilitating illness.

REFERENCES

1. Reynolds CF, Kupfer DJ. Depression and Aging: A look to the future. Psychiatr Serv 1999; 50:1167–1172.
2. Murray JL, Lopez AD, eds. Summary: The Global Burden of Disease. Boston, MA: Harvard School of Public Health; 1996
3. Centers for Disease Control and Prevention, National Center for Injury Prevention and Control. Web-based injury Statistics Query and Reporting System (WISQARS) [online] (2005). Accessed [March 28, 2008] available at http://www.cdc.gov/ncipc/dvp/Suicide/default.htm
4. Brent CY. Suicide and Aging I: Patterns of psychiatric diagnosis. International Psychogeriatrics 1995; 7(2):149–64.
5. Conwell Y. Suicide in elderly patients. In: Schneider LS, Reynolds CF, Lebowitz, BD. eds. Diagnosis and Treatment of Depression in Late Life. Washington D.C. American Psychiatric Press, 1996.
6. Center for Medicare and Medicaid Services. (2007). National Health Expenditure Projections 2007–2017.
7. Hartman M, Catlin A, Lassman D, et al. U.S. health spending by age, Selected Years Through 2004. Health Affairs 2008; 27(1):w1–w12.
8. Geriatric Depression Alliance: Diagnosis and Treatment of Late-Life Depression: Making a Difference. Bethesda, MD; American Association of Geriatric Psychiatry and Pfizer, Inc., 1996.
9. Simon GE, VonKroff M, Barlow W. Health care costs of primary care patients with recognized depression. Arch Gen Psychiatry 1995; 52:850–856.
10. Creed F, Morgan R, Fiddler M, et al. Depression and anxiety impair health-related quality of life and are associated with increased costs in general medical patients. Psychosomatics 2002; 43:302–309.
11. Unutzer J, Patrick DL, Simon G, et al.: Depressive symptoms and the cost of health services in HMO patients aged 65 years and older: A four year prospective study. JAMA 1997; 277:1618–1623.
12. Katon WJ, Lin E, Russo J, et al. Increased medical costs of a population based sample of depressed elderly patients. Arch Gen Psychiatry. 2003; 60:897–903.
13. Druss BG, Rohrbaugh RM, Rosenbeck RA. Depressive symptoms and health costs in older medical patients. Am J Psychiatry 1999; 156:477–479.
14. Luppa M, Heinrich S, Matschinger H, et al. Direct costs associated with depression in old age in germany. Journal of affective disorders. 2008; 105;195–204.
15. Noel PH, Williams JW, Unutzer J, et al. Depression and comorbid illness in elderly primary care patients: impact on multiple domains of health status and well-being. JAMA 2002; 287:1160–1170.
16. Arno PS, Levin C, Memmott MM. The economic value of informal caregiving. Health Affairs 1999; 18:182–188.
17. Gibson MJ, Houser A. Valuing the invaluable: A new look at the economic value of family caregiving. Public Policy Inst Am Assoc Retired Pers IB 2007; 82:1–12.
18. Scazufca M, Menezes PR, Almeida OP. Caregiver burden in an elderly population with depression in Sao Paulo, Brazil. Soc Psychiatry Psychiatr Epidemiol 2002; 37:416–422.
19. Wijeratne C, Lovestone S. A pilot study comparing psychological and physical morbidity in carers of elderly people with dementia and those with depression. Int J Geriatr Psychiatry 1996; 11:741–744.
20. Drinka TJ, Smith JC, Drinka PJ. Correlates of depression and burden for informal caregivers of patients in a geriatrics referral clinic. J Am Geriatr Soc 1987; 35:522–525.
21. Rosenvinge H, Jones D, Judge E, Martin A. Demented and chronic depressed patients attending a day hospital: Stress experienced by carers. Int J Geriatr Psychiatry 1998; 13:8–11.
22. Brodaty H, Luscombe G. Psychological morbidity in caregivers is associated with depression in patients with dementia. Alzheimer Dis Assoc Disord 1998; 12:62–70.

23. Leinonen E, Korpisammal, Pulkkinen L, et al. The comparison of burden between caregiving spouses of depressive and demented patients. Int J Geriatr Psychiatry 2001; 16:387–393.
24. Thompson A, Fan MY, Unutzer J, et al. One extra month of depression: The effects of caregiving on depression outcomes in the IMPACT trial. Int J Geriatr Psychiatry. 2008; 23; 511–516.
25. McCusker J, Latimer E, Cole M, et al. Major depression among medically ill elders contributes to sustained poor mental health in their informal caregivers. Age Ageing 2007; 36:400–406.
26. Schulz R, Beach SR. Caregiving as a risk factor for mortality: The caregiver health effects study. JAMA 1999; 282:2215–2219.
27. Boaz RF, Muller CF. Paid work and unpaid help by caregivers of the disabled and frail elders. Med Care 1992; 30:149–158.
28. Robinson KM. Family caregiving: Who provides the care, and at what cost? Nurs Econ 1997; 15:243–247.
29. Kingson ER, O'Grady-LeShane. The effects of caregiving on women's social security benefits. Gerontologist 1993; 33:230–239.
30. Langa KM, Velenstein MA, Fendrick M, et al. Extent and cost of informal caregiving for older americans with symptoms of depression. Am J Psychiatry 1997; 161:857–863.
31. Chapman DP, Perry GS. Depression as a major component of public health for older adults. Prev Chronic Dis 2008; 5(1). http://www.cdc.gov/pcd/issues/2008/jan/070150.htm. Accessed [March 28, 2008].
32. Lyness JM, Moonsberg J, Datto CJ, et al. Outcomes of minor and subsyndromal depression among elderly patients in primary care settings. Annals of Internal Medicine 2006; 144(4):496–504.
33. Sherbourne WK, Duan N, Unutzer J, et al. Quality improvements for depression in primary care. Do patients with subthreshold depression benefit in the long run. Am J Psychiatry 2005; 162:1149–57.
34. Engels GI, Vermey M. Efficacy of nonmedical treatments of depression in elders: A quantitative analysis. J Clin Geropsychological 1997; 3:17–35.
35. Klausner EJ, Clarkin JF, Spielman L. Late-life depression and functional disability: The role of goal-focused group psychotherapy. Int J Geriat Psychiatry 1998; 13:707–716.
36. Koder D, Brodaty H, Anstey K. Cognitive therapy for depression in the elderly. Int J Geriatr Psychiat 1996; 11:97–107.
37. Latour D, Cappeliez P. Pretherapy training for group cognitive therapy with depressed older adults. Can J Aging 1994; 13:221–235.
38. Cuijpers P, Van Straten A, Smit F. Psychological treatment of late-life depression: A meta analysis of randomized controlled trials. Int J Geriatr Psychiatry 2006; 21:1139–1149.
39. Issakidis AG, Sanderson K, Corry J, et al. Utilising survey data to inform public policy: Comparison of the cost-effectiveness of treatment of ten mental disorders. Br J Psychiatry 2004; 184:526–533.
40. Schoevers RA, Smit F, Deeg DJH, et al. Prevention of late-life depression in primary care. Am J Psychiatry 2006; 163:1611–1621.
41. Katon WJ, Lin E, Russo J, et al. Increased medical costs of a population based sample of depressed elderly patients. Arch Gen Psychiatry 2003; 60:897–903.
42. Andrews G, Sanderson K, Corry J, et al. Using epidemiological data to model efficiency in reducing the burden of depression. J Mental Health Policy Econ 2000; 3:175–186.
43. Mynor-Wallis LM, Gath DH, Lloyd-Thomas AF, et al. Randomised controlled trial comparing problem solving treatment with amitriptyline and placebo for major depression in primary care. BMJ 1995; 310(3977):441–445.
44. Katon WD, Shoenbaum M, Fan MY, et al. Cost-effectiveness of improving primary care treatment of late-life depression. Arch Gen Psyciatry 2005; 62:1313–1320.
45. Unutzer J, Katon WJ, Fan MY, et al. Long-term cost effects of collaborative care for late-life depression. Am J Manag Care 2008; 14:95–100.
46. Bosworth HB, Corrine I, Potter GG, et al. The effects of antidepressant medication adherence as well as psychosocial and clinical factors on depression outcome among older adults. Int J Geriatr Psychiatry 2008; 23:129–134.

47. Snowden M, Steinman L, Fredrick J. Treating depression in older adults: Challenges to implementing the recommendations of an expert panel. Prev Chronic Dis 2008; 5(1). http://www.cdc.gov/pcd/issues/2008/jan/07 0154.htm. Accessed [March 31, 2008].
48. Bambauer KZ, Safran DG, Ross-Degnan D, et al. Depression and cost related medication nonadherence in Medicare beneficiaries. Arch Gen Psychiatry 2007; 64:602–608.
49. Roblin DW, Platt R, Goodman MJ, et al. Effect of increased cost-sharing on oral hypoglycemic use in five managed care organizations: How much is too much? Med Assoc 2005; 43:951–959.
50. Huskamp HA, Deverka PA, Epstein AM, et al. The effect of incentive based formularies on prescription drug utilization and spending. N Engl J Med 2004; 349:2224–2232.
51. Goldman DP, Joyce GF, Escarce JJ, et al. Pharmacy benefits and the use of drugs by the chronically ill. JAMA 2004; 291:2344–2350.
52. Medicare Prescription Drug Improvement and Modernization Act of 2003. Available at http://cms.hhs.gov/medicarereform/MMAactFullText.pdf Accessed [March 28, 2008].
53. Briesacher SB, Shea DG, Cooper B, et al. Riding the roller coaster: The ups and downs in out-of-pocket spending under the standard Medicare drug benefit. Health Affairs 2005; 24:1022–1031.
54. DeNavas-Walt C, Proctor BD, Lee CH. Income poverty, and health insurance coverage in the United States: 2004 Current Population reports. Washington, D.C.: U.S. Census Bureau, 2005.
55. Frakt AB, Pizer SD. A first look at the new medicare prescription drug plans. Health Affairs 2006; 25(4):252–261.
56. Huskamp HA, Keating NL. The new medicare drug benefit: Formularies and their potential effects on access to medications. J Gen Inter Med. 2005; 20(7):662–665.
57. Verma K, and Verma S. Is the cheapest drug always the best alternative? Primary Psychiatry 2004; 11(1):66–71.

7 Late-Life Suicide

Ashok J. Bharucha

Western Psychiatric Institute and Clinic, University of Pittsburgh School of Medicine, Pittsburgh, Pennsylvania, U.S.A.

Suicide remains an all too common response to intolerable psychological and physical suffering in the elderly. Havens described this multidetermined process as "the final common pathway of diverse circumstances, of an interdependent network rather than an isolated cause, a knot of circumstances tightening around a single time and place"(1). No other segment of the population epitomizes this description more clearly than the elderly. It is the objective of this chapter to highlight the high rates, the interdependent network of physical, psychiatric, and personality dimensions that contribute to late-life suicide, as well as potential assessment and intervention strategies, particularly in primary care practices.

EPIDEMIOLOGY

According to the latest report of the National Center for Health Statistics (2004), the suicide rate for the general population is 11.1/100,000(2). The rate is higher for persons aged 65 years and older (14.3/100,000), and even more notably so for those aged 85 years and older (16.4/100,000) (2). Put another way, the elderly accounted for 16.0% of the suicides while constituting only 12.4% of the population (3). Of the demographic factors, disparity along gender lines is the most striking, with males being at consistently higher risk of completing suicide than females. Historically, suicide risk is incremental with advancing age in white males, and consistent with this trend, white males aged 85 years and older completed suicide nearly five times more frequently than the age-adjusted national rate in 2004, making them the highest risk group (2). In contrast, suicide rates for nonwhite males (Hispanic, African-American, and Native Americans) tend to peak in early adulthood and decline thereafter (4). Although they encompass multiple distinct ethnicities, older Asian-Americans (particularly Chinese- and Japanese-Americans) commit suicide at rates that are intermediate between those for Caucasian and African-Americans (2). Among all females residing in the United States, East Asian women have the highest proportional rate of suicide older than 65 years (5). Moreover, in a recent investigation of older primary care patients with depression, anxiety, and at-risk alcohol use, Asian-Americans expressed the greatest amount of suicide or death ideation, while it was the least for African Americans and intermediate for Caucasian Americans (6). Clearly, disparities in suicide rates along gender, racial, and ethnic lines have important implications for both clinical assessment as well as future research directions (7).

Marital status has also been linked to suicide risk (8). Age adjusted studies have reported that married persons have lower suicide rates than people who have never married. Those who are divorced, separated, or recently widowed have the highest rates of suicide. Divorce, especially, is strongly linked with increased suicide related mortality among men. To our knowledge, no specific conceptual synthesis of the interactions between age, marital status, race, and ethnicity-specific risk and protective factors for suicide currently exists in the literature (7).

Firearms are the most common method of suicide among the elderly. In 2004, 62.1% of elderly suicides were completed with firearms compared with 33.4% of all U.S. suicides (2). While males used firearms three times more frequently than females, evidence over the last decade indicates that suicide by firearms is becoming the preferred method for elderly females as well (2). The more violent and definitive nature of late-life suicide explains in part the finding that the ratio of attempted to completed suicide drops precipitously from 200:1 in the young to 4:1 in the elderly (9). The first suicide attempt in the elderly may well be the last given their compromised physical functioning, social isolation, and lack of communication of suicidal intent (4). Indirect self-destructive behaviors such as refusal of medication and food may also be suicidal in nature, however, such factors are infrequently taken into account in the medical examiners' determination of cause of death, thus substantially underestimating the actual number of late-life suicide deaths (10). The urgent need for the development and implementation of effective interventions is evident in the fact that demographers expect the elderly to account for one-third of all suicides in the United States by the year 2030 if current trends continue (4).

PHYSICAL ILLNESS

Age-related variations in recent life events preceding suicide suggest family, occupational, and financial problems to be most salient in the younger age groups, while physical illness has been noted to be a more common and critical element in both late-life suicide completers as well as attempters (11–14). However, the evidence pointing to an association between physical illness and suicide comes largely from studies which lack (a) age- and sex-specific control groups, (b) standardized measures of physical illness burden, (c) assessment of functional impairment and actual disability, and (d) statistical control for the confounding effect of depression and other psychiatric conditions (15). Indeed, the suicide risk conferred by physical illness is likely mediated by depression, hopelessness, and other psychological factors as indicated by the fact that the mere perception of physical illness is associated with a higher risk of completed suicide (16). Moreover, alcoholism is over-represented in the older studies that attempt to establish an association between physical illness and suicide (17).

Conwell et al. recently reported their findings from a case-control study in which psychological autopsy data on those primary care patients who had completed suicide within a month of visiting their primary physician ($N = 42$) were compared with prospective data on a representative control sample of older primary care patients from the same region ($N = 196$) (18). The authors noted significantly higher rates of physical and functional deficits and disability in individuals completing suicide. However, physical and functional measures no longer distinguished cases from controls after statistical adjustments were made for the presence of depressive symptoms or syndromes. Given the complex interplay between physical and mental disorders, and the fact that a vast majority (>70%) of elderly who complete suicide visit their primary care physician within the last month of their life, primary care practices appear to be a natural site for collaborative preventative strategies targeting both physical and mental health (19).

PSYCHOPATHOLOGY

Axis I Psychopathology

The ubiquitous presence of psychiatric illness (>90% of cases) in those who complete suicide is well documented, with the nature of the psychopathology varying with age (20–22). Older persons who commit suicide are most often in the midst of their first lifetime episode of nonpsychotic major depression (23). Unlike the younger age groups, primary psychotic illnesses, substance abuse (other than alcohol), and personality disorders are infrequent in late-life suicide; anxiety disorders are however commonly present (21,23). Conwell et al.'s controlled study of completed suicide among older primary care patients sheds more light on the salient issues at hand (18). Consistent with prior reports, major depression was not only significantly more common in suicide completers, but was also more severe according to the Hamilton Depression Rating Scale (21,23). When only the depressed subgroup of suicide completers and the prospective control subjects were examined, physical health measures failed to distinguish the groups. In spite of the fact that antidepressants were prescribed at significantly greater rates to the suicide completers than the prospective cohort, only 14.6% were receiving antidepressant pharmacotherapy at the time of death. The depressed subgroup of subjects in both cohorts was prescribed antidepressants with equal frequency despite the greater severity of mental illness in the suicide completers. After major depression, alcohol abuse and dependence are noted to be the most strongly associated Axis I risk factors for late-life suicide (24). The association is likely to be underestimated since an overwhelming majority of the studies that have investigated this risk factor have considered only persons meeting diagnostic criteria for alcohol abuse and dependence, and not the much larger proportion of elderly who engage in at-risk drinking (24). In addition to exacerbating depressive symptoms and comorbid medical conditions, at-risk alcohol use also potentially contributes to drug–drug interactions in a cumulative fashion that results in heightened suicide risk (24).

Axis II Psychopathology

Axis I psychopathology in late-life suicide has been described with considerable consistency in the literature (21,23). In contrast, there is a dearth of controlled studies using standardized personality inventories to determine personality traits that may confer vulnerability to late-life suicide. While categorical personality disorders are thought to be rare, certain traits may be instrumental in the biopsychosocial pathway leading to suicide. Geriatric specialists and psychological autopsy studies have long posited narcissistic personality (NP) as conferring vulnerability to suicide (25). Using a retrospective database analysis, Heisel et al. (2007) recently reported significantly higher scores on the Hamilton Rating Scale for Depression (HAM-D) suicide item for those with NP compared with those without NP, controlling for age, sex, depression, and cognitive functioning (26). In addition, the most methodologically rigorous investigations to date by Duberstein and colleagues have reported greater levels of Neuroticism (N) and lower "Openness to Experience" (OTE) in suicide completers compared to age-matched controls using the NEO personality inventory (27,28). Low openness to experience may indicate diminished adaptive capacity in a season of losses coupled with potential lack of communication of internal affective and cognitive states. It is well known that the elderly rarely communicate suicidal intent (29).

An important cognitive stance that is thought to be predictive of suicidal ideation and eventual suicide is hopelessness, defined by Beck as a state of negativism and pessimism unrelated to medical or psychiatric prognosis per se (30–32). Although Beck's sample consisted largely of younger individuals, similar impact of hopelessness on suicidal ideation and completed suicide has been reported in the elderly as well (33,34). Even after resolution of depressive symptoms, high levels of hopelessness may persist in depressed elderly with a history of suicide attempt(s) and may contribute to treatment noncompliance and eventual suicide (35). Independent of depression, hopelessness has been found to be a significant predictor of desire for physician-assisted suicide in a sample of terminally ill cancer patients treated in an academic facility specializing in the management of cancer patients (36). In contrast, an emerging body of literature suggests positive affect and future orientation to be potential protective factors against suicide (37,38).

Identification of individual factors that confer vulnerability to late-life suicide is an important starting point. However, the ultimate goal must be to elucidate the mechanisms by which the complex interplay of these biopsychosocial factors results in this tragic outcome.

Reciprocal Interplay of Suicidality and Depression Treatment Outcomes

Just as depression is a major independent risk factor for completed suicide, the presence of suicidal ideation is also associated with poorer course and outcome of depression treatment. Szanto and colleagues (2007) have recently published findings regarding the course of suicidality during depression treatment that merit mention (39). Based on the course of suicidal ideation (SI) during 12 weeks of antidepressant treatment (234 subjects with paroxetine; 203 subjects with nortriptyline), the authors classified the elderly subjects as either nonsuicidal or as having "emergent," "persistent," or "resolved" suicidality. At the end of the study, rates of emergent, persistent, and resolved suicidality were 7.8%, 12.6%, and 15.6%, respectively. Emergent suicidality was not associated with akathisia, and its occurrence did not differ between the selective serotonin reuptake inhibitor (paroxetine) and tricyclic antidepressant (nortriptyline). Subjects with emergent or persistent suicidality were more likely to maintain higher depression scores and experienced higher levels of anxiety and agitation during treatment, possibly denoting a more difficult-to-treat depression.

CLINICAL ASSESSMENT OF SUICIDE RISK

The assessment of suicide risk for an older person is particularly challenging since many do not communicate suicidal intent (29). However, a comprehensive assessment should begin with a review of the previously discussed demographic and mental health risk factors. Particular attention should be paid to older white males with depressive symptoms and alcohol use (even if these do not reach clinical diagnostic thresholds) with inflexible personalities who are recently widowed, socially isolated, in possession of a firearm, and who may be coping with medical and/or psychosocial stressors. A brief depression-screening instrument such as the Geriatric Depression Scale (GDS) (40) should be routinely completed in the waiting room of a primary care physician's office. For individuals who are deemed to be at high risk for suicide, specific direct inquiries into suicidal ideation, intent, or plan should be made. Nonadherence to a medical care regimen, progressive withdrawal from historically important social connections, and evidence that they are "wrapping up loose ends" (e.g., financial matters, insurance policies, estate planning, etc.), should raise further concern regarding suicide risk. Please refer also to the specific chapters within this book that provide detailed guidance regarding the assessment and management of depression, alcohol abuse and dependence, and review barriers to assessment and treatment of older adults with mood disorders, since these are additional aspects of the management of suicidal individuals.

PREVENTION

Primary Care Practice

The scenario of late-life suicide most often involves an elderly white, widowed male in the midst of his first episode of nonpsychotic major depression who has access to firearms. Of the modifiable risk factors, early and accurate diagnosis and treatment of major depression in the primary care setting appears to (41,42) offer an opportunity for meaningful intervention. The fact that a vast majority of older suicide victims have visited their primary care physician within a month of their death highlights, the importance of this treatment setting in averting late-life suicide (19,43). Furthermore, most older adults do not seek treatment from mental health professionals or utilize general suicide hotlines (44,45). The underdiagnosis and subtherapeutic treatment of depression by primary care physicians is however well recognized (46,47). The scope of the problem may be vastly underestimated considering the functional impairments and morbidity associated with even subthreshold depression which is likely to elude the primary care physician (48).

Providing primary care physicians with the knowledge and skills to effectively diagnose and manage depression, recognize ageist biases, and resist negative countertransference must become a high priority. Moreover, positive countertransference must also not go unnoticed since undue reverence, respect, and positive regard for the at-risk elder is likely to blind the clinician to the very real suicide potential. In addition, implementation of depression practice guidelines and the routine use of short depression screening instruments such as the GDS and the Center for Epidemiologic Studies-Depression Scale (CES-D), which have been validated in the primary care setting, appear prudent (49,40,50). Heisel et al. (2005) have recently demonstrated that a set of five GDS items assessing hopelessness, worthlessness, emptiness, an absence of happiness, and absence of the perception that it is "wonderful to be alive" is highly associated with suicidal ideation in a heterogeneous sample of older adults (51). Moreover, the same group of investigators has recently developed the Geriatric Suicide Ideation Scale (GSIS) that addresses limitations of prior suicide assessment scales that were neither developed nor validated with older adults (52). Although a Chinese version of the GSIS has demonstrated robust psychometric properties, the original instrument awaits further psychometric examination in diverse ethnic and cultural groups, and its predictive validity for future suicidal thoughts and behavior has not been established (53).

Collaborative care models in which mental health professionals provide on-site or telephone consultation show promise in optimizing management of depression in primary care practices (41,42). The IMPACT (Improving Mood: Promoting Access to Collaborative Treatment) study is a randomized, controlled trial involving 18 diverse primary care settings in which participants randomized to collaborative care had access to a depression care manager who supported antidepressant medication management prescribed by their primary care physician and offered a course of problem solving therapy for 12 months (41). Participants in the control arm received care as usual. At baseline, 139 (15.3%) intervention subjects and 119 (13.3%) controls reported thoughts of suicide. Intervention subjects had significantly lower rates of suicidal ideation than controls at six months (7.5% vs. 12.1%) and 12 months (9.8% vs. 15.5%), and even after intervention resources were no longer available at 18 months (8.0% vs. 13.3%) and 24 months (10.1% vs. 13.9%). There were no completed suicides in either group.

Similarly, PROSPECT (Prevention of Suicide in Primary Care Elderly: Collaborative Trial) is a randomized controlled trial involving patients from 20 primary care practices, in which the intervention consisted of services of trained depression care managers who offered algorithm-based recommendations to physicians and helped patients with treatment adherence over 18 months (42). Rates of suicidal ideation declined faster in intervention patients compared with usual care patients. The degree and speed of depressive symptom reduction was also more favorable for the intervention group. While the findings of these two collaborative care models are encouraging, they await replication in real-world settings, and cost-effectiveness analyses that will be critical to coverage by third-party payors have not yet been undertaken.

In addition to depression screening and initial management, the primary care physician operating within such a collaborative care model is in an opportune position to minimize the functional impairments, dependence, and demoralization associated with chronic medical conditions. However, referral to a psychiatrist should be strongly considered under the following conditions: atypical presentation, vague symptoms or multiple somatic complaints not well accounted for by a comprehensive medical workup, comorbid psychiatric conditions, polypharmacy, and active substance abuse. Most importantly, primary care physicians should seek urgent psychiatric consultation for those patients expressing suicidal ideation since vast majority of these individuals who experience dire emotional distress rarely communicate suicidal ideation to their primary care physicians (29).

Community Interventions

Several innovative community outreach programs have been developed to address the fact that older adults rarely utilize general crisis prevention hotlines or seek mental health treatment. Life Crisis Services of St. Louis, Missouri has instituted a Link-Plus component that receives referrals targeting depressed elderly in crisis from medical and mental health professionals (54). Case management and ongoing telephone contact is then provided. The Spokane Community Mental Health Center has developed the Gatekeepers Program which casts a broader net by instructing community members who routinely have contact with older adults in the recognition of at-risk elderly. Once a referral is made, in-home assessment and comprehensive case-management services are arranged (55). Similarly, the San Francisco Suicide Prevention Center has organized a Center for Elderly Suicide Prevention and

Grief Related Services. The center provides 24-hour crisis intervention, home visits, networking within local agencies, and volunteer assistance with social services (54). The longitudinal impact and cost-effectiveness of these innovative programs on curbing late-life suicide rates awaits critical examination.

De Leo et al.'s intervention model, the Tele-Help/Tele-Check service, combines both telephone assistance and twice a week visits with the clients to ascertain their needs and offer emotional support (56). In spite of the fact that the 12135 participants in this program were "old-old" (mean age 79 years), only one suicide was completed over a 4-year span. In a previous study of the Tele-Check service, the same group reported improved mood scores, fewer general practitioner home visits and fewer hospitalizations among those who had participated in the program for at least six months compared to those awaiting the service or who had just been enrolled (57). However, significant suicide risk reduction was observed for female service users only, and the study lacked a control group.

Psychoeducational Interventions

The assumption that training primary care physicians to appropriately diagnose and treat geriatric depression will have a positive impact on late-life suicide rates lacks critical analysis and affirmation. Preliminary support for this assumption comes from an uncontrolled study from the Swedish island of Gotland which reported notable declines in suicide rates in the year following a depression education program for primary care physicians (58). The result however was not sustained at 3-year follow-ups, leading the authors to conclude that such educational activities must be offered at frequent intervals (59). Further concern regarding the primary care management of depression stems from the limited time allotted to patient visits and fiscal disincentives directed at nonprocedural care, particularly with the proliferation of managed care organizations. The extent to which primary care clinicians can address both physical and psychiatric issues under these constraints is a matter worthy of thoughtful debate.

Pratt et al. have developed a 3-hour educational program on depression and suicide that is appropriate for both professional and lay audiences (60). The workshop combines an 18-minute slide show entitled *The Final Course*, a story of Mrs. Murphy, aged 72 years, with didactics and discussions. Compared to controls, participants at postcourse examination demonstrated significant gains in knowledge about late-life depression and suicide and interventions that would be appropriate and applicable to older adults experiencing such distress. A host of psychoeducational curricula exist and should be used to train health care professionals, employees of social service agencies, those who interact with the elderly on a routine basis, and the American population in general (61,62).

CONCLUSION

Medical advances of the last century have made little impact on suicide rates of the U.S. general population. Late-life suicide remains particularly problematic, and demographers expect further increases both in the rates and absolute numbers of elder suicide if current trends continue. While some optimism is engendered by the political and social activism of the "baby boomer" generation, suicide rates are higher for this generation than prior cohorts. The urgent need for biomedical, psychosocial and health care delivery research cannot be overly emphasized. Future research on late-life suicide should focus on (a) investigating the age, gender, race, and ethnicity-specific risk and protective factors for suicidal behavior (b), determining the mechanisms by which neurobiology of the aging process contributes to affective vulnerability (c), delineating the biological correlates of late-life suicidal behavior (d). elucidating the complex reciprocal interactions between physical and psychiatric illness (e), identifying personality traits that may confer vulnerability or resistance to suicidal behavior (f), developing and validating measures of suicidal ideation that are both specific for at-risk older adults and distinguish suicidal ideation from passive death ideation (g), designing therapeutic approaches that address hopelessness (h), conducting randomized controlled trials to ascertain the impact of psychoeducational programs for primary care clinicians (i), examining the impact of various collaborative primary care/mental health treatment models targeting the elderly specifically, and (j) examining the effectiveness of innovative community outreach programs in reducing late-life suicide rates. In the final analysis, the sustainability and dissemination of innovative care-management programs will depend on coverage by third-party payors.

REFERENCES

1. Havens L. The anatomy of a suicide. N Engl J Med 1965; 272:401–406.
2. http://www.cdc.gov/ncipc/wisqars/ (Accessed December 30, 2007).
3. http://www.suicidology.org/associations/1045/files/2004datapgv1.pdf (Accessed December 30, 2007).
4. McIntosh JL, Santos JF, Hubbard RW, et al. Elder Suicide: Research, Theory, and Treatment. Washington, D.C.: American Psychological Association, 1994.
5. McKenzie K, Serfaty M, Crawford M. Suicide in ethnic minority groups. Br J Psychiatry 2003; 183:100–101.
6. Bartels SJ, Coakley E, Oxman TE, et al. Suicidal and death ideation in older primary care patients with depression, anxiety, and at-risk alcohol use. Am J Geriatr Psychiatry 2002; 10:417–427.
7. Leong FTL, Leach MM. Ethnicity and suicide in the United States: Guest editors' introduction. Death Stud 2007; 31:393–398.
8. Kposowa AJ. Marital status and suicide in the National Longitudinal Mortality Study. J Epidemiol Community Health 2000; 54:254–261.
9. Parkin D, Stengel E. Incidence of suicidal attempts in an urban community. BMJ 1965; 2:133–138.
10. Osgood NJ, Brant BA. Suicidal behavior in long-term care facilities. Suicide Life Threat Behav 1990; 20:113–122.
11. Carney SS, Rich CL, Burke PA. Suicide over 60: The San Diego Study. J Am Geriatr Soc 1994; 42:174–180.
12. Heikkinen ME, Lonnqvist JK. Recent life events in elderly suicide: A nationwide study in Finland. Int Psychogeriatr 1995; 7:287–300.
13. Lyness JM, Conwell Y, Nelson JC. Suicide attempts in elderly psychiatric inpatients. J Am Geriatr Soc 1992; 40:320–324.
14. Lester D, Beck AT. Age differences in patterns of attempted suicide. Omega 1974; 5:317–322.
15. Quan H, Arboleda-Florez J, Fick GH, et al. Association between physical illness and suicide among the elderly. Soc Psychiatry Psychiatr Epidemiol 2002; 37:190–197.
16. Turvey CL, Conwell Y, Jones MP, et al. Risk factors for late-life suicide: A prospective, community-based study. Am J Geriatr Psychiatry 2002; 10:398–406.
17. Mackenzie TB, Popkin MK. Suicide in the medical patient. Int J Psychiatry Med 1987; 17:3–22.

18. Conwell Y, Lyness JM, Duberstein P, et al. Completed suicide among older patients in primary care practices: A controlled study. J Am Geriatr Soc 2000; 48:23–29.
19. Conwell Y. Suicide in elderly patients. In: Schneider LS, Reynolds CF III, Lebowitz BD, Friedhoff AJ, eds. Diagnosis and Treatment of Depression in Late Life: Results of the NIH Consensus Development Conference. Washington, D.C.: American Psychiatric Press Inc, 1994:397–418.
20. Dorpat TL, Ripley HS. A study of suicide in the Seattle area. Compr Psychiatry 1960; 1:349–359.
21. Waern M, Runeson BS, Allebeck P, et al. Mental disorder in elderly suicide: A case-control study. Am J Psychiatry 2002; 159:450–455.
22. Conwell Y, Olsen K, Caine ED, et al. Suicide in later life: Psychological autopsy findings. Int Psychogeriatr 1991; 3:59–66.
23. Conwell Y, Duberstein PR, Cox C, et al. Relationships of Axis-I diagnoses in victims of completed suicide: A psychological autopsy study. Am J Psychiatry 1996; 153:1001–1008.
24. Blow FC, Brockmann LM, Barry KL. Role of alcohol in late-life suicide. Alcohol Clin Exp Res 2004; 28:48S–56S.
25. Clark DC. Narcissistic crises of aging and suicidal despair. Suicide Life Threat Behav 1993; 23:21–26.
26. Heisel MJ, Links PS, Conn D, et al. Narcissistic personality and vulnerability to late-life suicidality. Am J Geriatr Psychiatry 2007; 15:734–741.
27. Duberstein PR. Openness to experience and completed suicide across the second half of life. Int Psychogeriatr 1995; 7:183–198.
28. Duberstein PR, Conwell Y, Seidlitz L, et al. Personality traits and suicidal behavior and ideation in depressed inpatients 50 years of age and older. J Gerontol 2000; 55B:P18–P26.
29. Pitkala K, Isometsa ET, Henriksson MM, et al. Elderly suicide in Finland. Int Psychogeriatr 2000; 12:209–220.
30. Beck AT, Schuyler D, Herman I. Development of suicide intent scales. In: Beck AT, Resnick HLP, Lettieri DJ, eds. The Prediction of Suicide. Bowie, MD: Charles, 1974:45–56.
31. Beck AT, Steer RA, Kovacs M, et al. Hopelessness and eventual suicide: Ten year prospective study of patients hospitalized with suicidal ideation. Am J Psychiatry 1985; 142:559–563.
32. Beck AT, Brown G, Berchick RJ, et al. Relationship between hopelessness and ultimate suicide: A replication with psychiatric outpatients. Am J Psychiatry 1990; 147:190–195.
33. Hill RD, Gallagher D, Thompson LW, et al. Hopelessness as a measure of suicide intent in the depressed elderly. Psychol Aging 1988; 3:230–232.
34. Ross RK, Bernstein L, Trent L, et al. A prospective study of risk factors for traumatic death in the retirement community. Prev Med 1990; 19:323–334.
35. Szanto K, Reynolds CF III, Conwell Y, et al. High levels of hopelessness persist in geriatric patients with remitted depression and a history of suicide attempt. J Am Geriatr Soc 1998; 46:1401–1406.
36. Breitbart W, Rosenfeld B, Pessin H, et al. Depression, hopelessness and desire for hastened death in terminally ill patients with cancer. JAMA 2000; 284:2907–2911.
37. Hirsch JK, Duberstein PR, et al. Positive affect and suicide ideation in older adult primary care patients. Psychiatry Aging 2007; 22:380–385.
38. Hirsch JK, Duberstein PR, Conner KR, et al. Future orientation and suicide ideation and attempts in depressed older adults ages 50 and over. Am J Geriatr Psychiatry 2006; 14:752–757.
39. Szanto K, Mulsant BH, Houck PR, et al. Emergence, persistence, and resolution of suicidal ideation during treatment of depression in old age. J Affect Disord 2007; 98:153–161.
40. Sheikh A, Yesavage JA. Geriatric Depression Scale (GDS): Recent evidence and development of a shorter version. Clin Gerontol 1986; 5:165–173.
41. Unutzer J, Tang L, Oshi S, et al. Reducing suicidal ideation in depressed older primary care patients. J Am Geriatr Soc 2006; 54:1550–1556.

42. Bruce ML, Ten Have TR, Reynolds CF, et al. Reducing suicidal ideation and depressive symptoms in depressed older primary care patients: A randomized controlled trial. JAMA 2004; 291:1081–1091.
43. Chiu HFK, Yip PSF, Chi I, et al. Elderly suicide in Hong Kong: A case-controlled psychological autopsy study. Acta Psychiatr Scand 2004; 109:299–305.
44. Felton BJ. The aged: settings, services and needs. In: Snowden LR, ed. Reaching the Underserved: Mental Health Needs of Neglected Populations. Beverly Hills, CA: Sage, 1982:23–42.
45. Gatz M, Smyer MA. The mental health system and older adults in the 1990s. Am Psychol 1992; 47:741–751.
46. Ben-Arie O, Welman M, Teggin AF. The depressed elderly living in the community: A follow-up study. Br J Psychiatry 1990; 157:425–427.
47. Diekstra RFW, Van Egmond M. Suicide and attempted suicide in general practice, 1979–1986. Acta Psychiatr Scand 1989; 79:268–275.
48. Johnson J, Weissman MM, Klerman GL. Service utilization and social morbidity associated with depressive symptoms in the community. JAMA 1992; 267:1478–1483.
49. Depression Guidelines Panel. Depression in Primary Care. Vol 1. Clinical Practices Guidelines. Rockville, MD: US DHHS, PHS, AHCPR, publication 1993; #93–0550.
50. Radloff LS. The CES-D scale: A self-report depression scale for research in the general population. Appl Psychol Measurement 1992; 7:343–351.
51. Heisel MJ, Flett GL, Duberstein PR, et al. Does the Geriatric Depression Scale (GDS) distinguish between older adults with high versus low levels of suicidal ideation? Am J Geriatr Psychiatry 2005; 13:876–883.
52. Heisel MJ, Flett GL. The development and initial validation of the Geriatric Suicide Ideation Scale. Am J Geriatr Psychiatry 2006; 14:742–751.
53. Chou KL, Jun LW, Chi I. Assessing Chinese older adults' suicidal ideation: Chinese version of the Geriatric Suicide Ideation Scale. Aging Ment Health 2005; 9:167–171.
54. McIntosh JL. Suicide prevention in the elderly (age 65–99). Suicide Life Threat Behav 1995; 25:180–192.
55. Florio ER, Rockwood TH, Hendryx MS, et al. A model gate-keeper program to find the at-risk elderly. J Case Manag 1996; 5:106–114.
56. De Leo D, Carollo G, Buono MD. Lower suicide rates associated with a tele-help/tele-check service for the elderly at home. Am J Psychiatry 1995; 152:632–634.
57. De Leo D, Rozzini R, Bernardini M, et al. Assessment of quality of life in the elderly assisted at home through a tele-check service. Qual Life Res 1992; 1:367–374.
58. Rutz W, Von Knorring L, Walinder J. Long-term effects of an educational program for general practitioners given by the Swedish Committee for the Prevention and Treatment of Depression. Acta Psychiatr Scand 1992; 85:83–88.
59. Rutz W, Von Knorring L, Pihlgren H, et al. Prevention of male suicides: Lessons from the Gotland study. Lancet 1995; 345:524.
60. Pratt CC, Schmall VL, Wilson W, et al. A model community education program on depression and suicide in later life. Gerontologist 1991; 31:692–695.
61. Butler RN, Lewis MI. Late-life depression: When and how to intervene. Geriatrics 1995; 50:44–55.
62. Osgood NJ. Prevention of suicide in the elderly. J Geriatr Psychiatry 1991; 24:293–306.

8 Neurobiologic Aspects of Late-Life Mood Disorders

Vladimir Maletic

Department of Neuropsychiatry and Behavioral Sciences, University of South Carolina School of Medicine, Greer, South Carolina, U.S.A.

INTRODUCTION

Major Depressive Disorder (MDD) and Cyclical Mood Disorders, including Bipolar Disorder (BD) type I and II are among the more prevalent psychiatric conditions (1–3). They are associated with considerable morbidity, mortality, and functional impairment (3–5). Mood disorders are highly recurrent conditions, possibly associated with a progressive course. Recent epidemiologic studies suggest that repeated mood episodes and residual symptoms enhance the risk of future recurrence (6,7). Both a greater number of episodes and the longer duration of mood disorders may be risk factors for structural changes in the brain and systemic consequences (8,9). Although the prevalence of mood disorders appears to be lower in the elderly than in younger age groups, absolute numbers may be dramatically increasing due to an aging population (10). A recent Australian study (11), for example, noted that the relative frequency of bipolar disorder in individuals older than 65 years, increased from 1% to 11% between 1980 and 1998. Enhanced understanding of the neurobiologic specificities of late-life mood disorders may help us address this growing need.

It is important to differentiate mood disorders present during late life (late-life major depressive disorder or MDD, late-life bipolar disorder or LLBD) from mood disorders with onset in late life (late-onset mood disorders or LOMD). Although definitions of late onset vary and cutoff age tends to be arbitrary, ranging from 30 to 65 years, 60 is the most commonly used demarcation point. Mood disorders starting in late life represent a particular clinical challenge. Normal brain aging, genetic predisposition, frequent polypharmacy, multiple medical, and neurological comorbidities, all converge to make late-life mood disorders a daunting diagnostic and treatment task.

If one accepts mood disorders as a consequence of complex interaction between a genetic vulnerability and environmental adversity (12,13), it follows that clinical symptoms may be a proxy for underlying biological processes (14). In contrast to our previous beliefs, even a euthymic state does not appear to bring complete restitution. Neuropsychological studies point out significant impairments in memory, attention, and executive function, even in "successfully treated" euthymic patients (15). These "minor" subsyndromal symptoms tend to be accompanied by shortcomings in familial, social, and occupational functioning (16,17). Based on our more recent insights into neurobiology of mood disorders, a revised treatment goal may surpass the current definition of remission (18) as the "gold standard," replacing it with full and sustained asymptomatic recovery attained as soon as possible.

Comprehensive understanding of etiology and pathophysiology of late-life mood disorders might assist us in choosing the most effective treatment strategies. An integrated review of neuroimaging, neuroendocrinological, pathohistological, and molecular–genetic research may well serve our purpose.

NEUROIMAGING STUDIES OF MOOD DISORDERS

Neuroimaging studies of mood disorders are occasionally characterized by equivocal findings and lack of replication. Manic patients are notoriously challenging subjects for neuroimaging research. In some studies, patients were medicated, in others not. Quite often, subjects' mood states are poorly characterized and lack homogeneity.

Despite these limitations, neuroimaging studies provide a very useful "window" into the nature of mood disorders. Strakowski, et al. utilized MRI to compare ventricular volumes of healthy volunteers to those of bipolar patients with one or multiple episodes (9). Patients who have suffered multiple episodes had significantly larger lateral ventricles than the ones experiencing the first episode or healthy subjects. Number of manic episodes was directly correlated with the volume of lateral ventricles. Brambilla et al. also noted an association between ventricular volume and the number of all previous mood disorder episodes (19). Studies such as these, pointing out global cerebral morphological alterations in patients suffering from mood disorders, have prompted research into more specific regional functional and structural differences.

Prefrontal cortical abnormalities are a common finding in mood disorders. Since subregions of the prefrontal cortex (PFC) have vastly different functional roles, they deserve a more focused discussion. Ventromedial prefrontal cortex (VMPFC) tends to have increased activity in both unipolar and bipolar depression, as well as in mania (20,21). VMPFC has rich reciprocal connections with limbic formations and the hypothalamus (8,13,22). Hypothetically, this prefrontal subregion, together with Anterior Cingulate Cortex (ACC) and limbic areas serves as an integrated network involved in processing emotionally relevant information, for the purpose of guiding behavior and orchestrating adaptive, autonomic, and endocrine responses (23). VMPFC is not only a major recipient of limbic projections, it also modulates amygdalar and hippocampal activity through complex feedback connections (13,24). Blumberg et al. have found both functional and structural changes in VMPFC of bipolar, adolescent and young adult patients. These alterations may be reflected in compromised ability to adapt to social and emotional challenges (14,25). Manic patients tend to be excessively preoccupied by hedonic interests, while depressed ones demonstrate impaired mental flexibility (26). VMPFC is also involved in regulation of appetitive drives and pain response (27). Increased VMPFC activity in MDD patients has been associated with melancholy ruminations (28). It is therefore very intriguing that several authors noted a significant reduction in VMPFC volume (up to 32%) in MDD patients compared to healthy controls (29,30).

Lateral orbital prefrontal cortex (LOPFC) appears to have a role in suppressing maladaptive and perseverative emotional responses. Its activity is enhanced in the depressive state but appears decreased in bipolar mania. Altshuler et al. have found that decreased LOFC activation correlates with duration of mania (31). Apparent disinhibition in manic patients may be a consequence of impaired LOPFC function. Lacerda et al. have found a significant reduction in LOPFC gray matter volume of MDD patients compared to healthy subjects (30). It is intriguing to speculate about the relationship between delayed treatment response in patients with repeated mood episodes and prefrontal cortical structural alterations.

Dorsolateral prefrontal cortex (DLPFC), together with dorsal ACC, and parts of the parietal cortex is considered a component of the executive function network (28). It tends to have a "top-down" regulatory influence over limbic formations (31). Decreased activity in DLPFC, in bipolar disorder, and MDD, may be reflected in compromised working memory, impaired sustained attention, and executive dysfunction (32,33). Lyoo et al. have found thinning of DLPFC in bipolar patients that correlated with duration of illness (33).

Subgenual ACC (sgACC) has a role in assessing salience of emotional and motivational information and making necessary adjustments in behavior. It is also involved in modulation of sympathetic and neuroendocrine responses. Functional imaging studies suggest increased metabolism in this area, both in manic and depressed patients (when corrected for reduced volume) (34). Metabolic activity in sgACC was substantially more prominent in manic than depressed state (34). Structural studies have noted significantly decreased volume of sgACC in bipolar and MDD population. Drevets et al. noted that sgACC had a 48% lesser volume in individuals with familial depression and a 39% reduction in gray matter volume of BD patients (35). These alterations may be implicated in disturbances of motivation and neuroendocrine function, a common feature of mood disorders (34). Additionally, a MRI study by Chen and colleagues, focusing on MDD patients, reported a negative correlation between gray matter volumes of dorsal ACC and DLPFC and symptom severity in MDD patients (36). This finding lends credence to the hypothesis that these "executive network" areas have a role in "top-down" limbic modulation (36). Diminished function and volume of pregenual ACC in MDD patients has also been associated with a delayed treatment response (37).

Limbic structures appear to be differently affected by bipolar disorder (BD) than by MDD. Hippocampus is a key limbic area located at "crossroads" of circuitry regulating stress response, mood, memory, and neuroendocrine function (8). This central location may render it vulnerable to functional dysregulation that accompanies extreme stress and mood disorders (8). The results of morphometric studies of hippocampal volume in bipolar patients are inconsistent—some have found enlargement, some have found loss of volume, many have noted no difference in size—compared to controls (14,38). Bearden and colleagues have reported a beneficial effect of chronic lithium treatment on preserving and even restoring hippocampal volume in BD subjects (39). By contrast, alterations in hippocampal volume are commonly reported in MDD patients. Sheline et al. have characterized an inverse relationship between the days of untreated depression and hippocampal volume (40). Furthermore, Colla and colleagues noted a negative correlation between duration of depression and volume of hippocampus, corrected for age and intracranial volume (41). Only one post hoc analysis (42) has found a significant increase in hippocampal volume (21%, $p = 0.004$) after six to seven months of antidepressant treatment in a small subset of patients with atypical depression.

Structural studies of the amygdala may reflect the progression of illness. Bipolar children and adolescents have a smaller volume of the amygdala, while adults tend to have a larger volume, compared to matched controls (43). Functional studies have, for the most part, found increased activity in amygdala of bipolar and depressed patients (44). Amygdala plays a role in rapidly assessing and assigning emotional value to surprising and ambiguous stimuli. Functional studies have detected increased amygdala "reactivity" to angry and fearful faces, both in BD and MDD. It is intriguing to consider that amygdala "overactivity" may translate into increased anxiety and emotional misattribution, a common characteristic of mood disorders. Since limbic structures have significant bidirectional connections with the hypothalamus and brainstem, it is not surprising that sympathetic and neuroendocrine dysregulation, have been noted in mood disorders (45).

Several other structures appear to be affected by mood disorders. Functional and structural changes have been noted in basal ganglia and thalamus of patients with mood disorders (38). Many, but not all, studies have found alterations in cerebellar function in patients with MDD (38,46). Limited studies support midline cerebellar atrophy in bipolar population. Vermal size appears to be associated with the number of previous mood episodes (47). This is of particular interest since the vermis of cerebellum has been implicated in generating automatic emotional responses, such as empathy to facial expressions.

Several studies have found altered connectivity between limbic and paralimbic prefrontal areas in MDD and bipolar patients (48,49). Combined with the studies that have found white matter abnormalities in patients with mood disorders (50), evidence points to a compromised integrity of fronto-subcortical and prefrontal-limbic circuits (48,49) (Fig. 1). Additional involvement of fronto-cerebellar-thalamic

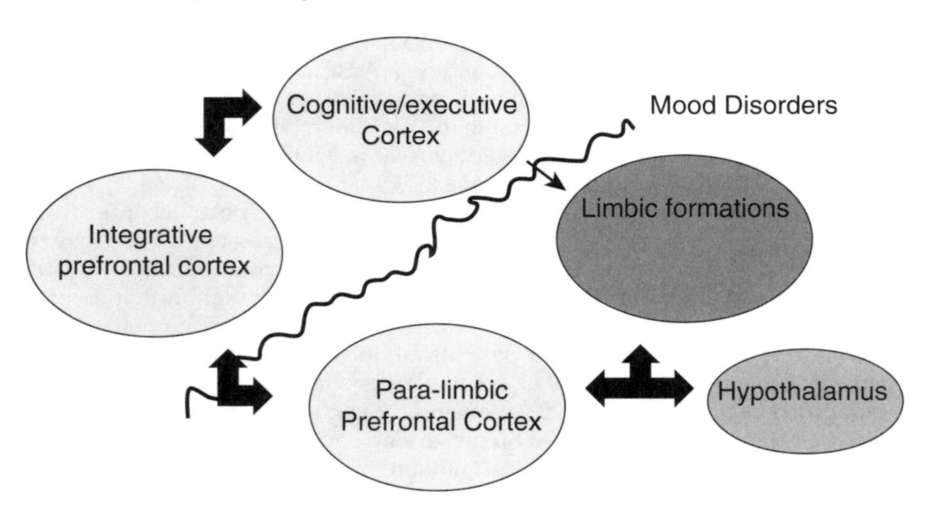

FIGURE 1 Mood disorders alter the dynamic connectivity among neuroanatomic structures involved in regulation of mood and stress response. Limbic structures (amygdala, hippocampus, and nucleus accumbens) have reciprocal connections with "para-limbic" cortical areas, subgenual anterior cinuglate and ventro-medical prefrontal cortex (VMPFC). Hypothetically, disrupted "connectivity" between limbic/paralimbic areas and rostral integrative prefrontal formations results in compromised feedback regulation of limbic activity. Consequently, the dorsal cognitive/ executive network is hypoactive, while excessively active limbic areas continue to stimulate the hypothalamus and brainstem areas, leading to neuroendocrine dysregulation and sympathetic hyperactivity. *Source:* From Ref. 13.

circuitry is likely (48). In summary, structural and functional studies support an organic basis for emotional (34), cognitive (50), and neuroendocrine (45) symptomatology of affective illness. In some instances, there is evidence of cumulative effect of prior episodes.

NEUROENDOCRINE, SYMPATHETIC, AND NEUROIMMUNE DYSREGULATION IN MOOD DISORDERS

Disruption of hypothalamic-pituitary-adrenal axis (HPA) function in BD and MDD is well documented. Amygdala overactivity combined with compromised hippocampal regulatory role, are often cited as casual factors (8,45). Increased release of CRF contributes to greater ACTH secretion and eventual elevation of circulating glucocorticoids. Glucocorticoid receptors in hippocampus and hypothalamus appear to have diminished sensitivity in mood disorders, therefore disrupting physiologic feedback regulation (51). A significant proportion of patients with melancholic depression and BD have persistently elevated cortisol levels (51). Notably, individuals suffering from atypical depression tend to have lower corticosteroid levels, compared to healthy controls (52). This discrepancy in corticosteroid levels may bear witness to genetic heterogeneity among depressive disorders.

In addition to HPA dysregulation, mood disorders may be associated with excessive sympathetic nervous system (SNS) activation. Some authors hypothesize that the constellation of SNS overactivity and glucocorticoid receptor insufficiency may contribute to activation of innate immune response and subsequent release of inflammatory cytokines from macrophages.

Inflammatory cytokines can not only alter synthesis of neurotrophic factors (especially BDNF) in the CNS, but also interfere with monoaminergic transmission (52,53). Cytokines may diminish sensitivity of glucocorticoid and insulin receptors, further disrupting endocrine control (51,52,53) (Fig. 2). Increased SNS activity, inflammatory dysregulation, enhanced platelet/endothelial aggregation, and unhealthy lifestyle, may all contribute to a significantly greater risk of cerebrovascular and cardiovascular disease in the population with mood disorders (54,55). MDD patients appear to have approximately 50% greater mortality due to endocrine, cerebrovascular, and cardiovascular disease, compared to normative sample. The risk in bipolar individuals is almost doubled (4). HPA dysregulation combined with compromised glucocorticoid and insulin receptor sensitivity, mediated by inflammatory cytokines, might also explain the high rate of diabetes, dyslipidemia, and osteoporosis in the bipolar population (51–55).

Elevated glucocorticoids have been associated with suppressed TSH secretion and compromised enzymatic conversion of relatively inactive T4 to T3 (51). Ensuing low-grade thyroid dysfunction has been noted in BPD, and probably impacts both the clinical presentation of mood disorders and their response to treatment. Similar thyroid abnormalities have also been described in MDD patients (56).

PATHOHISTOLOGIC AND GENETIC ALTERATIONS IN MOOD DISORDERS

Bipolar disorder and MDD appear to be associated with significant cell pathology. Several postmortem studies have established reductions in glia cell numbers and density in BPD and MDD. Glial cell pathology was noted in the sgACC, DLPFC, orbitofrontal cortex, and amygdala of unmedicated bipolar and MDD patients

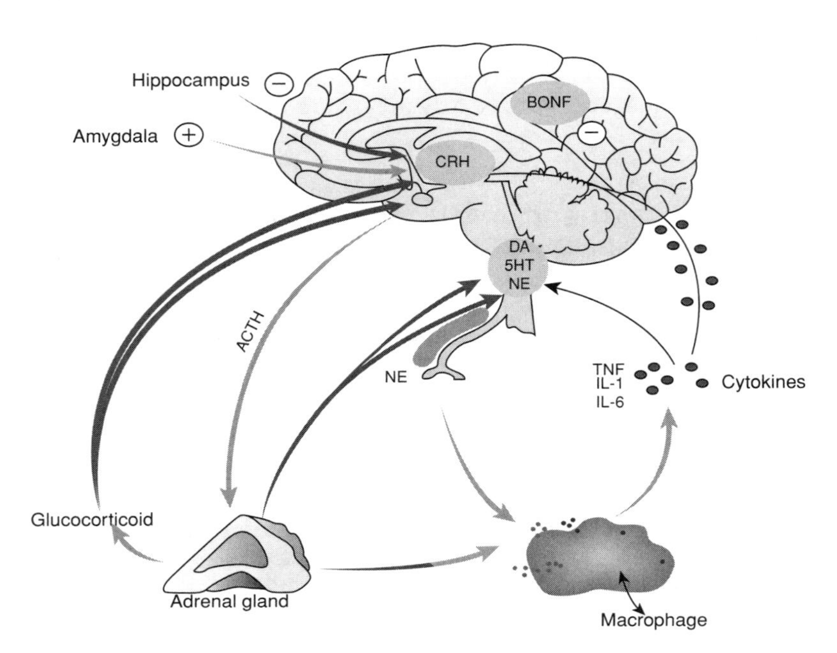

FIGURE 2 Mood disorders have systemic consequences. Limbic dysregulation results in compromised neuroendocrine control. Stress leads to release of CRH, ACTH, and glucocorticoids. Sympathetic overactivity contributes to immune activation and release of proinflammatory cytokines (TNF, IL-1, IL-6). In depression, disruption of 5HT, NE, and DA transmission may impair the regulatory feedback loops that "turn off" the stress response. Inflammatory cytokines further interfere with monoaminergic and neurotrophic signaling. They may also diminish central corticosteroid receptor sensitivity, leading to further disruption of feedback control. *Abbreviations*: CRH, corticotropin-releasing hormone; ACTH, adrenocorticotropic hormone; 5HT, serotonin; NE, norepinephrine; DA, dopamine. *Source*: Adapted from Ref. 52.

(57–59). It appears that at least two types of glia cells may have been affected, astroglia and oligodendroglia. Uranova et al. described a prominent 29% reduction in oligodendroglia of bipolar and 19% reduction in DLPFC (BA 9) of MDD patients (59). Having in mind the crucial role that DLPFC plays in executive function and "top-down" limbic regulation, this finding is striking. Hamidi et al. have described reductions in oligodendroglia density in amygdala of MDD patients (60). Rajkowsa et al. have noted a significant reduction of glia density in DLPFC and OPFC of MDD subjects (61). Ongur et al. (62) have noted a 41% glial reduction in sgACC of individuals suffering from familial BPD. Further supporting glial involvement in mood disorders, Stockmaier et al. characterized a significant decrease in glial density in hippocampal dentate gyrus of MDD subjects (63). Distribution of cellular pathology remarkably coincides with findings of structural and functional imaging studies, hinting at the association with clinical manifestations of bipolar illness and MDD.

Findings of neuronal alterations in mood disorders have been much more equivocal. A recent study of DLPFC found 16% to 22% decrease in neuronal density in BPD. These large pyramidal neurons correspond with glutaminergic excitatory neurons (58). Additionally, Bezchlibnyk et al. have reported decreased neuronal size in the amygdala of BD subjects (64). Benes et al. described morphologic changes in nonpyramidal hippocampal neurons of BD patients (65). Since amygdala and ACC both receive regulatory input from DLPFC, one would wonder about the clinical consequences of these histologic alterations. Neuronal changes appear to be more discrete in MDD. Some authors have noted decreased pyramidal somal size in hippocampus (63), in ACC (66), DLPFC (BA 9), and OPFC (BA 47) in postmortem studies of MDD patients (67).

In contrast to these cortical and limbic findings, bipolar patients appear to have a higher number of noradrenergic neurons in the locus coeruleus compared to MDD subjects (68). Subtle morphologic differences of serotoninergic dorsal raphae neurons were observed in patients suffering from mood disorders (68).

Age is inversely correlated with gray matter volume in bipolar patients but not in healthy controls (69). Additionally, an age-dependant decrement in astroglial markers was reported in a group of MDD subjects (70). Accelerated telomere shortening found in mood disorders may be a consequence of stress-related oxidative damage. One recent study suggests that changes in telomere length may represent as much as 10 years of accelerated aging (71). Lung et al. have described similar reduction in telomeres of MDD patients, related to MAO polymorphism (72).

Until recently, glia cells have been cast in the supportive role in the CNS. Approximately 90% of the brain tissue is composed of glia cells. In dramatic contrast to our prior belief, contemporary research has established astroglia and oligodendroglia as full-fledged neuronal partners in neurotransmission (57). The novel concept of the tripartite synapse emphasizes the role of astroglial processes in encapsulating and containing the contents of the synaptic cleft. Astroglia virtually surround neurons and may have a role in synchronizing their activity (73). Almost all classes of serotonin, norepinephrine, dopamine, cholinergic, GABA, glutamate, neurotrophin, and cytokine receptors are expressed on glia cell membranes (57,73,74). Additionally, they have monoamine (5HTT, NAT, DAT) and glutamate transporters. Evidence suggests that neurotrophic factors, brain-derived and glia-derived neurotrophic factors (BDNF and GDNF), as well as cytokines (tumor necrosis factor-alpha, TNF-α) are synthesized within glia cells (57,74). Unlike neurons that release neurotransmitters in response to action potential, glia cells empty glutamate vesicles in response to graded increase in cytoplasmatic Ca^{2+}. Astroglia have a role in regulating neuronal energy supply, for example, by releasing lactate to ameliorate increased energy needs at the time of peak neuronal activity. Cerebral perfusion is significantly influenced by astroglia; on one end astroglial appendages "sense" the synaptic activity, on the other hand, their distal processes "feet" modulate vascular tone and capillary permeability (75,76).

In summary, histologic evidence does not support mood disorders as a typical neurodegenerative diseases. Conventional neurodegenerative disorders are associated with neuronal loss and prominent gliosis. In contrast, mood diseases tend to manifest glial loss, morphologic changes in neurons, and thinning of interneuronal neuropil (57). Given the histologic evidence, one can hypothesize that mood disorders may be a consequence of disrupted neuron–glia relationship, resulting in compromised neurotransmission (57,77). Studies also support a role for accelerated aging, most likely due to oxidative stress (70,71). The relationship between cell pathology and clinical manifestations of mood disorders has yet to be definitively established.

GENETICS AND MOLECULAR NEUROBIOLOGY OF MOOD DISORDERS

Mood disorders are most likely genetically heterogeneous diseases, associated with alterations in a multitude of polymorphic genes (20,78,79). Dozens of different genes have been implicated in various genetic studies of MDD. Most consistent evidence supports the role for 5HTTPR, 5HT2A, COMT, MAO, and val66met BDNF polymorphism as propagating vulnerability for MDD (80–84). Genes regulating synthesis of CRF and glutamate receptors have also been implicated (78,20). A study by Caspi et al. established an association among the short allele of 5HTTPR (less functional polymorphism), vulnerability to stress, as a precipitant of MDD, severity of symptoms, and suicidality in MDD patients (84). Short allele has also been associated with lesser ACC, amygdala, and hippocampal volumes (83). Structural changes are associated with aberrant "connectivity" between ACC and amygdala, possibly interfering with adaptive emotional modulation (83,85,86). The combination of the 5HTTPR short allele and 5HT1A, less competent allele, has also been associated with exaggerated reactivity of amygdala in medicated MDD patients. Gotlib et al. have postulated a relationship among the 5HTT short allele, response to stress, HPA reactivity, and susceptibility to MDD (87). Kendler et al. have described an interaction among 5HTTPR short variant, stressful life events, female gender, and risk of developing MDD. Women with short 5HTTPR allele had a sevenfold greater hazard ratio of developing a depressive episode when exposed to stress (12).

Recent evidence has implicated the val66met polymorphism of the BDNF gene in the pathogenesis of mood disorders. The lower functioning met-allele has been associated with lesser gray matter volume in DLPFC, LOPFC (81), and hippocampus (88). In a groundbreaking study, Kaufman et al. have described an interaction between childhood mistreatment, short variant of 5HTTPR allele, met BDNF allele and lack of social support, resulting in increased depression scores in children (80). This study provides true "proof of concept," supporting the validity of a biopsychosocial model of affective disease. Similar studies have reported that 5HTT, COMT, and MAOA polymorphism and gender have a convergent effect on endocrine stress response (82). MAOA polymorphism may also interact with maltreatment, adversely impacting childrens' mental health. In summary, genes regulating monoamine receptors, transporters, and enzymes involved in their metabolism, all seem to contribute to vulnerability toward MDD (89). These genes combined with those regulating corticosteroid signaling also influence structure and connectivity of areas involved in generating an adaptive stress response (20,48,78). Genetic modulation of neurotrophic factors, involved in regulating cellular resilience, neuroplasticity, and neurogenesis, may also be compromised in MDD and bipolar patients (20,48,78,79).

Much as in MDD, genes regulating serotonin receptors, transporter, COMT, and BDNF have been implicated in conveying susceptibility towards BD (79,90). A recent comprehensive review concluded that complex genetic alterations in bipolar disorder interact with each other and may impact an integrated intracellular signaling network (79). Affected gene networks regulate synthesis of growth and neuroprotective factors, stress-activated kinase pathways, circadian rhythms, and synaptic activity. Phosphoinositide-3-kinase (PI3K)/AKT pathway is general signal transduction pathway for growth factors, including BDNF and consequently BCL-2. Glycogen Synthase Kinase-3 (GSK-3) signaling pathway modulates apoptosis and synaptic plasticity (20,48,78,79,91). Increased activity in GSK pathway supports apoptosis. Attenuation of GSK-3 activity leads to upregulation of BCL-2 and β-catenin, with consequent enhancement of neuroplasticity and cellular resilience (48,91,92). This pathway is also involved in circadian regulation (79).

Interestingly enough inhibition of GSK-3 pathway produces both antimanic and antidepressant effects. Many agents with mood stabilizing properties such as lithium, valproate, and atypical antipsychotics, directly and indirectly, modulate PI3K, GSK-3, and Wnt signaling pathways, further supporting their involvement in pathogenesis of bipolar disorder (48,78,79,91,92). A recent study noted that MDD patients who had aberrant genetic regulation of GSK-3 function tended to have limited benefit from conventional antidepressants but improved significantly with adjunctive mood-stabilizer treatment (93).

There is another surprising indication from genetic studies of bipolar disorder; the affected stress-activated kinase pathways do not appear to directly affect neurotransmitter trafficking, they are funneled toward regulating oligodendroglia function (79). Oligodendroglia have a principle role in myelination of central neuronal pathways. It is very intriguing that recent functional neuroimaging studies imply that lack of "connectivity" between limbic and prefrontal structures (48) may be the underpinning of bipolar symptomatology.

INTEGRATION OF NEUROBIOLOGIC FINDINGS

Before attempting an integration of complex and diverse neurobiological research material, a review of inherent limitations may be warranted. Mood disorders are phenomenologically, genetically, and biologically heterogeneous conditions (78,79,94). Research correlating findings from different areas (e.g., imaging genetics) is relatively scarce. Other studies characterizing associations between clinical phenomena and biological indicators are not capable of ascertaining the direction of association, let alone establishing causality. Given these limitations, any attempt at integration of neurobiological findings is by necessity, speculative, relative, and probabilistic. Clinical and epidemiologic studies have consistently identified stress as a precipitant and a perpetuant of mood disorders (6,95,96). In the later course of illness, the relationship between stress and mood episodes dissipates, and recurrence seems to be facilitated by a different set of biological factors (6,96). Functional and structural neuroimaging studies have implicated limbic areas (especially amygdala and hippocampus) and PFC in the pathophysiology of mood disorders (24–26,30,32,34,46). As a rule, limbic and paralimbic prefrontal areas (sgACC, VMPFC, and LOPFC) tend to have increased activity, accompanied by volumetric alterations (23,29,30,46). Dorsal, prefrontal areas (DLPFC, dACC), usually considered components of the executive function network, have diminished activity, also accompanied by structural changes (33,46,97). Ventral (more affective) and dorsal (more cognitive) areas, under physiologic conditions tend to have reciprocal activity (97,98). Limbic structures, PFC, ACC, and hypothalamus, function as components of a highly integrated circuitry, regulating emotional, cognitive, endocrine, sympathetic, and neuroimmune responses as an adaptation to stress. In circumstances when repeated stress overwhelms genetically vulnerable substrate, a mood episode may ensue (8,13,14,20,48,51,78,99,100).

On the synaptic and cellular level, insufficient monoaminergic signaling may lead to dysregulation of glutaminergic and GABAergic transmission (101,102). Disruption of endocrine regulation, due to limbic-prefrontal dysfunction, combined with excessive sympathetic activation, triggers innate immune response (8,52). Proinflammatory cytokines, excessive glutamate, glucocorticoids, and CRF,

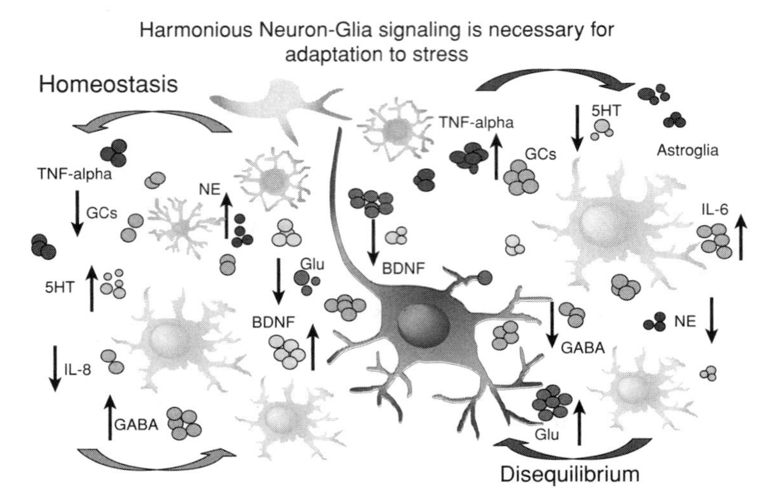

FIGURE 3 Compromised neuron-glia signaling in affective disorders. The combination of repeated stress and genetic vulnerability may create disturbance in monoamine, GABA, and glutamate signaling. Mood disorders are often associated with disruption in neuroendicrine, sympathetic, and neuroimmune regulation. The confluence of excessive excitatory/ diminished inhibitory neurotransmission, inadequate monoaminergic signaling, elevated glucocorticoids, CRF, and proinflammatory cytokines may compromise neurotrophic support. Disruption of neuron-glia communication may lead to apoptotic cellular alterations creating a breach in neural connectivity.

together with inadequate GABAergic and monoaminergic modulation impact genetically vulnerable neurons and glia cells (52,57,99–106) (Fig. 3). Their mutual regulation starts breaking down: calcium currents, neurotrophic signaling, regulation of transmitters trafficking, perfusion, and energy regulation are disrupted. Glia cells release excessive glutamate, which binds to extrasynaptic NMDA receptors (57,99). Neurons become flooded with Ca^{2+} (57,99,107). The process of apoptosis may begin (99). Glia cells are reduced and functionally incapacitated neurons undergo morphological changes (57,107). Due to pathologic processes, synapses are no longer functioning well (99). Intracellular signaling is out of balance: proapoptotic factors and reactive oxygen species accumulate, neurotrophic synthesis/signaling becomes insufficient (99–104). Consequently, skeletal protein synthesis is compromised and synaptic processes retract (99). Connectivity between limbic and prefrontal areas becomes further disrupted, thus perpetuating the vicious cycle (32,48,57,61,107). This multileveled dysregulation may in part be manifested by complex clinical symptoms of a mood episode. Although this hypothetical scenario is fairly well supported by empirical evidence, it should be considered as provisional, pending ongoing research.

BIOLOGICAL SPECIFICITY OF LATE-ONSET MOOD DISORDERS

The existence of late-life mood disorders, as a separate entity, is a topic of controversy. Some authors believe that age of onset of mood disorders is a continuous variable, with unimodal distribution (10,108); others claim a specific neurobiological distinction characterizing the late-onset disease (109). Both views may have merit. A group of authors have conceptualized late-life mood disorders as a consequence of interaction between somewhat lesser genetic diathesis and cerebrovascular/white matter changes associated with the aging process (10,110,111,112). In further support of this hypothesis, Godin et al. have noted that a greater volume of white matter lesions may be a predictor of a future depressive episode (111). Sheline et al. have recently reported significant white matter changes in the tracts connecting brain regions critical for emotional processing and executive function (50). In this group of elderly depressed patients, whole brain white matter hyperintensities correlated with executive function, while whole brain gray matter correlated with processing speed. Other authors have found biophysical changes, even in normal appearing white matter, in late-life depressed patients (113). They speculated about the impact of white matter changes on neural connectivity between the areas involved in emotional regulation. Density of glia cells in DLPFC is reduced in an age-dependant manner (70). Sweet et al. have posited that astroglial changes combined with cerebrovascular alterations may mediate the relationship between late-onset depression and dementia (112). More than half of the individuals with late-onset depression also had prominent problems with executive function and information processing. In late onset MDD, the reported reduction in hippocampal volume may be a contributor to cognitive difficulties. Systemic factors may also contribute to late-life mood disorders. Bremmer et al. have noted that late-life depression was associated with both hyper- and hypocortisolemia (another contribution of hippocampal alterations?), as well as with cardiovascular disease (114). The same author, in a separate study, reported an association between elevated proinflammatory cytokines (IL-6) and MDD in elderly (115).

Some of the same factors have been associated with the late-life onset BD. Greater cerebrovascular risk/burden (116), white matter hyperintensities (117), greater cortical atrophy, and less prominent family history of depression (10) have all been noted as distinguishing features of late onset BD. Kennedy et al. have proposed a model that takes into account genetic heterogeneity of BD and potential genetic specificities of late-onset BD. Individuals with more penetrant genetic variants, involving genes with a greater effect are more susceptible and may develop the disease earlier in their life (118). Combinations of genes with weaker effect may result in different manifestations (pleiotrophy) (118). These discrete, low-grade manifestations are likely to avoid early detection. Only later, with convergence of multiple psychosocial and biological factors (e.g., cellular and vascular changes associated with aging, medical disease, lifelong substance abuse, multiple medications), would this, more subtle genetic vulnerability, become "unmasked" and manifest itself as a late-life mood disorder.

SUMMARY

- Residual symptoms of mood disorders represent an active state of disease and may be associated with an increased risk of recurrence.
- Persistent functional changes may be translated into structural alterations. Compromised activity of neurotrophic/neuroprotective factors may underlie this transformation.
- Mood disorders affect not only affective and cognitive functioning, but also have far reaching effects on the regularion of neuroendocrine, autonomic, and neuroimmune processes, resulting in metabolic disturbances, vascular disease, osteoporosis, and immune deficiency.

- Neurobiological understanding of mood disorders may prompt earlier diagnosis and emphasis on effective treatment, recognizing that residual symptoms may be a proxy for smoldering biological processes.
- Late-life mood disorders may be either a manifestation of the cumulative effect of life-long mood disorder with its sequelae, or possibly, a product of lesser genetic diathesis and convergent psychosocial and biological factors associated with aging.

REFERENCES

1. Remick RA. Diagnosis and management of depression in primary care: A clinical update and review. Can Med Assoc J 2002; 167:1253–1260.
2. Kessler RC, Chiu WT, Demler O. Prevalence, severity and comorbidity of 12-month DSM-IV disorders in the National Comorbidity Survey Replication. Arch Gen Psychiatry 2005; 62:617–627.
3. Akiskal H.S. The bipolar spectrum in psychiatry and general medical practice. Primary Psychiatry 2004; 11(9):30–35.
4. Osby U, Brandt B, Correia N, et al. Excess mortality in bipolar and unipolar disorder in Sweden. Arch Gen Psychiatry 2001; 58:844–850.
5. Judd LL, Akiskal HS, Schettler PJ, et al. Psychosocial disability in the course of bipolar I and II disorders: A prospective, comparative, longitudinal study. Arch Gen Psychiatry 2005; 62:1322–1330.
6. Kendler KS, Thornton LM, Gardner CO. Stressful life events and previous episodes in the etiology of major depression in women: An evaluation of the "kindling" hypothesis. Am J Psychiatry 2001; 158:582–586.
7. Judd LL, Akiskal HS, Maser JD, et al. Major depressive disorder: A prospective study of residual subthreshold depressive symptoms as predictor of rapid relapse. J Affect Disord 1998; 50:97–108.
8. Sheline YI. 3D MRI studies of neuroanatomic changes in unipolar major depression: The role of stress amd medical comorbidity. Biol Psychiatry 2000; 48:791–800.
9. Strakowski SM, DelBello MP, Zimmerman ME, et al. Ventricular and periventricular structural volumes in first- versus multiple-episode bipolar disorder. Am J Psychiatry 2002; 159:1841–1847.
10. Depp CA, Jeste DV. Bipolar disorder in older adults: A critical overview. Bipolar Disord 2004; 6:343–367.
11. Almeida OP, Fenner S. Bipolar Disorder: Similarities and differences between patients with illness onset before and after 65 years of age. Inter Psychogeriatr 2002; 14(3):311–322.
12. Kendler KS, Kuhn JW, Vittum J, et al. The interaction of stressful life events and a serotonin transporter polymorphism in the prediction of episodes of major depression. Arch Gen Psychiatry 2005; 62:529–535.
13. Maletic V, Robinson M, Oakes T, et al. Neurobiology of depression: An integrated view of key findings. Int J Clin Pract 2007; 61(12):2030–2040.
14. Maletic V, Neuroprotective issues in bipolar disorder, in managing bipolar disorder from urgent situations to maintenance therapy, Part 2: Focus on maintenance. J Clin Psychiatry 2007; 68(8):1295–1300.
15. Mur M, Portella MJ, Martinez-Aran A, et al. Persistent neuropsychological deficit in euthymic bipolar patients: Executive function as a core deficit. J Clin Psychiatry 2007; 68:1078–1086.
16. Vieta E, Sanchez-Moreno J, Lahuerta J, et al. Subsyndromal depressive symptoms in patients with bipolar and unipolar disorder during clinical remission. J Affect Disord 2008; 107:169–174.
17. Altshuler LL, Post RM, Black DO, et al. Subsyndromal depressive symptoms are associated with functional impairment in patients with bipolar disorder: Results of a large, multisite study. J Clin Psychiatry 2006; 67:1551–1560.

18. American Psychiatric Association. Diagnostic and Statistical Manual of Mental Disorders, 4th ed. Text Revision. Washington, D. C.: American Psychiatric Association, 2000.
19. Brambilla P, Harenski K, Nicoletti M, et al. MRI study of posterior fossa structures and brain ventricles in bipolar patients. J Psychiatr Res 2001; 35:313–322.
20. Manji HK, Drevets WC, Charney DS. The cellular neurobiology of depression. Nat Med 2001; 7:541–547.
21. Killgore WD, Yurgelun-Todd DA. Ventromedial prefrontal activity correlates with depressed mood in adolescent children. Neuroreport 2006; 17:167–171.
22. Milad MR, Wright CI, Orr SP, et al. Recall of fear extinction in humans activates ventromedial prefrontal cortex and hippocampus in concert. Biol Psychiatry 2007; 62(10):446–454.
23. Drevets WC, Öngür D, Price JL. Neuroimagery abnormalities in the subgenual prefrontal cortex: Implications for the pathophysiology of familial mood disorders. Mol Psychiatry 1998; 3:220–226.
24. Drevets WC, Bogers W, Raichle ME. Functional anatomical correlates of antidepressant drug treatment assessed using PET measures of regional glucose metabolism. Eur Neuropsychopharmacol 2002; 12:527–544.
25. Blumberg HP, Krystal JH, Bansal R, et al. Age, rapid-cycling, and pharmacotherapy effects on ventral prefrontal cortex in bipolar disorder: A cross-sectional study. Biol Psychiatry 2006; 59:611–618.
26. Blumberg HP, Leung HC, Skudlarski P, et al. A functional magnetic resonance study of bipolar disorder. Arch Gen Psychiatry 2003; 60:601–609.
27. Ongur D, Price JL. The organization of networks within the orbital and medial prefrontal cortex of rats, monkeys and humans. Cereb Cortex 2000; 10(3):206–219.
28. Drevets WC. Functional neuroimaging studies of depression: The anatomy of melancholia. Annu Rev Med 1998; 49:341–361.
29. Bremner JD, Vythilingam M, Vermetten E, et al. Reduced volume of orbitofrontal cortex in major depression. Biol Psychiatry 2002; 51:273–279.
30. Lacerda ALT, Keshavan MS, Hardan AY, et al. Anatomic evaluation of the orbitofrontal cortex in major depressive disorder. Biol Psychiatry 2004; 55:363–368.
31. Altshuler LL, Bookheimer SY, Townsend J, et al. Blunted activation in orbitofrontal cortex during mania: A functional magnetic resonance imaging study. Biol Psychiatry 2005; 58:763–769.
32. Mayberg HS. Modulating dysfunctional limbic-cortical circuits in depression: Towards development of brain-based algorithms for diagnosis and optimized treatment. Br Med Bull 2003; 65:193–207.
33. Lyoo IK, Sung YH, Dager SR, et al. Regional cerebral cortical thinning in bipolar disorder. Bipolar Disord 2006; 8:65–74.
34. Drevets WC. Neuroimaging and neuropathological studies of depression: Implications for the cognitive-emotional features of mood disorders. Curr Opin Neurobiol 2001; 11:240–249.
35. Drevets WC, Price JL, Simpson JR. Subgenual prefrontal cortex abnormalities in mood disorders. Nature 1997; 386:824–827.
36. Whittle S, Allen NB, Lubman DI, et al. The neurobiological basis of temperament: Towards a better understanding of psychopathology. Neurosci Biobehav Rev 2005; 30:511–525.
37. Chen CH, Ridler K, Suckling J, et al. Brain imaging correlates of depressive symptom severity and predictors of symptom improvement after antidepressant treatment. Biol Psychiatry 2007; 62:407–414.
38. Beyer JL, Krishnan KR. Volumetric brain imaging findings in mood disorders. Bipolar Disord 2002; 4:89–104.
39. Bearden CE, Thompson PM, Dalwani M, et al. Greater cortical gray matter density in lithium-treated patients with bipolar disorder. Biol Psychiatry 2007; 63(8):7–16.
40. Sheline YI, Gado MH, Kraemer HC. Untreated depression and hippocampal volume loss. Am J Psychiatry 2003; 160;1516–1518.
41. Colla M, Kronenberg G, Deuschle M, et al. Hippocampal volume reduction and HPA-system activity in major depression. J Psychiatr Res 2007; 41:553–560.

42. Vythilingam M, Vermetten E, Anderson GM, et al. Hippocampal volume, memory, and cortisol status in major depressive disorder: Effects of treatment. Biol Psychiatry 2004; 56:101–112.
43. Blumberg HP, Fredericks C, Wang F, et al. Preliminary evidence for persistent abnormalities in amygdala volumes in adolescents and young adults with bipolar disorder. Bipolar Disord 2005; 7:570–576.
44. Sheline YI, Barch DM, Donnelly JM, et al. Increased amygdala response to masked emotional faces in depressed subjects resolves with antidepressant treatment: An MRI study. Biol Psychiatry 2001; 50:651–658.
45. Drevets WC, Price JL, Bardgett ME, et al. Glucose metabolism in the amygdala in depression: Relationship to diagnostic subtype and plasma cortisol levels. Pharmacol Biochem Behav 2002; 71:431–447.
46. Fitzgerald PB, Laird AR, Maller J, et al. A meta-analytic study of changes in brain activation in depression. Hum Brain Mapping 2008; 29:683–695.
47. Mills NP, Delbello MP, Adler CM, et al. MRI analysis of cerebellar vermal abnormalities in bipolar disorder. Am J Psychiatry 2005; 162:1530–1532.
48. Carlson PJ, Singh JB, Zarate CA, et al. Neural circuitry and neuroplasticity in mood disorders: Insights for novel therapeutic targets. NeuroRx 2006; 3:22–41.
49. Yurgelun-Todd DA, Silveri MM, Gruber SA, et al. White matter abnormalities observed in bipolar disorder: A diffusion tensor imaging study. Bipolar Disord 2007; 9:504–512.
50. Sheline YI, Price JL, Vaishnavi SN, et al. Regional white matter hyperintensity burden in automated segmentation distinguishes late-life depression subjects from comparison subjects matched for vascular risk factors. Am J Psychiatry 2008; 165(4):524–532.
51. Tsigos C, Chrousos GP. Hypothalamic-pituitary-adrenal axis, neuroendocrine factors and stress. J Psychosom Res 2002; 53:865–871.
52. Raison CL, Capuron L, Miller AH. Cytokines sing the blues: Inflammation and the pathogenesis of depression. Trends Immunol 2006; 27:24–31.
53. Raison CL, Miller AH. When not enough is too much: The role of insufficient glucocorticoid signaling in the pathophysiology of stress-related disorders. Am J Psychiatry 2003; 160:1554–1565.
54. Musselman DL, Evans DL, Nemeroff CB. The relationship of depression to cardiovascular disease: Epidemiology, biology and treatment. Arch Gen Psychiatry 1998; 55(7):580–592.
55. Taylor V, MacQueen G. Associations between bipolar disorder and metabolic syndrome: A review. J Clin Psychiatry 2006; 67:1034–1041.
56. Pfennig A, Frye MA, Koberle U, et al. The mood spectrum and hypothalamic-pituitary-thyroid axis. Prim Psychiatry 2004; 11:42–47.
57. Rajkowska G, Miguel-Hidalgo JJ. Gliogenesis and glial pathology in depression. CNS & Neuro Dis Drug Targets 2007; 6:219–233.
58. Rajkowska G, Halaris A, Selemon LD. Reductions in neuronal and glial density characterize the dorsolateral prefrontal cortex in bipolar disorder. Biol Psychiatry 2001; 49:741–752.
59. Uranova NA, Vostrikov VM, Orlovskaya DD, et al. Oligodendroglial density in the prefrontal cortex in schizophrenia and mood disorders: A study from the Stanley Neuropathology Consortium. Schizophr Res 2004; 67:269–275.
60. Hamidi M, Drevets WC, Price JL. Glial reduction in amygdala in major depressive disorder is due to oligodendrocytes. Biol Psychiatry 2004; 55:563–569.
61. Rajkowska G, Miguel-Hidalgo JJ, Wei J, et al. Morphometric evidence for neuronal and glial prefrontal cell pathology in major depression. Soc Biol Psychiatry 1999; 45:1085–1098.
62. Ongur D, Drevets WC, Price JL. Glial reduction in the subgenual prefrontal cortex in mood disorders. Proc. Natl Acad Sci U S A 1998; 95:13290–13295.
63. Stockmeier CA, Mahajan GJ, Konick LC, et al. Cellular changes in the postmortem hippocampus in major depression. Biol Psychiatry 2004; 56:640–650.

64. Bezchlibnyk YB, Sun X, Wang JF, et al. Neuron somal size is decreased in the lateral amygdalar nucleus of subjects with bipolar disorder. J Psychiatry Neurosci 2007; 32(3):203–210.
65. Benes FM. The role of apoptosis in the neuronal pathology in schizophrenia and bipolar disorder. Curr Opin Psychiatry 2004; 17(3):189–190.
66. Chana G, Landau S, Beasley C, et al. Two-dimensional assessment of cytoarchitecture in the anterior cingulated cortex in major depressive disorder, bipolar disorder, and schizophrenia: Evidence for decreased neuronal somal size and increased neuronal density. Biol Psychiatry 2003; 53:1086–1098.
67. Rajkowska G. Histopathology of the prefrontal cortex in major depression: What does it tell us about dysfunctional monoaminergic circuits? Prog Brain Res 2000; 126:397–412.
68. Bauman B, Bogerts B, Neuroanatomical studies on bipolar disorder. Br J Psychiatry 2001; 178(suppl 41):s142–s147.
69. Moorhead TW, McKirdy J, Sussman JED, et al. Progressive gray matter loss in patients with bipolar disorder. Biol Psychiatry 2007; 62(8):894–900.
70. Si X, Miguel-Hidalgo JJ, O'Dwyer G, et al. Age-dependent reductions in the level of glial fibrilary acidic protein in the prefrontal cortex in major depression. Neuropsychopharmacology 2004; 29:2088–2096.
71. Simon NM, Smoller JW, McNamara,et al. Telomere shortening and mood disorders: Preliminary support for a chronic stress model of accelerated aging. Biol Psychiatry 2006; 60:432–435.
72. Lung FW, Chen NC, Shu BC. Genetic pathway of major depressive disorder in shortening telometric length. Psychiatr Genet 2007; 17:195–199.
73. Murai KM, Van Meyel DJ. Neuron-glial communication at synapses: Insights from vertebrates and invertebrates. Neuroscientist 2007; 13(6):657–666.
74. Pav M, Kovaru H, Fiserova A, et al. Neurobiological aspects of depressive disorder and antidepressant treatment: Role of glia. Physiol Res 2008; 57:151–164.
75. Volterra A, Meldolesi J. Astrocytes, from brain glue to communication elements: The revolution continues. Nature Rev Neurosci 2005; 6:626–640.
76. Haydon PG, Caramignoto G. Astrocyte control of synaptic transmission and neurovascular coupling. Physiol Res 2006; 86:1009–1031.
77. Elmariah SB, Hughes EG, Oh EJ, et al. Neurotrophin signaling among neurons and glia during formation of tripartate synapses. Neuron Glia Biology 2004; 1:339–349.
78. Charney DS, Manji HK. Life stress, genes and depression: Multiple pathways lead to increased risk and new opportunities for intervention. Sci STKE 2004; 225(re5):1–11.
79. Carter CJ. Multiple genes and factors associated with bipolar disorder converge on growth factor and stress activated kinase pathways controlling translation initiation: Implications for oligodendrocyte viability. Neurochem Int 2007; 50:461–490.
80. Kaufman J, Yang BZ, Douglas-Palumberi H, et al. Brain-derived neurotrophic factor—5HHLPR gene interactions and environmental modifiers of depression in children. Biol Psychiatry 2006; 59:673–680.
81. Pezwas L, Verchinski BA, Mattay VS, et al. The brain-derived neurotrophic factor val66met polymorhism and variation in human cortical morphology. J Neurosci 2004; 24(45):10099–10102.
82. Jabbi M, Korf J, Kema IP, et al. Convergent genetic modulation of the endocrine stress response involves polymorphic variations of 5HTT, COMT, MAO. Mol Psychiatry 2007; 12:483–490.
83. Pezawas L, Meyer-Lindberg A, Drabant E, et al. 5HTTLPR polymorphism impacts human cingulated amygdala interactions: A genetic susceptibility mechanism for depression. Nature Neurosci 2005; 8(6):828–834.
84. Caspi A, Sugden K, Moffitt TE, et al. Influence of life stress on depression: Moderation by a polymorphism in the 5-HTT gene. Science 2003; 301:386–389.
85. Hariri AR, Drabant EM, Munoz KE, et al. A susceptibility gene for affective disorders and the response of the human amygdala. Arch Gen Psychiatry 2005; 62:146–152.
86. Heinz A, Braus DF, Smolka MN, et al. Amygdala-prefrontal coupling depends on a genetic variation of the serotonin transporter. Nature Neurosci 2005; 8(1):20–21.

87. Gotlib IH, Joormann J, Minor KL, et al. HPA axis reactivity: A mechanism underlying the association among 5-HTLPR, stress and depression. Biol Psychiatry 2007; doi: 10.1016/j.biopsych.2007.07.023
88. Frodl T, Schüle C, Schmitt G, et al. Association of the brain-derived neurotrophic factor Val66Met polymorphism with reduced hippocampal volumes in major depression. Arch Gen Psychiatry 2007; 64:410–416.
89. Kim-Cohen J, Caspi A, Taylor A, et al. MAOA, maltreatment, and gene-environment interaction predicting children's mental health: New evidence and a meta-analysis. Mol Psychiatry 2006; 11:903–913.
90. Glolghari VM, Sponheim SR. Divergent backward masking performance in schizophrenia and bipolar disorder: Association with COMT. Am J Med Genet B Neuropsychiatr Genet 2008; 147(2):223–227.
91. Bachmann RF, Schloesser RJ, Gould TD, et al. Mood stabilizers target cellular plasticity and resilience cascades. Mol Neurobiology 2005; 32:173–202.
92. Manji HK, Quiroz JA, Payne JL, et al. The underlying neurobiology of bipolar disorder. World Psychiatry 2003; 2(3):136–146.
93. Adli M, Hollinde DL, Stamm T, et al. Response to lithium augmentation in depression is associated with the glycogen synthase kinase 3-beta-50 T/C single nucleotide polymorphism. Biol Psychiatry 2007; 62(11):1295–1302.
94. Manji HK, Quiroz JA, Sporn J, et al. Enhancing neuronal plasticity and cellular resilience to develop novel improved therapeutics for difficult to treat depression. Biol Psychiatry 2003; 53:707–742.
95. Parker G, Willhelm K, Mitchell P, et al. Predictors of 1-year outcome in depression. Aust N Z J Psychiatry 2000; 34:56–64.
96. Johnson L, Andersson-Lundman G, Aberg-Wistedt A, et al. Age of onset in affective disorder: Its correlation with hereditary and psychosocial factors. J Affect Disord 2000; 59:139–148.
97. Mayberg HS. Positron emission tomography imaging in depression: A neural system perspective. Neuroimag Clin N Am 2003; 13:805–815.
98. Mayberg HS, Liotti M, Brennan SK, et al. Reciprocal limbic-cortical function and negative mood: Converging PET findings in depression and normal sadness. Am J Psychiatry 1999; 156:675–682.
99. Pittenger C, Duman RS. Stress, depression and neuroplasticity: A convergence of mechanisms. Neuropsychopharmacology 2008; 13:88–109.
100. Mitoma M, Yoshimura R, Sugita A, et al. Stress at work alters serum brain-derived neurotrophic factor (BDNF) levels and plasma 3-methoxy-4-hydroxyphenylglycol (MHPG) levels in healthy volunteers: BDNF and MHPG as possible biological markers of mental stress? Prog Neuro-Psychopharmacol Biol Psychiatry 2008; 32:679–85.
101. Nestler EJ, Barrot M, DiLeone RJ, et al. Neurobiology of depression. Neuron 2002; 34:13–25.
102. Kugaya A, Sanacora G. Beyond monoamines: Glutaminergic function in mood disorders. CNS Spectrums 2005; 10:808–819.
103. Brietzke E, Kapczinski F. TNF-alpha as a molecular target in bipolar disorder. Prog Neuro-Psychopharm Biol Psychiatry 2008; doi: 10.1016/j.pnpbp.2008.01.006.
104. Schloesser RJ, Huang J, Klein PS, et al. Cellular plasticity cascades in the pathophysiology and treatment of unipolar disorder. Neuropsychopharmacology 2008; 33:110–133.
105. Weidenfeld J, Newman ME, Itzik A, et al. Adrenocortical axis response to adrenergic and glutamate stimulation are regulated by the amygdala. NeuroReport 2005; 16(11):1245–1249.
106. Rajkowska G, O'Dwyer G, Teleki Z, et al. GABAergic neurons immunoreactive for calcium binding proteins are reduced in the prefrontal cortex in major depression. Neuropsychopharmacology 2007; 32:471–482.
107. Anand A, Li Y, Wang Y, et al. Activity and connectivity of brain mood regulating circuit in depression: A functional magnetic resonance study. Biol Psychiatry 2005; 57:1079–1088.

108. Zisook S, Lesser I, Stewart JW, et al. Effect of age at the onset on the course of major depressive disorder. Am J Psychiatry 2007; 164:1539–1546.
109. Leboyer H, Henry C, Paillere-Martinot M-L, et al. Age of onset in bipolar affective disorders: A review. Bipolar Disorders 2005; 7:111–118.
110. Alexopoulos GS, Meyers BS, Young RC, et al. Clinically defined vascular depression. Am J Psychiatry 1997; 154:562–565.
111. Godin O, Dufouil C, Maillard P, et al. White matter lesions as a predictor of depression in the elderly: The 3 C-Dijon study. Biol Psychiatry 2008; 63:663–669.
112. Sweet RA, Hamilton RL, Butters MA, et al. Neuropathologic correlates of late-onset major depression. Neuropsychopharmacology 2004; 29:2242–2250.
113. Kumar A, Gupta RC, Thomas A, et al. Biophysical changes in normal-appearing white matter and subcortical nuclei in late-life major depression detected using magnetization transfer. Psychiatry Res Neuroimaging 2004; 130:131–140.
114. Bremmer MA, Deeg DJH, Beekman ATF, et al. Major depression in late life associated with both hypo- and hypercortisolemia. Biol Psychiatry 2007; 62(5):479–486.
115. Bremmer MA, Beekman ATF, Deeg DJH, et al. Inflammatory markers in late-life depression: Results from a population-based study. J Affect Disord 2008; 106(3):249–255.
116. Wylie ME, Benoit HM, Pollock BG, et al. Age at onset in geriatric bipolar disorder. Am J geriatr Psychiatry 1999; 7(1):77–83.
117. Zanetti MV, Cordeiro Q, Busatto GF. Late onset bipolar disorder associated with white matter hyperintensities: A pathophysiological hypothesis. Prog Neuro-Psychopharm Biol Psychiatry 2007; 31:551–556.
118. Kennedy JL, Farrer LA, Andreasen NC, et al. The genetics of adult-onset neuropsychiatric disease: Complexities and conundra? Science 2003; 302:822–826.

9 The Interface Between Depression and Dementia

Donald A. Davidoff

Neuropsychological and Psychodiagnostic Testing Service, McLean Hospital, Belmont, and Department of Psychiatry, Harvard Medical School, Boston, Massachusetts, U.S.A.

Manjola Ujkaj

Geriatric Psychiatry Program, McLean Hospital, Belmont, and Department of Psychiatry, Harvard Medical School, Boston, Massachusetts, U.S.A.

INTRODUCTION

In recent years, increasing attention has been directed toward the complex relationships between depression and dementia in the elderly. The predominant research hypothesis has been that depression is a risk factor or even a prodrome for dementia. It is also possible that dementia is a risk factor for depression, that the two disorders share a common etiology, that they are mutually influencing despite separate etiologies, or that their co-occurrence is simply coincidental (1,2). Beyond these theoretical considerations, even the clinical task of distinguishing mood from cognitive symptoms can be a challenge when working with patients whose multiple symptoms, advanced age, medical disease burden, and functional impairment complicate the assessment process. Because both memory complaints and mood complaints are so prevalent among the elderly, a careful and informed process of evaluation and treatment planning is important. This chapter will attempt to shed light on the interrelationships of mood and cognitive disturbances in later life by reviewing normative cognitive changes that occur with aging, examining the varied presentations of depression across the age span and considering biologic, neuroanatomical, and clinical variables affecting the interface between depression and cognition.

HETEROGENEITY OF DEPRESSION IN THE GERIATRIC POPULATION

As individuals age, their unique personality and cognitive characteristics are sculpted by life events, social interactions, work experiences, and medical health, thus magnifying the differences among them. In the same way, clinical presentations of mental disorders become increasingly individualized and heterogeneous. The DSM-IV TR, which provides criteria for diagnosing depression in all age groups (3), recognizes that older individuals present with more prominent cognitive and/or somatic symptoms than younger ones. The DSM requirement that either depressed mood or anhedonia be present in order to diagnose a major depressive episode, however, obstructs identification of those older adults unable to experience or to express these complaints. Thoughts of death, in an older adult, may be associated with a reality-based process of life review and planning, and may not be necessarily indicative of a depressive disorder. In depressed elders characterized by somatic rather than mood symptoms, the focus can erroneously turn to somatic diagnoses and away from recognition of a depressive disorder. Fatigue, pain, insomnia, and appetite changes are all nonspecific symptoms, common, and nondiagnostic in the elderly and potentially associated with either depression, dementia, or neither of these diagnoses. Similarly, cognitive complaints such as memory slips are not necessarily indicative of a dementing process in the elderly. It is not uncommon to observe stability at follow-up in older adults with the mild difficulties considered to represent Age-Related Cognitive Decline.

COGNITIVE DIFFERENCES BETWEEN NORMAL AGING, DEPRESSION, AND DEMENTIA

In typical cognitive aging, there is preservation through the eighth decade of life of crystallized intelligence, defined as the utilization of previously stored information in familiar ways. In contrast, fluid intelligence, which is the use of novel information in unfamiliar or complex ways, begins to decline as early as the fifth decade of life (4,5). In light of evidence that fluid intelligence relies primarily on the efficiency of frontal systems, it would appear that a subclinical "dysexecutive syndrome" manifested by a decline in fluid intelligence may well be common in individuals regarded as aging normally. This change in executive function is likely to form the basis of Age-Related Cognitive Decline encountered in otherwise well-functioning older adults. When subtle changes in executive function are exacerbated by the slowed processing speed typically associated with aging, cognitive impairment may become apparent even though interference with functioning is negligible. Because of the wide range of normative values in older adults, however, caution must be exercised in assigning a diagnosis. These symptoms may represent nonpathologic findings rather than the presence of either a mood disorder or even the cognitive syndrome that sometimes precedes dementia, mild cognitive impairment (MCI).

Dysexecutive function similar to that observed with normal aging or Age-Related Cognitive Decline is also seen in both younger depressed adults and, with greater severity, in older depressed adults. Veiel's meta-analysis of studies of depressed adults younger than 60 years concluded that their depression was associated with reduced mental flexibility, impaired executive function, and a slowed reaction time (4). Consistent findings were more recently reported by Grant et al. (6), who compared healthy nongeriatric controls to nongeriatric patients who met DSM-IV TR criteria for major depressive disorder without psychotic features. In addition, this group reported an association of prolonged reaction time with increasing severity of depression. Lockwood et al. confirmed the presence of a dysexecutive syndrome in depressed older adults and noted its greater severity in this group relative to comparison groups of normal and depressed younger adults and normal elders.

Although slowed reaction time and executive dysfunction may be the symptoms most truly linked with depression, older depressed patients also express concern about memory difficulties that can raise family's and clinicians' concerns about the presence of dementia. Depression does indeed objectively impair memory performance through the effects of abulia, apathy, impaired organization of information, and decreased effort and engagement. Cognitive complaints including forgetfulness in the context of depression were at one time referred to as "depressive pseudodementia" and thought to be reversible with treatment of the underlying mood disorder (7,8). Cummings (9), however, cautioned that the cognitive disturbances associated with depression may not be "pseudo" at all and may, in fact, signify both a genuine impairment in the present as well as an enhanced risk for the subsequent development of dementia that is not depression related. To indicate the significant import of the cognitive symptoms in late-life depression, which can be viewed as a "secondary dementia" to differentiate them from specific primary dementia diagnoses, he recommended the use of the term "dementia syndrome of depression" (DSD) in place of the potentially misleading "pseudodementia."

When a patient reports or shows both mood changes and cognitive symptoms too severe to be explained by normal aging, how best can we determine the presence of depression, dementia, or the combination of these disorders? First, the overlapping cognitive changes of depression and dementia (10) differ in the greater severity of cognitive impairment in demented elders (11) across a range of imposed demands. The depressed patient, whose cognitive dysfunction owes much to abulia or apathy, may reply "I don't know" to less challenging tasks but engage more fully and respond more effectively to tasks of greater difficulty (12). In contrast, cognitive deficits in patients with dementia appear more uniform and less colored by the demand characteristics of the task. Furthermore, the pattern of cognitive deficits between depression and dementia differs in other ways, including the prominence of demonstrable memory impairment in either Alzheimer or Vascular Dementia. In Alzheimer disease (AD), the problem is primarily one of storage of new information, while in vascular dementia difficulties with retrieval predominate. In either type of dementia, however, patients show a higher rate of forgetting over time than do patients with depression (13). Furthermore, patients with dementia tend to make many false-positive errors (incorrectly claiming recall of what never occurred or what was not presented), in contrast to patients with depression, who tend toward false-negative errors (failing to recall what occurred or was presented) (14). Compared to the difference in memory difficulties between normal and depressed elders, the difference between depressed and demented elders' memory impairment is of greater magnitude.

Several nonmemory cognitive domains, too, are significantly more impaired in dementia than in depression in older adults, further aiding differentiation of these two syndromes. In demented patients, characteristic failures are seen on tasks assessing language, visuospatial functioning, executive functioning, and praxis (11). Depressed, nondemented individuals, however, show no measurable differences from healthy elders in regard to expressive and receptive language. While Emery and Breslau (15) did document subtle differences in language functions between depressed and healthy elders, they also noted that such differences were quite small in comparison to the differences between depressed and demented elders. In addition, language difficulties in depression may appear similar but arise from a different source than language difficulties in dementia; for example, productive naming in depressed elders may result from reduced processing speed while the impairment in demented elders may owe more to diminished ability to utilize semantic knowledge (16). Such findings give additional credence to the observation that performance of depressed individuals varies with the demand characteristics of the task.

THE INTERFACE BETWEEN DEPRESSION AND DEMENTIA

While looking through a cognitive lens helps to clarify some similarities and differences between depression and dementia, additional understanding can be gained by exploring several other aspects of the interface between these two illnesses. We will note here observations arising from the comparisons between early-onset and late-onset depression in the elderly, epidemiologic studies of late life depression, neuroimaging studies of atrophy or white matter lesions, and findings regarding the hypothalamic-pituitary-adrenal axis's possible role in depression and dementia.

The possibility that dementia is more closely linked with depression that begins later in life has been raised by studies that distinguish early-onset depression (EOD) from late-onset depression (LOD) and show both clinical and biologic differences between EOD and LOD (1). The diagnosis of late-life depression is assigned when a first episode has occurred at a relatively advanced age, but the threshold age has varied between 45 and 65 years among studies (17). Though findings also vary to some extent, individuals with LOD in comparison with EOD in general less likely to have comorbid psychiatric illnesses (18); more likely to have medical comorbidity (18–21). Of most interest in the present discussion, the cognitive profile of individuals with LOD has been shown to differ from that of individuals with EOD. Greater cognitive impairment in LOD as compared to EOD has been suggested by the preponderance of studies in this area (22–24) indicate that those elders with LOD are more likely to develop dementia than those with EOD. Furthermore, LOD subjects eventually diagnosed with dementia presented with symptoms characterized by motivation-related difficulties including apathy, abulia, decreased energy, and decreased concentration (1). As mentioned earlier, it is those individuals with LOD who are most likely to have such a presentation (21) again supporting the possibility of a relationship between LOD and the subsequent development of dementia. Although two studies fail to confirm the association of LOD with greater severity of cognitive impairment (25,26), these studies were carried out in small cohorts and may have lacked sufficient power to detect differences that would nonetheless be meaningful (27).

Epidemiologic studies including both cross-sectional and longitudinal cohorts also support the notion of a relationship between late-life depression and cognitive impairment or development of dementia. A number of studies suggest that a history of depression is associated with increased risk of developing dementia (28,29). Steffens et al. (29), in particular found that the risk for developing dementia was strengthened significantly when the depressive episode occurred during the two years prior to the diagnosis of dementia. In contrast, Dufouil et al. (30), in a large French community-based study of elders older than 65 years, found no initial relationship between depressive symptoms and cognitive impairment yet documented an association between cognitive impairment and severity of depression at 3-year follow-up. Chen et al. (31), in a U.S.-based elderly sample, suggested that depressive symptoms might be an early manifestation of dementia rather than a predictor.

Neuroimaging studies provide an additional vantage point for examining the interface between depression and dementia. Cerebral atrophy and ventricular enlargement; the well-known findings in dementia (27) have been noted to be present (although less prominent) in depressed elders by Elkis et al. (32) in a meta-analysis of 29 studies. Alexopoulos et al. (33) reported the consistent finding of greater ventricular atrophy in LOD than EOD subjects. This group also noted that the pattern of atrophy in LOD closely resembled that of subjects with AD. Rabins et al. (34) reported confirmatory findings of increased cortical atrophy in subjects with LOD.

Temporal lobe and hippocampal atrophy, findings associated with AD, have been noted in some studies of late-life depression patients as well. Greenwald et al.

(35), for example, found that patients with LOD had significantly more left medial temporal and left caudate atrophy than subjects of similar age with EOD. They also found that greater medial temporal atrophy correlated with later age of depression onset and greater cognitive impairment in these depressives. A larger subsequent study by Ashtari et al. (36), however, did not bear out the original findings despite the incorporation of Greenwald et al.'s (35) data. Kumar et al. (37), furthermore, reported no association between age of onset of depression and cortical atrophy. Thus, reports of the association between cortical atrophy and either the presence of depression or its age of onset are not consistent.

White matter lesions have been associated both with dementia and depression. Deep white matter lesions, in particular, have been reported frequently as a neuroimaging finding characteristic of late-life depression (27). Increased severity of subcortical white matter changes have been associated with LOD but not with EOD (38,39). Salloway et al. (40), found both a greater severity of subcortical white matter changes and more cognitive impairment in LOD than EOD. Lesser et al. (41) demonstrated similar findings and noted that the severity of white matter changes was associated with executive dysfunction. Hickie et al. (42) also found a relationship between white matter changes and age of onset of depression as well as an association between white matter changes and slowed processing speed. In another longitudinal study, Hickie et al. (43), found that 29% of his sample came to develop a probable vascular dementia that was predicted by age of depression onset and severity of white matter changes.

It appears therefore that, in general, white matter changes are positively associated with depression during old age. Severity of the depression is positively correlated with the number of lesions. Depressed patients with white matter changes exhibit greater levels of cognitive impairment than those without such changes (44). Alexopoulos (45) proposed that the cognitive impairments seen in older depressed patients stem from ischemic damage to frontostriatal and frontolimbic circuits. It is well known that damage to these circuits results in a dysexecutive syndrome. White matter changes have also been noted in vascular dementia, and vascular risk factors have been recognized increasingly as relevant to the development of AD (46). The significance of white matter changes in late-onset depression, vascular dementia, and AD, appears worthy of further investigation.

Some additional light may be shed on the interface of depression and dementia by examining the role of the hypothalamic-pituitary-adrenal (HPA) axis. Dysregulation of the HPA axis with consequent hypercortisolemia has been observed in patients both with depression (48) and with AD (49). High levels of circulating glucocorticoids are associated with hippocampal atrophy in humans and with effects on prefrontal cortex in animal studies (50). Both the hippocampi and the prefrontal cortex are recognized as important in learning, and memory and impairment of these areas is implicated in AD. Both depressed and nondepressed (50) patients with hypercortisolemia have been shown to perform more poorly on tests of declarative memory when compared with normal controls. It would appear that involvement of the HPA axis and presence of elevated circulating glucocorticoids might provide a mechanism by which depression could increase cognitive impairment and even serve as a risk factor for vascular dementia or AD.

To sum up, it appears that there is a relationship between late-life, particularly late-onset, depression and dementia. Individuals with LOD are more likely to have cortical atrophy and white matter changes. Individuals with positive findings on neuroimaging are more likely to show cognitive impairment on formal testing than those without such findings. Individuals with positive findings, both on neuroimaging and cognitive testing, may be those at greatest risk for the development of a dementing illness. Thus, depressed individuals with late onset, neuroimaging findings, and impaired cognitive test performance may well have a higher risk of developing dementia than those with EOD, although late-life depression in general is likely correlated with an increased risk for developing dementia.

INTERFACE BETWEEN DEPRESSION AND MCI

MCI represents a clinical entity that has been referred to as an intermediate category between normal cognitive aging and dementia. Several different criteria sets have been used to define MCI, but the currently favored definition criteria are those of Petersen et al. (51) as revised by the Stockholm Consensus Group, (i) presence of cognitive complaint from either the subject and/or family member; (ii) absence of dementia; (iii) change from normal functioning; (iv) decline in any area of cognitive functioning; (v) preserved overall general functioning, but possibly with increasing difficulty in the performance of activities of daily living. These criteria further classify MCI into amnestic and nonamnestic subtypes, each subclassified according to the presence of impairments in single or multiple domains. Despite the increasing literature on the relationship between MCI and dementia, only a few studies have investigated the relationship between MCI and depression. The heterogeneity of both MCI and of late-life depression has contributed to some variability in findings, but several general conclusions are emerging.

One important principle is that depressive symptoms and MCI often coexist and that subjects with MCI have a high prevalence of depressive symptoms (52–54). The very first population-based study investigating the prevalence of neuropsychiatric symptoms in MCI (52) found a prevalence of depressive symptoms of 20%, which was significantly higher than in the general population. In a longitudinal study of older Mexican Americans, Raji et al. (53) found that subjects with clinically relevant depressive symptoms had significantly lower MMSE scores, cross-sectionally. Recently, data from the Italian Longitudinal Study on Aging (54) showed that 87 (63.3%) of the 139 MCI subjects had mild or severe depression as determined by a higher score on the 30-item Geriatric Depression Scale (GDS > 10).

Some studies have shown that depression is a clear risk factor for the development of MCI. Findings from the Cardiovascular Health Study (52,55) showed that subjects with higher prevalence of depressive symptoms at baseline were more likely to develop MCI at 6-year follow-up. The risk of developing MCI increased proportionally with the severity of baseline depressive symptoms from 10.0% to 13.3% to 19.7%, for no-, low-, and moderate- to high-depressive symptoms, respectively. Another prospective study (56) followed a cohort of 840 cognitively normal subjects for a period of 3.5 years and reported that patients who developed depression had more than double the risk of developing MCI during the follow-up. In contrast to the findings of the Cardiovascular Health Study, however, the risk for MCI was not associated with the severity of baseline depressive symptoms. Similarly, data from the Italian Longitudinal Study on Aging (54) failed to show an association between higher symptoms of depression at baseline and risk of incident MCI development at follow-up after 3.5 years.

A related question is whether progression from MCI to dementia is affected by the presence of depression. So far, no clear consensus has emerged from studies that report a variety of findings. In their longitudinal study of seven years, Raji et al. (53) found that subjects with clinically relevant depressive symptoms at baseline, when compared to those without, had a greater and steeper decline in MMSE score during the follow-up. The findings of another longitudinal study (57) showed that MCI subjects with depression were more than twice as likely to develop AD over the three years follow-up as those without depression at baseline. A recent prospective cohort study (54), however, failed to link the presence of baseline depressive symptoms with greater risk for progression of MCI to dementia after a 3.5-year follow-up. Further investigations into this question should focus on the characteristics of the MCI definition, the advantages and disadvantages of instruments used to assess cognitive and mood symptoms, and the relevance of different study populations and designs to outcome.

CONCLUSIONS

In answer to the questions posed at this chapter's beginning, the precise nature of the interface between depression and dementia remains uncertain. Each of the hypotheses proposed there is supported by at least some convincing evidence. Chodosh et al. (47), for example, concluded that depressive symptomatology can predict which older adults will experience cognitive decline in the future, suggesting that depression is a risk factor for dementia; Steffens et al. (29) noted that some late-life depressive symptoms are early manifestations of dementia, indicating a prodromal relationship; Sachs-Ericsson (58) sees the relationship as mutually influencing, noting both that depressive symptoms predict subsequent cognitive decline and that awareness of cognitive decline may provoke reactive depression; Wright and Persad (1) review the relationship between the HPA axis and depression and dementia underscoring the possibility of shared pathophysiology; Butters (59) has investigated the possibility of genetic factors (ApoE) suggesting that such factors may influence the age-of-onset of depression; and Lockwood et al. (60) conclude that the relationship between depression and dementia may be merely coincidental.

Further elucidation of the depression/dementia interface can be aided by use of clear and less ambiguous terminology. In the interest of facilitating communication about the various syndromes in which both cognitive impairment and mood symptoms are seen concomitantly, we propose the following as a nosology for these conditions:

1. Reserve the term "*major depressive disorder*" for those elders who meet DSM-IV TR criteria for that disorder and who have no objective cognitive findings on formal cognitive testing, even if they complain of slowness, forgetfulness, or executive dysfunction. Consider specifying whether the depression is of late or early onset in order to facilitate understanding of the relationships between age of onset and various concomitant or prognostic features of depression.
2. Reserve the term "*mild cognitive impairment with depression*" for those elders who meet diagnostic criteria for major depressive disorder and show evidence of cognitive impairment on neuropsychologic evaluation.
3. Reserve the term "*dementia with depression*" for individuals with the dual diagnoses of a dementia and major depressive disorder whether of late or early onset.
4. Discontinue the use of the terms "*pseudodementia*" and "*dementia syndrome of depression*" as confusing and noncontributory to our understanding.

REFERENCES

1. Wright SL, Persad C. Distinguishing between depression and dementia in older persons: Neuropsychological and neuropathological correlates. J Geriatr Psychiatry Neurol 2007; 20(4):189–198.
2. Jorm AF. Is depression a risk factor for dementia or cognitive decline? A review. Gerontology 2000; 46(4):219–227.
3. American Psychiatric Association. Diagnostic and Statistical Manual of Mental Disorders, 4th ed. Text Revision. Washington, D.C.: American Psychiatric Association, 2000.
4. Veiel HO. A preliminary profile of neuropsychological deficits associated with major depression. J Clin Exp Neuropsychol 1997; 19(4):587–603.
5. Lawrence J, Davidoff D, Berlow J. Diagnosing depression in later life. In: Ellison JM, Verma S, eds. Depression in Later Life: A multidisciplinary Psychiatric Approach. New York, NY: Marcel Dekker, 2003:55–78.
6. Grant MM, Thase ME, Sweeney JA. Cognitive disturbance in outpatient depressed younger adults: Evidence of modest impairment. Biol Psychiatry 2001; 50(1):35–43.
7. Lamberty GJ, Bieliauskas LA. Distinguishing between depression and dementia in the elderly: A review of neuropsychological findings. Arch Clin Neuropsychol 1993; 8(2):149–170.
8. Kiloh LG. Pseudo-dementia. Acta Psychiatr Scand 1961; 37:336–351.
9. Cummings JL. Dementia and depression: An evolving enigma. J Neuropsychiatry Clin Neurosci 1989; 1(3):236–242.
10. Bäckman L, Jones S, Berger AK, et al. Cognitive impairment in preclinical Alzheimer's disease: A meta-analysis. Neuropsychology 2005; 19(4):520–531.
11. Crowe SF, Hoogenraad K. Differentiation of dementia of the Alzheimer's type from depression with cognitive impairment on the basis of a cortical versus subcortical pattern of cognitive deficit. Arch Clin Neuropsychol 2000; 15(1):9–19.
12. Bazin N, Perruchet P, De Bonis M, et al. The dissociation of explicit and implicit memory in depressed patients. Psychol Med 1994; 24(1):239–245.
13. King DA, Caine ED, Conwell Y, et al. The neuropsychology of depression in the elderly: A comparative study of normal aging and Alzheimer's disease. J Neuropsychiatry Clin Neurosci 1991 Spring; 3(2):163–168.
14. Budson AE, Todman RW, Schacter DL. Gist memory in Alzheimer's disease: Evidence from categorized pictures. Neuropsychology 2006; 20(1):113–122.
15. Emery OB, Breslau LD. Language deficits in depression: Comparisons with SDAT and normal aging. J Gerontol 1989; 44(3):M85–M92.
16. Hart RP, Kwentus JA, Taylor JR, et al. Productive naming and memory in depression and Alzheimer's type dementia. Arch Clin Neuropsychol 1988; 3(4):313–22.
17. Lyness JM, Noel TK, Cox C, et al. Screening for depression in elderly primary care patients. A comparison of the Center for Epidemiologic Studies—Depression Scale and the Geriatric Depression Scale. Arch Intern Med 1997; 157(4):449–454.
18. Lyness JM, Conwell Y, King DA, et al. Age of onset and medical illness in older depressed inpatients. Int Psychogeriatr 1995; 7(1):63–73.
19. Emery VO, Oxman TE. Update on the dementia spectrum of depression. Am J Psychiatry 1992; 149(3):305–317.
20. Krishnan KR, Hays JC, Tupler LA, et al. Clinical and phenomenological comparisons of late-onset and early-onset depression. Am J Psychiatry 1995; 152(5):785–788.
21. Heun R, Kockler M, Papassotiropoulos A. Distinction of early- and late-onset depression in the elderly by their lifetime symptomatology. Int J Geriatr Psychiatry 2000; 15(12):1138–1142.
22. Alexopoulos GS, Young RC, Meyers BS. Geriatric depression: Age of onset and dementia. Biol Psychiatry 1993; 34(3):141–145.
23. van Ojen R, Hooijer C, Jonker C, et al. Late-life depressive disorder in the community, early onset and the decrease of vulnerability with increasing age. J Affect Disord 1995; 33(3):159–166.

24. van Reekum R, Simard M, Clarke D, et al. Late-life depression as a possible predictor of dementia: Cross-sectional and short-term follow-up results. Am J Geriatr Psychiatry 1999 Spring; 7(2):151–159.
25. Baldwin B. Age of onset of depression in the elderly. Br J Psychiatry 1990; 156:445–446.
26. Holroyd S, Duryee JJ. Differences in geriatric psychiatry outpatients with early- vs. late-onset depression. Int J Geriatr Psychiatry 1997; 12(11):1100–1106.
27. Schweitzer I, Tuckwell V, O'Brien J, et al. Is late onset depression a prodrome to dementia? Int J Geriatr Psychiatry 2002; 17(11):997–1005.
28. Jorm AF, van Duijn CM, Chandra V, et al. Psychiatric history and related exposures as risk factors for Alzheimer's disease: A collaborative re-analysis of case-control studies: EURODEM Risk Factors Research Group. Int J Epidemiol 1991; 20:S43–S47.
29. Steffens DC, Plassman BL, Helms MJ, et al. A twin study of late-onset depression and apolipoprotein E e4 as risk factors for Alzheimer's disease. Biol Psychiatry 1997; 41:851–856.
30. Dufouil C, Fuhrer R, Dartigues JF, Alpérovitch A. Longitudinal analysis of the association between depressive symptomotology and cognitive deterioration. Am J Epidemiol 1996; 144:634–641.
31. Chen P, Ganguli M, Mulstan BH, et al. The temporal relationship between depressive symptoms and dementia. Arch Gen Psychiatry 1999; 56:261–266.
32. Elkis H, Friedman L, Wise A, et al. Meta-analyses of studies of ventricular enlargement and cortical sulcal prominence in mood disorders. Comparisons with controls or patients with schizophrenia. Arch Gen Psychiatry 1995; 52(9):735–746.
33. Alexopoulos GS, Young RC, Shindledecker RD. Brain computed tomography findings in geriatric depression and primary degenerative dementia. Biol Psychiatry 1992; 31(6):591–599.
34. Rabins PV, Pearlson GD, Aylward E., et al. Cortical magnetic resonance imaging changes in elderly inpatients with major depression. Am J Psychiatry 1991; 148:617–620.
35. Greenwald BS, Kramer-Ginsberg E, Krishnan KRR, et al. MRI signal hyperintensities in geriatric depression. Am J Psychiatry 1996; 153:1212–1215.
36. Ashtari M, Greenwald BS, Kramer-Ginsberg E, et al. Hippocampal/amygdala volumes in geriatric depression. Psychol Med 1999; 29(3):629–638.
37. Kumar R, Parslow RA, Jorm AF, et al. Clinical and neuroimaging correlates of mild cognitive impairment in a middle-aged community sample: The personality and total health through life 60 + study. Dement Geriatr Cogn Disord 2006; 21(1):44–50.
38. Figiel GS, Krishnan KR, Koraiswamy PM, et al. Subcortical hyperintensities on brain magnetic resonance imaging: A comparison between late age onset and early onset elderly depressed subjects. Neurbiol Aging 1991; 12:245–247.
39. O'Brien JT, Ames D. White matter lesions in depression and Alzheimer's disease. Br J Psychiatry 1996; 169(5):671.
40. Salloway S, Malloy P, Kohn R. MRI and neuropsychological differences in early- and late-life-onset geriatric depression. Neurology 1996; 46(6):1567–1574.
41. Lesser IM, Boone KB, Mehringer CM. Cognition and white matter hyperintensities in older depressed patients. Am J Psychiatry 1996; 153:1280–1287.
42. Hickie I, Scott E, Mitchell P, et al. Subcortical hyperintensities on magnetic resonance imaging: Clinical correlates and prognostic significance in patients with severe depression. Biol Psychiatry 1995; 37:151–160.
43. Hickie I, Scott E, Wilhelm K, et al. Subcortical hyperintensities on magnetic resonance imaging in patients with severe depression: A longitudinal evaluation. Biol Psychiatry 1997; 42(5):367–374.
44. Baldwin RC, Walker S, Simpson SW, et al. The prognostic significance of abnormalities seen on magnetic resonance imaging in late life depression: Clinical outcome, mortality and progression to dementia at three years. Int J Geriatr Psychiatry 2000; 15:1097–1104.
45. Alexopoulos GS. The vascular depression hypothesis: 10 years later. Biol Psychiatry 2006; 60(12):1304–1305.
46. Breteler MM. Vascular risk factors for Alzheimer's disease: An epidemiologic perspective. Neurbiol Aging 2000; 21:153–160.

47. Chodosh J, Kado DM, Seeman TE, et al. Depressive symptoms as a predictor of cognitive decline: MacArthur Studies of Successful Aging. Am J Geriatr Psychiatry 2007; 15(5):406–415.
48. Davis KL, Davis BM, Greenwald BS, et al. Cortisol and Alzheimer's disease: I: Basal studies. Am J Psychiatry 1986; 143:300–305.
49. Belanoff JK, Gross K, Yager A, et al. Corticosteroids and cognition. J Psychiatric Res 2001; 35:127–145.
50. O'Brien JT, Schweitzer I, Ames D, et al. Cortisol suppression by dexamethasone in the healthy elderly: Effects of age, dexamethasone levels, and cognitive function. Biol Psychiatry 1994; 36:389–394.
51. Petersen RC, Winblad B, Palmer K, et al. Mild cognitive impairment–beyond controversies, towards a consensus: Report of the International Working Group on Mild Cognitive Impairment. J Intern Med 2004; 256(3):240–246.
52. Lyketsos CG, Lopez O, Jones B, et al. Prevalence of neuropsychiatric symptoms in dementia and mild cognitive impairment: Results from the cardiovascular health study. JAMA 2002; 288(12):1475–1483.
53. Raji MA, Reyes-Ortiz CA, Kuo YF, et al. Depressive symptoms and cognitive change in older Mexican Americans. J Geriatr Psychiatry Neurol 2007; 20(3):145–152.
54. Solfrizzi V, D'Introno A, Colacicco AM, et al. Italian Longitudinal Study on Aging Working Group. Incident occurrence of depressive symptoms among patients with mild cognitive impairment: The Italian longitudinal study on aging. Dement Geriatr Cogn Disord 2007; 24(1):55–64.
55. Barnes DE, Alexopoulos GS, Lopez OL, et al. Depressive symptoms, vascular disease, and mild cognitive impairment: Findings from the Cardiovascular Health Study. Arch Gen Psychiatry 2006; 63(3):273–279.
56. Geda YE, Knopman DS, Mrazek DA, et al. Depression, apolipoprotein E genotype, and the incidence of mild cognitive impairment: A prospective cohort study. Arch Neurol 2006; 63(3):435–440.
57. Modrego PJ, Ferrández J. Depression in patients with mild cognitive impairment increases the risk of developing dementia of Alzheimer type: A prospective cohort study. Arch Neurol 2004; 61(8):1290–1293.
58. Sachs-Ericsson N, Joiner T, Plant EA, et al. The influence of depression on cognitive decline in community-dwelling elderly persons. Am J Geriatr Psychiatry 2005; 13(5):402–408.
59. Butters MA, Sweet RA, Mulsant BH, et al. APOE is associated with age-of-onset, but not cognitive functioning, in late-life depression. Int J Geriatr Psychiatry 2003; 18(12):1075–1081.
60. Lockwood KA, Alexopoulos GS, van Gorp WG. Executive dysfunction in geriatric depression. Am J Psychiatry 2002; 159(7):1119–1126.

10 The Vascular Depression Concept and Its Implications

Robert Emmett Kelly, Jr.* **and George S. Alexopoulos**
Weill Medical College of Cornell University, New York, New York, U.S.A.

INTRODUCTION

The vascular depression hypothesis, as stated by Alexopoulos et al., a decade ago, was that cerebrovascular disease may predispose, precipitate, or perpetuate some geriatric depressive syndromes (1). The hypothesis called attention to the possibility that vascular factors may contribute to depression. This broad hypothesis was not meant to be tested explicitly in research studies; rather, it was meant to serve as a conceptual platform on which to build specific hypotheses that can be tested experimentally. The hypothesis has served as a guide in the generation of studies of the epidemiology, pathogenesis, clinical presentation, outcomes, and treatment of a large subgroup of geriatric patients with depression. In this chapter we examine vascular depression–related research and developments, with an eye to clinical implications and possible future research.

DEFINITION OF VASCULAR DEPRESSION

The past decade of vascular depression research has involved a search for useful definitions of depression whose etiology is thought to be closely linked to vascular issues. Because the precise biological mechanisms leading to depression are unknown (1), any definition of vascular depression will necessarily be both overly inclusive and not inclusive enough to perfectly identify a homogeneous group sharing common etiology and pathogenesis. However, preliminary diagnostic categories are necessary in order to guide hypothesis testing and provide a common ground on which to compare study findings. These categories can and should be modified or discarded as dictated by the weight of contemporary research findings, continually reflecting our refined understanding of the relationship between cerebrovascular disease and depression.

In addition to the broad vascular depression hypothesis, Alexopoulos et al. proposed a working clinical definition of vascular depression (1) involving two cardinal features: (*i*) depression onset after 65 years of age or change in the course of depression (development of more frequent and persistent depressive episodes) after the onset of vascular disease in patients with early-onset depression; and (*ii*) clinical and/or laboratory evidence of vascular disease or vascular risk factors. Examples of

*This work was supported by NIMH grants RO1 MH079414, RO1 MH075897, P30 MH068638, T32 MH19132, the Sanchez Foundation, and the TRU Foundation, US.

clinical manifestations included history of stroke or transient ischemic attacks, focal neurologic signs, atrial fibrillation, angina, history of myocardial infarction, carotid bruit, hypertension, and hyperlipidemia. Examples of pertinent laboratory findings included evidence of infarcts or carotid occlusion or stenosis of the Willis Circle arteries and significant white matter intensities at the territory of the perforating arteries. Secondary vascular depression features (features expected to be present in most, but not all patients with vascular depression) included in the definition were (*i*) cognitive impairment consisting of, but not limited to, disturbance of executive functions, i.e., planning, organizing, sequencing, and abstracting; (*ii*) psychomotor retardation; (*iii*) limited depressive ideation, e.g., guilt; (*iv*) poor insight; (*v*) disability; and (*vi*) absence of family history of mood disorders.

This definition of vascular depression attempts to identify individuals with depression consequent to cerebrovascular disease, with good sensitivity and specificity. It is overly inclusive because for some individuals with late-onset depression and signs of cerebrovascular disease (or conditions associated with cerebrovascular disease) the depression might not actually be related to cerebrovascular disease. It is not inclusive enough because for some individuals late-onset depression may be caused, at least in part, by cerebrovascular disease without clinical or laboratory evidence of cerebrovascular disease and without any signs of cardiovascular disease, hypertension, or hyperlipidemia.

THE EVIDENCE LEADING TO THE VASCULAR DEPRESSION HYPOTHESIS

The rationale for the vascular depression hypothesis was based on a combination of epidemiologic data, clinical correlates, and neuroimaging findings supporting the view that there exists a relationship between cerebrovascular disease and depression.

Epidemiologic Data

Depression is common in patients with vascular and cerebrovascular disease. A temporal connection between cerebrovascular disease and admission to a psychiatric hospital was noted in early studies, where cerebrovascular disease occurred two to three years prior to admission (2,3). Stroke is often accompanied by depression (4–9). Hackett et al. (10) reported that approximately 33% of stroke survivors suffered from depression. One study of 248 coronary bypass patients found that depressive symptoms were present in 43% of the patients before surgery and in 68% after (1,11). Also, vascular and cerebrovascular disease is frequent in elderly patients with depression (12). In a large study of primary care patients, vascular disease was more common among depressed than nondepressed patients (13). A large recent prospective study (14) found a significant association between depression and increased risk of ischemic stroke, even after adjusting for inflammatory markers (C-reactive protein).

A natural consequence of the vascular depression hypothesis is that one would expect a higher incidence of cerebrovascular disease with late-life depression. This expectation is supported by previous studies. Depression is highly prevalent in patients with conditions associated with cerebrovascular disease, including hypertension (15), coronary artery disease (16), and vascular dementia (17). Patients with late-onset depression were found to have more vascular risk factors than elderly patients with early-onset depression (18), although negative findings also exist (19). Late-onset bipolar disorders often are associated with vascular and degenerative brain disease and negative family history of mood disorders (20).

Alexopoulos et al. have also proposed that late-onset depression includes a group of patients with neurologic disorders that may not be clinically evident when the depression first appears (1). This position has been supported by studies showing that patients with late-onset depression have more neuropsychological (21,22) and neuroradiologic abnormalities (23–25), higher morbidity and mortality (26,27), greater disability (28), and lower familial prevalence of mood disorders (29) than elderly patients with early-onset depression. Some studies have not supported the association between late-onset depression and high neurologic morbidity, possibly due to study limitations (e.g., inclusion of nonvascular depression patients in the late-onset samples) (1).

Clinical Findings

Vascular depression tends to manifest itself differently than nonvascular depression. Patients with late-onset major depression and vascular risk factors appear to have more psychomotor retardation, less agitation and guilt, poorer insight, greater impairment in frontal functions, and more disability than elderly patients with early-onset depression without vascular risk factors (30,31). In general, treatment response (particularly to antidepressant medications) has been poorer in the vascular depression group (24,32–38), but negative findings also exist (33,39,40). As noted below, the responses to specific classes of medication and psychotherapy may also differ in the vascular depression group.

Neuroimaging Findings

A number of neuroimaging findings support the vascular depression hypothesis. In a Japanese sample, silent cerebral infarcts were observed in 59 (94%) of 63 patients with late-onset depression (41). In a study of 35 depressed elderly patients without neurologic history, 14 (40%) were found to have lesions of the thalamus and basal ganglia, whereas only 1 of 22 normal elderly volunteers had such lesions (42).

In some cases, depression may be the only manifestation of stroke. "Silent" stroke is far more common than manifest stroke in the elderly, occurring five times more often than brain infarcts with peripheral neurologic signs according to a Dutch study by Vermeer et al. (43). In a U.S. elderly, noninstitutionalized population sample, the Cardiovascular Health Study (44) of 3327 people aged 65 years and older without previous history of transient ischemic attack or stroke, 28% showed MRI-evidence of previous infarcts; 81% of these had lacunes only (45). Those with silent lacunes had more cognitive dysfunction than those without any brain infarcts.

White Matter Hyperintensities

White matter hyperintensities (WMHs) are areas of increased intensity on T2-weighted magnetic resonance imaging (MRI). They represent areas of demyelination and/or enlargement of perivascular spaces, and are often associated with evidence of ischemia (cellular loss, glial and macrophage response) on post-mortem histologic analysis (46). Nonvascular causes of WMHs, such as demyelinating disorders also occur. WMHs are often classified by location as being either periventricular white matter hyperintensities (PWMHs) or deep white matter hyperintensities (DWMHs). PWMHs differ from DWMHs in that they are usually due to ependymal loss, with associated subependymal demyelination and gliosis (46). DWMHs (in the dorsolateral prefrontal cortex) were more frequently found to be of ischemic nature among depressed elderly patients (47), while PWMHs were not (48), and DWMHs, but not PWMHs were associated with depressive symptoms (49).

The relationship between atherosclerosis and ischemic WMHs has not been clearly established due to limited sample sizes in post-mortem histologic analyses, but WMHs have been more common in patients with cerebrovascular disease (50) and have been associated with factors related to cerebrovascular disease, such as cardiac disease (51), hypertension (50,52,53), smoking (53), and reduced cerebral blood flow (51). Executive dysfunction (54–56) and disability (57,58) have been associated with WMHs, and worsening of WMHs in a sample of 1919 elderly subjects from the Cardiovascular Health Study who had two MRIs over a 5-year period was associated with cognitive decline over the same period compared with subjects who had no worsening in WMH grade (59).

Whether WMHs are a cause of or a marker for vascular depression is not yet clear, but a number of studies have found that elderly patients with depression have WMHs more often than nondepressed patients (24,42,60–64), especially in frontal and temporal regions (65), although negative findings exist (66). Depressed elderly with late-onset depression had significantly larger subcortical white matter lesions than elderly with early-onset depression (67). Two studies of fractional anisotropy (a measure of white matter integrity) found significantly lower fractional anisotropy in specific frontal regions of elderly depressed subjects compared with elderly controls. Those regions were the right superior frontal gyrus (68) and the anterior cingulate cortex, left middle frontal gyrus and the superior frontal gyri, bilaterally (69).

Some studies have documented an association between MR-signs of white matter damage and poorer remission of depression and response to antidepressant medication. Increases in WMH volume over a 2-year period were associated with significantly lower rates of sustained remission of late-life depression over the same period; (70) lower fractional anisotropy in distributed cerebral networks was associated with poor antidepressant response in geriatric depression; (71,72) and dilatation of Virchow-Robin spaces (indicating damage in white matter) predicted nonresponse to antidepressant monotherapy with 80% sensitivity and 62% specificity (73).

DISEASES AND SYNDROMES RELATED TO VASCULAR DEPRESSION

Since 1997, two main disorders related to the general vascular depression concept (not the specific working definition described above) have received considerable attention—subcortical ischemic depression (SID) and depression-executive dysfunction syndrome (DED). Neither definition is sensitive enough to include all individuals whose late-life depression is related to cerebrovascular disease or specific enough to exclude individuals whose depression is not related to cerebrovascular disease. However, each of these syndromes identifies a group of depressed individuals whose clinical characteristics, prognosis, and treatment response as a group differ from those found for other depressed elderly individuals. There is considerable overlap between the two groups in the patients identified by each of the definitions. Not surprisingly, the clinical characteristics and treatment implications for each group are similar. Below follows a description of each of the syndromes and some advantages that each definition offers in describing and understanding vascular depression.

Subcortical Ischemic Depression

Subcortical ischemic depression, proposed by Krishnan et al. (52), is a condition defined by the combination of depression and MRI-evidence of subcortical ischemic changes. It is a type of vascular depression. This definition comprises patients with reliable indications of ischemia: diffuse (score 3 on the Coffey classification system) subcortical grey matter hyperintense lesions (SGMHLs) and DWMHs scored as 2 (beginning confluence of foci) or 3 (large confluent areas). Punctate (score 1) DWMHs and SGMHLs as well as multipunctate (score 2) SGMHLs are not counted toward the diagnosis of SID as they are not considered reliable enough indications of ischemia, even though they can represent ischemia. In a post-mortem histopathologic study by Thomas et al. (74), all of the punctate DWMHs found in the brains of elderly depressed individuals were assessed as ischemic, but this only represented nine punctate lesions found in four depressed individuals—too small a sample to draw conclusions concerning the rate of ischemia in punctate lesions in the depressed elderly population. The same study found only one-third of punctate DWMHs to be ischemic in a corresponding sample of nondepressed elderly subjects.

Rationale for the Focus on Subcortical Regions

The search for a relationship between depression and lesions in specific areas of the brain has given mixed results. A meta-analysis by Carson et al. including 35 studies (out of 143 studies of poststroke depression and lesion location) did not find any difference between the rate of depression for left compared with right hemispheric lesions (75). Among the fewer studies that also reported where lesions occurred (anterior, intermediate, or posterior areas of the brain) no differences were found in the rates of depression based on location; but as Roman (76) points out, in most of those studies, stroke location was determined using anatomically inaccurate methods (CT-scan estimates of the distances from the frontal poles) and subcortical lesions were not included. Studies focusing on subcortical lesions have found an increased rate of depression for lesions in the basal ganglia, particularly the caudate and putamen, regions involved with frontal-subcortical circuits (42,77,78). The subcortical disorders, Parkinson disease and Huntington disease, show elevated incidence of depression beyond what would be expected in other equally disabling disorders, with depression frequently preceding the disorders (79). Subcortical vascular dementia results in depression more often than cortical dementias; subcortical dementias result in depression more often than Alzheimer dementia; (80) and Alzheimer patients with subcortical atrophy are more likely to become depressed than those without (81). These findings support the view that subcortical lesions, even more so than lesions in other regions of the brain, increase the risk of depression.

Advantages and Limitations of the SID Definition

A main advantage of the SID definition, as argued by Taylor et al. (82), is that in addition to describing a disease in phenomenological terms (largely the current approach in psychiatry today), it describes disease in terms of pathology presumed to be involved in the etiology of the disease. Thus, SID represents a movement from the nominalist to the essentialist method for describing disease—a movement toward understanding the underlying causes of a disease rather than merely describing its manifestations. Taylor et al. point out that the 2-tier system involving one axis for disease manifestation and another for disease etiology forms the basis for the World Health Organization (WHO) classification of diseases, and that the general approach of directing treatments toward underlying causes has become the mainstay of modern medicine. Thus, although the SID definition has its limitations and may well be replaced as our knowledge grows, it represents one step toward an essentialist approach for psychiatry, following examples from other medical disciplines. SID involves a measurable biological abnormality, so it may lend itself readily to verification of treatment effects (aimed at improving cerebrovascular integrity).

One limitation of the SID definition is that it excludes types of vascular depression caused by damage to other areas of the brain. Besides subcortical areas, geriatric depression has also been associated with left frontal lesions (83), WMHs in the medial orbitofrontal cortex, abnormalities in neurons of the dorsolateral prefrontal cortex, and low brain volumes in the hippocampus, subgenual anterior cingulate, and orbitofrontal cortex (81). Subcortical regions interact with the frontal cortex through numerous pathways and damage anywhere along these pathways might predispose an individual toward the development of depression.

Another limitation of the SID definition is that it must necessarily be overly inclusive: The coexistence of depression and ischemic brain lesions does not mean that the two are related to each other in every case. As ischemic lesions are often found in the nondepressed elderly, it stands to reason that some elderly patients with depression due to nonvascular causes will also have unrelated ischemic brain lesions.

Depression-Executive Dysfunction Syndrome

Depression-executive dysfunction syndrome, proposed by Alexopoulos et al. (84), is a condition defined by the combination of depression and evidence of executive dysfunction. In their paper on DED, Alexopoulos et al., evaluated executive dysfunction using the initiation/perseveration domain of the Dementia Rating Scale (DRS). Specifically, executive dysfunction was defined by a score of one standard deviation below the mean DRS score for a group of 31 elderly subjects without history or presence of psychiatric disorders (mean 36.04; standard deviation 1.81). Depression was defined by meeting research diagnostic criteria and DSM-IV criteria for unipolar major depression, and scoring 18 or higher on the 24-item Hamilton Rating Scale for Depression (Ham-D). With DED, the focus is on functional rather than on physical or biological abnormalities. DED extends beyond the vascular depression concept because the functional abnormalities can be caused by vascular insults or any pathology that compromises the integrity of brain circuitry involved in executive brain function.

Rationale for the Focus on Executive Dysfunction

Executive dysfunction and late-onset depression are frequently comorbid conditions (85–88). Although cognitive functions are frequently compromised in both young and elderly depressed patients compared with normal controls, the executive tasks of response inhibition and sustained effort are more frequently impaired in geriatric depression, as reflected by abnormal initiation/perseveration scores in approximately 40% of elderly depressed patients (81). Baseline executive dysfunction and long latency of the P300 auditory evoked potential (a measure of prefrontal function) predicted poor response to six weeks of antidepressant treatment (36). In another sample, executive function evaluated with initiation/perseveration or

Stroop Color-Word scores was associated with poor citalopram response in geriatric depression (89). Impaired response inhibition (a fundamental component of executive function), but not other neuropsychological dysfunctions, also predicted poor response to citalopram treatment (90). Baseline executive dysfunction also predicted greater rates of relapse and recurrence of major depression among elderly subjects in remission (91), while memory impairment, disability, medical burden, social support, and history of previous episodes were not significantly associated with the outcome of depression.

Executive dysfunction, like other symptoms and signs frequently associated with depression, improves as depression subsides, but generally persists even after remission of depression (92–95). For some depressed elderly patients, executive dysfunction is a stable clinical characteristic, accentuated during episodes of depression, but rarely returns to normal. The close relationship between geriatric depression and executive dysfunction is an indication that the impairments underlying executive dysfunction might be integral to mechanisms perpetuating depression, at least for some individuals. Those impairments may be due to damage of specific neural pathways.

Disorders of the basal ganglia and their prefrontal projections are frequently complicated by executive dysfunction and depression (84). Lesions to frontal and subcortical regions have been associated with executive dysfunction and with depression (96,97). A large recent meta-analysis (98) found a significant inverse correlation between severity of poststroke depression during the first six months after stroke and distance from the frontal pole among patients with left hemisphere stroke. The authors cited their focus on short-term symptom severity (first six months poststroke) as a possible reason for why their results were different than in the Carson et al. study, mentioned above; they also mentioned that a reappraisal of the Carson et al. study, adding some studies they felt met the Carson et al. inclusion criteria, resulted in finding that poststroke depression was significantly more common with left anterior lesions compared with left posterior lesions and compared with right anterior lesions. These studies support the view that damage to frontal regions, in addition to subcortical regions, is associated with vascular depression.

Elderly depressed patients with executive dysfunction have more pronounced psychomotor retardation and reduced interest in activities compared to depressed patients without executive dysfunction, a clinical presentation that resembles medial frontal lobe syndromes (84). Damage to fronto-striato-limbic networks is hypothesized to be related to both executive dysfunction and depression (1). Five such frontostriatal circuits have been described (79,99). These circuits run from the cortex to the basal ganglia, the globus pallidus, the thalamus, and back to the cortex again. Neurotransmitters involved in these circuits include GABA, enkephalins, and glutamate, with dopamine and acetylcholine serving a modulating role. As these circuits are involved in positive affect-guided anticipation, their loss could predispose to depression through failure to anticipate incentives (30).

Advantages and Limitations of the DED Definition

With DED, the focus is on measurement of a brain function rather than on a "physically" measurable quantity. As such, this approach involves more difficult measurement and quantification issues than SID, but it also offers some potential advantages. It is difficult, if not impossible, to predict whether or not a particular brain lesion will result in depression. This difficulty is due in part to brain plasticity and interindividual variations in brain function, as well as variations in environmentally and genetically determined resilience to depression. Rather than measuring extent of brain lesions as an approximation for loss of brain function that can predispose to depression, it may prove more fruitful in some cases to measure loss of brain function directly. Such measures could prove more relevant and might be flexible enough to encompass a wider range of pathologic mechanisms that can lead to loss of brain function and depression.

Common Elements of Disorders in the Vascular Depression Family

The literature on DED often refers to DED under the heading of "vascular depression" (100), but because DED does not require evidence of vascular disease, one might question the appropriateness of describing DED as a member of the "vascular depression family" of disorders. However, for the sake of this discussion, we will consider DED to belong to that family. Executive dysfunction is common in patients with vascular lesions (76), so there is considerable overlap in patients meeting criteria for DED and other definitions of vascular depression. DED shares with other members of this family the concept of a form of depression that is associated with damage to specific neural pathways. As such, DED and the entire vascular depression family integrate well with biologically-oriented exploration of brain function.

Considerable evidence in the literature, as described above, supports the view that late-life depression, particularly if late in onset or accompanied by signs of vascular disease or executive dysfunction, includes a large subgroup of individuals whose depression differs from early-onset depression in its clinical characteristics and treatment response. These differences in clinical characteristics and treatment response as manifested in groupwise experimental comparisons are similar across studies despite differences in the definitions of vascular depression. For example, patients with vascular depression compared with nonvascular depression, as defined by a brain-MRI–based definition of vascular depression (58), more often had older age, late age at onset, anhedonia, and disability, and less often had psychosis or a family history of mental illness. A later case-control study (involving 139 depressed elderly subjects) of the SID variant of vascular depression (seen in 54% of the subjects) found a positive association for SID with older age, lassitude (from the Montgomery Asberg Depression Rating Scale (101), "difficulty in getting started or slowness initiating and performing everyday activities"), history of hypertension, and Instrumental Activities of Daily Living (IADL, a measure of executive function); and a negative association with loss of libido or a family history of mental illness (52). The relationship between SID and impaired IADL in that study no longer held after controlling for the other factors in a logistic regression. A clinical study involving 126 elderly subjects with major depression found that those who met criteria for DED significantly more often than those without DED had older age, loss of interest in activities, psychomotor retardation, reduced fluency, impaired visual naming, paranoia, and impaired IADL (84). Finally, a comparison of patients with late-onset depression with recurrent early-onset depression found more anhedonia, executive dysfunction, and cardiovascular disease, but better episodic memory among those with late-onset depression (102).

TREATMENT IMPLICATIONS

The generally poorer treatment response in vascular depression, at least for our usual first-line treatments (e.g., SSRIs), motivates the search for better and possibly different treatment strategies for this subgroup of depressed patients. However, no expert consensus on the subject exists and current data are too preliminary to draw fixed conclusions and offer sufficiently validated recommendations. The evaluation of an elderly patient with depression, possibly related to vascular issues, follows the same guidelines as for other geriatric psychiatry patients (30,81). Here, we mention certain issues that deserve attention due to the possibility of comorbid vascular disease in virtually any elderly patient (including "silent" cardiovascular disease).

A recent review on the relationship between vascular disease and depression (103) concluded that depression has a clear bidirectional relationship with vascular diseases, finding that preexisting vascular disease predicted the onset of depression and preexisting depression predicted the onset of cardiovascular disease and stroke in a great majority of studies. To break a potential vicious cycle, optimal treatment of elderly depression or cardiovascular disease should involve a two-pronged approach, addressing depression and cardiovascular disease simultaneously. Primary clinicians should screen for depression for the same reasons that they screen for high blood pressure, hypercholesterolemia, and other factors associated with cardiovascular disease. Likewise, psychiatrists should consider cardiovascular health in the assessment of their patients. At a minimum, primary care and psychiatry need to work together to insure that proper diagnostic workups and treatment issues in both areas are fully addressed (104).

Medication Side Effects and Interactions

Treatment of depression necessitates a continual evaluation of possible medication side effects and interactions. The reader is referred elsewhere for a comprehensive discussion of the topic (30,81). Here, we describe some issues that occur more commonly and require particular attention among the depressed elderly and those with cardiovascular disease and related conditions.

Some depressions can be caused by or exacerbated by medications, including some medications used to treat cardiovascular disease and associated conditions (such as hypertension). Such medications include β-blockers, clonidine, hydralazine, and reserpine. Conversely, some psychotropic medications can compromise the treatment of cardiovascular disease, for example, by increasing blood pressure (e.g., amphetamines, venlafaxine), by increasing body weight and blood cholesterol levels (e.g., mirtazapine, many antipsychotic drugs), by predisposing to heart-block, or possibly by increasing risk of cardiac arrhythmias (e.g., TCAs) (81).

Medications used for depression and cardiovascular disease can also produce unwanted side effects through pharmacodynamic synergism. Side effects common to both groups of medications, such as orthostatic hypotension, dry mouth, and sexual side effects can be significantly exacerbated through additive or synergistic effects. More serious conditions (e.g., Stevens-Johnson Syndrome) also occur with many medications in both groups. Another mechanism that frequently can lead to increasing side effects is one medication altering the pharmacokinetic properties of a second medication. For example, lithium levels can be increased by thiazides and enalapril, and metoprolol levels can be increased by 2D6-inhibitors (e.g., fluoxetine and paroxetine) (81).

Age-related renal changes result in an increased risk for hyponatremia among the elderly (105) and syndrome of inappropriate antidiuretic hormone (SIADH) is much more common in this population, particularly when taking medications that are known to have SIADH as a possible side effect, such as the SSRIs. Other psychotropic medications thought to increase the risk of SIADH include carbamazepine, MAOIs, TCAs, and phenothiazines (106). Diuretics, commonly used to treat hypertension (frequently observed with cardiovascular disease), also lower serum sodium, and thiazide diuretics are known as a possible cause of SIADH. Close coordination of treatment is necessary between the psychiatrist and other physicians involved in a patient's care to address potential synergistic effects of multiple medications predisposing toward hyponatremia, and to help identify which medications or medication combinations are most responsible for causing hyponatremia, when it occurs. For example, if a patient who has been successfully treated with an SSRI for years without hyponatremia should suddenly develop hyponatremia, the hyponatremia workup should include close attention to recent medication changes, in collaboration with the patient's other physicians, before concluding that the SSRI was solely responsible for the hyponatremia.

Treatment of Vascular Disease

The treatment of vascular disease usually lies outside of the psychiatrist's responsibilities. However, it is important nonetheless for the psychiatrist to be aware of what that treatment entails, both to encourage patients to adhere to their medical treatments and to participate in decisions about what medication changes to make when unwanted side-effects or interactions occur with a patient's medications. Some psychiatrists have taken on responsibilities ordinarily assigned to primary care practitioners, such as monitoring weight and blood pressure or prescribing medications like metformin, prophylactically, for patients taking medications associated with weight gain and increased risk of diabetes (e.g., olanzapine) (107). The fact that cerebrovascular disease is often silent means that for some patients depression may be the only manifestation of underlying cerebrovascular disease, and the high comorbidity with cardiovascular disease in general means that a thorough cardiovascular disease workup should be considered as part of the standard late-life depression evaluation, particularly for late-onset depression. Focusing on health habits such as smoking, diet, and exercise may help patients improve lifestyle choices that will lower the risk of cardiovascular disease as well as possibly have a direct impact on depression. Finally, while some psychiatric medications, as mentioned above, may increase the risk of cardiovascular disease others may reduce the risk. The increased platelet activation associated with depression (108) may be reduced by SSRIs (109) and potentially reduce the risk of heart attacks through a mechanism similar to that of aspirin. However, SSRIs may also increase bleeding risks, a possible side effect to keep in mind in patients taking aspirin or anticoagulation therapy.

Treatments Targeting Depression

Whyte and Mulsant (110) concluded that poststroke depression is multifactorial in origin, consistent with the biopsychosocial model of mental illness, and that conventional antidepressant treatments for this form of depression are effective. They found in their review of 10 antidepressant medication treatment trials for poststroke depression that more than 60% of patients responded to medication, with no clear advantage to any class of medication. However, one of the three randomized controlled trials that used standardized criteria for the diagnosis of depression (111) found treatment response to nortriptyline to be significantly higher than to both placebo and fluoxetine (which had a lower response rate than placebo). The other two randomized controlled trials found significantly better treatment response for fluoxetine and nortriptyline, respectively, than for placebo. Whyte and Mulsant concluded that the effects of psychostimulants with poststroke depression are unclear, but that they appear to be well tolerated and may have positive effects, based on one open-label and two chart-review studies of methylphenidate treatment of elderly depressed stroke patients. Finally, the authors concluded that electroconvulsive therapy (ECT) has been shown to be useful in treating poststroke depression, based on two retrospective chart reviews, the larger of which noted that 19 out of 20 elderly patients were markedly or moderately improved after ECT treatment.

In addition to the above-mentioned medications, citalopram (112), trazodone (113), amphetamine (114), and methylphenidate (115,116) have been found effective in poststroke depression. Escitalopram was superior to placebo for prevention of depression after stroke (117). Antidepressants promoting ischemic recovery (such as dopamine or norepinephrine enhancing agents) might prove useful in the treatment of vascular depression, while those inhibiting ischemic recovery (e.g., α-adrenergic blocking agents) might prove counterproductive (30). Also, augmentation with some medications normally used only to treat cerebrovascular disease may improve depression outcomes, as was the case in a recent study of nimodipine augmentation of fluoxetine treatment (118) for vascular depression (Alexopoulos' definition). Prophylactic treatment of nondepressed stroke patients was associated with significantly lower rate of development of depression in a recent meta-analysis of 10 randomized, placebo-controlled antidepressant medication trials (119).

Recent studies by Jorge et al. found that repetitive transcranial magnetic stimulation (rTMS) was well tolerated and effective in treating antidepressant medication resistant poststroke depression (120) and vascular depression (defined by depression with onset of major depressive disorder after age 50, history of subcortical stroke, and/or >2 of the cardiovascular risk factors arterial hypertension, diabetes mellitus, obesity, hyperlipidemia, and smoking) (121). When compared with sham stimulation, 10–15 sessions of active rTMS over the left dorsolateral prefrontal cortex were associated with a significant reduction of depressive symptoms. Future research attempting replication and comparing rTMS with other forms of treatment for poststroke or vascular depression might be helpful in elucidating the potential benefits of rTMS over other forms of treatment for these conditions.

Psychosocial interventions and rehabilitation programs may also play a vital role in treating or preventing vascular depression. In a preliminary study by Alexopoulos et al. (122) depressive symptoms in patients with DED responded significantly better to problem-solving therapy than to supportive therapy; and in a recent study (117) post-stroke patients receiving problem-solving therapy developed depression significantly less frequently than a placebo control group. In contrast, a study of 123 stroke patients (mean age 66 years) with depression (123) did not find any significant differences in outcomes of mood, function, or satisfaction with cognitive behavioral therapy compared to standard care or an attention placebo intervention. A poststroke rehabilitation intervention sponsored by the Finnish Heart Association described by Kotila et al. (124) was associated with significantly lower incidence of depression after stroke (42% vs. 55%). Research based on mechanisms hypothesized to contribute to vascular depression may lead to the discovery of effective therapeutic interventions (including psychologic and social) for vascular depression (104,125).

CONCLUSION

The vascular depression hypothesis has provided direction in characterizing the nature of some geriatric depressive syndromes, their relationships to damage in specific neural pathways, and effective treatment strategies, but the work in this area is in its early stages. Considerable evidence now suggests a bidirectional relationship between cardiovascular (including cerebrovascular) disease and late-life depression. This evidence underscores the importance of a close working relationship between primary care and psychiatric health care practitioners to ensure the proper evaluation and care for cardiovascular disease and comorbid depression among elderly patients. We hope that further research will elucidate mechanisms involved in the genesis of vascular depression, however defined, and result in corresponding treatment advances.

REFERENCES

1. Alexopoulos GS, Meyers BS, Young RC, et al. 'Vascular depression' hypothesis. Arch Gen Psychiatry 1997; 54(10):915–922.
2. Post F. The Significance of Affective Disorders in Old Age. London, England, UK: Institute of Psychiatry, 1962 Maudsley Monograph 10.
3. Post F, Schulman K. New views on old age affective disorder. In: Aire T, ed. Recent Advances in Psychogeriatrics. New York, NY: Churchill Livingstone Inc., 1985:119–140.
4. Starkstein SE, Robinson RG. Depression in cerebrovascular disease. In: Depression in Neurological Disease. Baltimore, MD: The Johns Hopkins University Press, 1993:28–49.
5. Folstein MF, Maiberger R, McHugh PR. Mood disorder as a specific complication of stroke. J Neurol Neurosurg Psychiatry 1977; 40(10):1018–1020.
6. Ebrahim S, Barer D, Nouri F. Affective illness after stroke. Br J Psychiatry 1987; 151:52–56.
7. Mendez MF, Adams NL, Lewandowski KS. Neurobehavioral changes associated with caudate lesions. Neurology 1989; 39(3):349–354.
8. Robinson RG. Neuropsychiatric consequences of stroke. Annu Rev Med 1997; 48:217–229.
9. Robinson RG. Poststroke depression: Prevalence, diagnosis, treatment, and disease progression. Biol Psychiatry 2003; 54(3):376–387.
10. Hackett ML, Yapa C, Parag V, et al. Frequency of depression after stroke: A systematic review of observational studies. Stroke 2005; 36(6):1330–1340.
11. Peterson JC, Charlson ME, Williams-Russo P, et al. New postoperative depressive symptoms and long-term cardiac outcomes after coronary artery bypass surgery. Am J Geriatr Psychiatry 2002; 10:192–198.
12. Whyte EM, Mulsant BH, Vanderbilt J, et al. Depression after stroke: A prospective epidemiological study. J Am Geriatr Soc 2004; 52(5):774–778.
13. Luber MP, Meyers BS, Williams-Russo PG, et al. Depression and service utilization in elderly primary care patients. Am J Geriatr Psychiatry 2001; 9:169–176.
14. Arbelaez JJ, Ariyo AA, Crum RM, et al. Depressive symptoms, inflammation, and ischemic stroke in older adults: A prospective analysis in the cardiovascular health study. J Am Geriatr Soc 2007; 55(11):1825–1830.
15. Rabkin JG, Charles E, Kass F. Hypertension and DSM-III depression in psychiatric outpatients. Am J Psychiatry 1983; 140(8):1072–1074.
16. Carney RM, Rich MW, Tevelde A, et al. Major depressive disorder in coronary artery disease. Am J Cardiol 1987; 60(16):1273–1275.
17. Sultzer DL, Levin HS, Mahler ME, et al. A comparison of psychiatric symptoms in vascular dementia and Alzheimer's disease. Am J Psychiatry 1993; 150(12):1806–1812.
18. Baldwin RC, Tomenson B. Depression in later life. A comparison of symptoms and risk factors in early and late onset cases. Br J Psychiatry 1995; 167(5):649–652.
19. Krishnan KR, Hays JC, Tupler LA, et al. Clinical and phenomenological comparisons of late-onset and early-onset depression. Am J Psychiatry 1995; 152(5):785–788.

20. Young RC, Klerman GL. Mania in late life: Focus on age at onset. Am J Psychiatry 1992; 149(7):867–876.
21. Alexopoulos GS, Meyers BS, Young RC, et al. The course of geriatric depression with "reversible dementia": A controlled study. Am J Psychiatry 1993; 150(11):1693–1699.
22. Alexopoulos GS, Young RC, Meyers BS. Geriatric depression: Age of onset and dementia. Biol Psychiatry 1993; 34(3):141–145.
23. Alexopoulos GS, Young RC, Shindledecker RD. Brain computed tomography findings in geriatric depression and primary degenerative dementia. Biol Psychiatry 1992; 31(6):591–599.
24. Coffey CE, Figiel GS, Djang WT, et al. Leukoencephalopathy in elderly depressed patients referred for ECT. Biol Psychiatry 1988; 24(2):143–161.
25. Jacoby RJ, Levy R. Computed tomography in the elderly. 3. Affective disorder. Br J Psychiatry 1980; 136:270–275.
26. Jacoby RJ, Levy R, Bird JM. Computed tomography and the outcome of affective disorder: A follow-up study of elderly patients. Br J Psychiatry 1981; 139:288–292.
27. Roth M, Kay DW. Affective disorders arising in the senium. II. Physical disability as an aetiological factor. J Ment Sci 1956; 102(426):141–150.
28. Alexopoulos GS, Vrontou C, Kakuma T, et al. Disability in geriatric depression. Am J Psychiatry 1996; 153(7):877–885.
29. Baron M, Mendlewicz J, Klotz J. Age-of-onset and genetic transmission in affective disorders. Acta Psychiatr Scand 1981; 64(5):373–380.
30. Alexopoulos GS. Depression in the elderly. Lancet 2005; 365(9475):1961–1970.
31. Alexopoulos GS, Meyers BS, Young RC, et al. Clinically defined vascular depression. Am J Psychiatry 1997; 154(4):562–565.
32. Steffens DC, Conway CR, Dombeck CB, et al. Severity of subcortical gray matter hyperintensity predicts ECT response in geriatric depression. J ECT 2001; 17(1): 45–49.
33. Sneed JR, Roose SP, Keilp JG, et al. Response inhibition predicts poor antidepressant treatment response in very old depressed patients. Am J Geriatr Psychiatry 2007; 15(7):553–563.
34. Simpson SW, Jackson A, Baldwin RC, et al. Subcortical hyperintensities in late-life depression: Acute response to treatment and neuropsychological impairment. Int Psychogeriatr 1997; 9(3):257–275.
35. Simpson S, Baldwin RC, Jackson A, et al. Is subcortical disease associated with a poor response to antidepressants? Neurological, neuropsychological and neuroradiological findings in late-life depression. Psychol Med 1998; 28(5):1015–1026.
36. Kalayam B, Alexopoulos GS. Prefrontal dysfunction and treatment response in geriatric depression. Arch Gen Psychiatry 1999; 56(8):713–718.
37. Smith GS, Gunning-Dixon FM, Lotrich FE, et al. Translational research in late-life mood disorders: Implications for future intervention and prevention research. Neuropsychopharmacology 2007; 32(9):1857–1875.
38. Almeida OP, Waterreus A, Hankey GJ. Preventing depression after stroke: Results from a randomized placebo-controlled trial. J Clin Psychiatry 2006; 67(7):1104–1109.
39. Salloway S, Correia S, Boyle P, et al. MRI subcortical hyperintensities in old and very old depressed outpatients: The important role of age in late-life depression. J Neurol Sci 2002; 203–204:227–233.
40. Janssen J, Pol HE, Schnack HG, et al. Cerebral volume measurements and subcortical white matter lesions and short-term treatment response in late life depression. Int J Geriatr Psychiatry 2007; 22(5):468–474.
41. Fujikawa T, Yamawaki S, Touhouda Y. Incidence of silent cerebral infarction in patients with major depression. Stroke 1993; 24(11):1631–1634.
42. Coffey CE, Figiel GS, Djang WT, et al. Subcortical hyperintensity on magnetic resonance imaging: A comparison of normal and depressed elderly subjects. Am J Psychiatry 1990; 147(2):187–189.
43. Vermeer SE, Koudstaal PJ, Oudkerk M, et al. Prevalence and risk factors of silent brain infarcts in the population-based Rotterdam Scan Study. Stroke 2002; 33(1):21–25.

44. Fried LP, Borhani NO, Enright P, et al. The Cardiovascular Health Study: Design and rationale. Ann Epidemiol 1991; 1(3):263–276.
45. Longstreth WT, Jr, Bernick C, Manolio TA, et al. Lacunar infarcts defined by magnetic resonance imaging of 3660 elderly people: The Cardiovascular Health Study. Arch Neurol 1998; 55(9):1217–1225.
46. Thomas AJ, Perry R, Barber R, et al. Pathologies and pathological mechanisms for white matter hyperintensities in depression. Ann N Y Acad Sci 2002; 977:333–339.
47. Thomas AJ, Perry R, Kalaria RN, et al. Neuropathological evidence for ischemia in the white matter of the dorsolateral prefrontal cortex in late-life depression. Int J Geriatr Psychiatry 2003; 18(1):7–13.
48. Thomas AJ, O'Brien JT, Barber R, et al. A neuropathological study of periventricular white matter hyperintensities in major depression. J Affect Disord 2003; 76(1–3):49–54.
49. Krishnan MS, O'Brien JT, Firbank MJ, et al. Relationship between periventricular and deep white matter lesions and depressive symptoms in older people. The LADIS Study. Int J Geriatr Psychiatry 2006; 21(10):983–989.
50. Breteler MM, van Swieten JC, Bots ML, et al. Cerebral white matter lesions, vascular risk factors, and cognitive function in a population-based study: The Rotterdam Study. Neurology 1994; 44(7):1246–1252.
51. Fazekas F, Niederkorn K, Schmidt R, et al. White matter signal abnormalities in normal individuals: Correlation with carotid ultrasonography, cerebral blood flow measurements, and cerebrovascular risk factors. Stroke 1988; 19(10):1285–1288.
52. Krishnan KR, Taylor WD, McQuoid DR, et al. Clinical characteristics of magnetic resonance imaging-defined subcortical ischemic depression. Biol Psychiatry 2004; 55(4):390–397.
53. Liao D, Cooper L, Cai J, et al. The prevalence and severity of white matter lesions, their relationship with age, ethnicity, gender, and cardiovascular disease risk factors: The ARIC Study. Neuroepidemiology 1997; 16(3):149–162.
54. Murphy CF, Gunning-Dixon FM, Hoptman MJ, et al. White-matter integrity predicts stroop performance in patients with geriatric depression. Biol Psychiatry 2007; 61(8):1007–1010.
55. van Swieten JC, Geyskes GG, Derix MM, et al. Hypertension in the elderly is associated with white matter lesions and cognitive decline. Ann Neurol 1991; 30(6):825–830.
56. Ylikoski R, Ylikoski A, Erkinjuntti T, et al. White matter changes in healthy elderly persons correlate with attention and speed of mental processing. Arch Neurol 1993; 50(8):818–824.
57. Steffens DC, Bosworth HB, Provenzale JM, et al. Subcortical white matter lesions and functional impairment in geriatric depression. Depress Anxiety 2002; 15(1):23–28.
58. Krishnan KR, Hays JC, Blazer DG. MRI-defined vascular depression. Am J Psychiatry 1997; 154(4):497–501.
59. Longstreth WT, Jr, Arnold AM, Beauchamp NJ, Jr, et al. Incidence, manifestations, and predictors of worsening white matter on serial cranial magnetic resonance imaging in the elderly: The Cardiovascular Health Study. Stroke 2005; 36(1):56–61.
60. Tupler LA, Krishnan KR, McDonald WM, et al. Anatomic location and laterality of MRI signal hyperintensities in late-life depression. J Psychosom Res 2002; 53(2):665–676.
61. Steffens DC, Krishnan KR, Crump C, et al. Cerebrovascular disease and evolution of depressive symptoms in the cardiovascular health study. Stroke 2002; 33(6):1636–1644.
62. Krishnan KR, Goli V, Ellinwood EH, et al. Leukoencephalopathy in patients diagnosed as major depressive. Biol Psychiatry 1988; 23(5):519–522.
63. Coffey CE, Figiel GS, Djang WT, et al. White matter hyperintensity on magnetic resonance imaging: Clinical and neuroanatomic correlates in the depressed elderly. J Neuropsychiatry Clin Neurosci 1989; 1(2):135–144.
64. Coffey CE, Wilkinson WE, Weiner RD, et al. Quantitative cerebral anatomy in depression. A controlled magnetic resonance imaging study. Arch Gen Psychiatry 1993; 50(1):7–16.
65. O'Brien JT, Firbank MJ, Krishnan MS, et al. White matter hyperintensities rather than lacunar infarcts are associated with depressive symptoms in older people: The LADIS Study. Am J Geriatr Psychiatry 2006; 14(10):834–841.

66. Rainer MK, Mucke HA, Zehetmayer S, et al. Data from the VITA Study do not support the concept of vascular depression. Am J Geriatr Psychiatry 2006; 14(6):531–537.
67. Janssen J, Hulshoff Pol HE, de Leeuw FE, et al. Hippocampal volume and subcortical white matter lesions in late life depression: Comparison of early and late onset depression. J Neurol Neurosurg Psychiatry 2007; 78(6):638–640.
68. Taylor WD, MacFall JR, Payne ME, et al. Late-life depression and microstructural abnormalities in dorsolateral prefrontal cortex white matter. Am J Psychiatry 2004; 161(7):1293–1296.
69. Bae JN, MacFall JR, Krishnan KR, et al. Dorsolateral prefrontal cortex and anterior cingulate cortex white matter alterations in late-life depression. Biol Psychiatry 2006; 60(12):1356–1363.
70. Taylor WD, Steffens DC, MacFall JR, et al. White matter hyperintensity progression and late-life depression outcomes. Arch Gen Psychiatry 2003; 60(11):1090–1096.
71. Alexopoulos GS, Murphy CF, Gunning-Dixon FM, et al. Microstructural white matter abnormalities and remission of geriatric depression. Am J Psychiatry 2008; 165(2):238–244.
72. Alexopoulos GS, Kiosses DN, Choi SJ, et al. Frontal white matter microstructure and treatment response of late-life depression: A preliminary study. Am J Psychiatry 2002; 159(11):1929–1932.
73. Patankar TF, Baldwin R, Mitra D, et al. Virchow-Robin space dilatation may predict resistance to antidepressant monotherapy in elderly patients with depression. J Affect Disord 2007; 97(1–3):265–270.
74. Thomas AJ, O'Brien JT, Davis S, et al. Ischemic basis for deep white matter hyperintensities in major depression: A neuropathological study. Arch Gen Psychiatry 2002; 59(9):785–792.
75. Carson AJ, MacHale S, Allen K, et al. Depression after stroke and lesion location: A systematic review. Lancet 2000; 356(9224):122–126.
76. Roman GC. Vascular depression: An archetypal neuropsychiatric disorder. Biol Psychiatry 2006; 60(12):1306–1308.
77. Starkstein SE, Robinson RG, Berthier ML, et al. Differential mood changes following basal ganglia vs. thalamic lesions. Archives of Neurology 1988; 45(7):725–730.
78. Vataja R, Leppavuori A, Pohjasvaara T, et al. Poststroke depression and lesion location revisited. J Neuropsychiatry Clin Neurosci 2004; 16(2):156–162.
79. Rogers MA, Bradshaw JL, Pantelis C, et al. Frontostriatal deficits in unipolar major depression. Brain Res Bull 1998; 47(4):297–310.
80. Alexopoulos GS. Late-life mood disorders. In: Sadavoy J, Jarvik LF, Grossberg GT, Meyers BS, eds. Comprehensive Textbook of Geriatric Psychiatry, 3rd ed. New York, NY: W. W. Norton, 2004:609–653.
81. Alexopoulos GS. Geriatric mood disorders. In: Sadock BJ, Sadock VA, eds. Kaplan & Sadock's Comprehensive Textbook of Psychiatry, 8th ed. Baltimore, MD: Lippincott Williams & Wilkins, 2005:3677–3687.
82. Taylor WD, Steffens DC, Krishnan KR. Psychiatric disease in the twenty-first century: The case for subcortical ischemic depression. Biol Psychiatry 2006; 60(12):1299–1303.
83. Robinson RG. Mood disorders secondary to stroke. Semin Clin Neuropsychiatry 1997; 2(4):244–251.
84. Alexopoulos GS, Kiosses DN, Klimstra S, et al. Clinical presentation of the "depression-executive dysfunction syndrome" of late life. Am J Geriatr Psychiatry 2002; 10(1):98–106.
85. Lockwood KA, Alexopoulos GS, van Gorp WG. Executive dysfunction in geriatric depression. Am J Psychiatry 2002; 159(7):1119–1126.
86. Elderkin-Thompson V, Kumar A, Bilker WB, et al. Neuropsychological deficits among patients with late-onset minor and major depression. Arch Clin Neuropsychol 2003; 18(5):529–549.
87. Sobin C, Sackeim HA. Psychomotor symptoms of depression. Am J Psychiatry 1997; 154(1):4–17.
88. Sheline YI, Barch DM, Garcia K, et al. Cognitive function in late life depression: Relationships to depression severity, cerebrovascular risk factors and processing speed. Biol Psychiatry 2006; 60(1):58–65.

89. Alexopoulos GS, Kiosses DN, Heo M, et al. Executive dysfunction and the course of geriatric depression. Biol Psychiatry 2005; 58(3):204–210.
90. Sneed JR, Keilp JG, Brickman AM, et al. The specificity of neuropsychological impairment in predicting antidepressant non-response in the very old depressed. Int J Geriatr Psychiatry 2008; 23(3):319–323.
91. Alexopoulos GS, Meyers BS, Young RC, et al. Executive dysfunction and long-term outcomes of geriatric depression. Arch Gen Psychiatry 2000; 57(3):285–290.
92. Nebes RD, Pollock BG, Houck PR, et al. Persistence of cognitive impairment in geriatric patients following antidepressant treatment: A randomized, double-blind clinical trial with nortriptyline and paroxetine. J Psychiatr Res 2003; 37(2):99–108.
93. Murphy CF, Alexopoulos GS. Longitudinal association of initiation/perseveration and severity of geriatric depression. Am J Geriatr Psychiatry 2004; 12(1):50–56.
94. Butters MA, Becker JT, Nebes RD, et al. Changes in cognitive functioning following treatment of late-life depression. Am J Psychiatry 2000; 157(12):1949–1954.
95. Bhalla RK, Butters MA, Mulsant BH, et al. Persistence of neuropsychologic deficits in the remitted state of late-life depression. Am J Geriatr Psychiatry 2006; 14(5):419–427.
96. Chemerinski E, Robinson RG. The neuropsychiatry of stroke. Psychosomatics 2000; 41(1):5–14.
97. Vataja R, Pohjasvaara T, Mantyla R, et al. Depression-executive dysfunction syndrome in stroke patients. Am J Geriatr Psychiatry 2005; 13(2):99–107.
98. Narushima K, Kosier JT, Robinson RG. A reappraisal of poststroke depression, intra- and inter-hemispheric lesion location using meta-analysis. J Neuropsychiatry Clini Neurosci 2003; 15(4):422–430.
99. Alexander GE, DeLong MR, Strick PL. Parallel organization of functionally segregated circuits linking basal ganglia and cortex. Annu Rev Neurosci 1986; 9:357–381.
100. Sneed JR, Roose SP, Sackeim HA. Vascular depression: A distinct diagnostic subtype? Biol Psychiatry 2006; 60(12):1295–1298.
101. Montgomery SA, Asberg M. A new depression scale designed to be sensitive to change. Br J Psychiatry 1979; 134:382–389.
102. Rapp MA, Dahlman K, Sano M, et al. Neuropsychological differences between late-onset and recurrent geriatric major depression. Am J Psychiatry 2005; 162(4):691–698.
103. Thomas AJ, Kalaria RN, O'Brien JT. Depression and vascular disease: What is the relationship? J Affect Disord 2004; 79(1–3):81–95.
104. Alexopoulos GS, Buckwalter K, Olin J, et al. Comorbidity of late life depression: An opportunity for research on mechanisms and treatment. Biol Psychiatry 2002; 52(6):543–558.
105. Larsen PD, Martin JH. Renal system changes in the elderly. AORN J 1994; 60(2):298–301.
106. Baylis PH. The syndrome of inappropriate antidiuretic hormone secretion. Int J Biochem Cell Biol 2003; 35(11):1495–1499.
107. Wu RR, Zhao JP, Guo XF, et al. Metformin addition attenuates olanzapine-induced weight gain in drug-naive first-episode schizophrenia patients: A double-blind, placebo-controlled study. Am J Psychiatry 2008; 165(3):352–358.
108. Whyte EM, Pollock BG, Wagner WR, et al. Influence of serotonin-transporter-linked promoter region polymorphism on platelet activation in geriatric depression. Am J Psychiatry 2001; 158(12):2074–2076.
109. Steffens DC, Chung H, Krishnan KR, et al. Antidepressant treatment and worsening white matter on serial cranial magnetic resonance imaging in the elderly: The Cardiovascular Health Study. Stroke 2008; 39(3):857–862.
110. Whyte EM, Mulsant BH. Post stroke depression: Epidemiology, pathophysiology, and biological treatment. Biol Psychiatry 2002; 52(3):253–264.
111. Robinson RG, Schultz SK, Castillo C, et al. Nortriptyline versus fluoxetine in the treatment of depression and in short-term recovery after stroke: A placebo-controlled, double-blind study. Am J Psychiatry 2000; 157(3):351–359.
112. Andersen G, Vestergaard K, Lauritzen L. Effective treatment of poststroke depression with the selective serotonin reuptake inhibitor citalopram. Stroke 1994; 25(6):1099–1104.

113. Reding MJ, Orto LA, Winter SW, et al. Antidepressant therapy after stroke. A double-blind trial. Arch Neurol 1986; 43(8):763–765.
114. Masand P, Murray GB, Pickett P. Psychostimulants in post-stroke depression. J Neuropsychiatry clin Neurosci 1991; 3(1):23–27.
115. Lazarus LW, Winemiller DR, Lingam VR, et al. Efficacy and side effects of methylphenidate for poststroke depression. J Clin Psychiatry 1992; 53(12):447–449.
116. Lingam VR, Lazarus LW, Groves L, et al. Methylphenidate in treating poststroke depression. J Clin Psychiatry 1988; 49(4):151–153.
117. Robinson RG, Jorge RE, Moser DJ, et al. Escitalopram and problem-solving therapy for prevention of poststroke depression: a randomized controlled trial. JAMA 2008; 299:2391–2400.
118. Taragano FE, Bagnatti P, Allegri RF. A double-blind, randomized clinical trial to assess the augmentation with nimodipine of antidepressant therapy in the treatment of "vascular depression". Int psychogeriatr 2005; 17(3):487–498.
119. Chen Y, Patel NC, Guo JJ, et al. Antidepressant prophylaxis for poststroke depression: A meta-analysis. Int Clin Psychopharmacol 2007; 22(3):159–166.
120. Jorge RE, Robinson RG, Tateno A, et al. Repetitive transcranial magnetic stimulation as treatment of poststroke depression: A preliminary study. Biol Psychiatry 2004; 55(4):398–405.
121. Jorge RE, Moser DJ, Acion L, et al. Treatment of vascular depression using repetitive transcranial magnetic stimulation. Arch Gen Psychiatry 2008; 65:268–276.
122. Alexopoulos GS, Raue P, Arean P. Problem-solving therapy versus supportive therapy in geriatric major depression with executive dysfunction. Am J Geriatr Psychiatry 2003; 11(1):46–52.
123. Lincoln NB, Flannaghan T. Cognitive behavioral psychotherapy for depression following stroke: A randomized controlled trial. Stroke 2003; 34(1):111–115.
124. Kotila M, Numminen H, Waltimo O, et al. Depression after stroke: Results of the FINNSTROKE Study. Stroke 1998; 29(2):368–372.
125. Alexopoulos GS, Schultz SK, Lebowitz BD. Late-life depression: A model for medical classification. Biol Psychiatry 2005; 58(4):283–289.

11 Mood Disorders and Medical Illness in the Elderly

David S. Harnett
Lawrence Memorial Hospital of Medford/Hallmark Health System, Medford, Massachusetts, U.S.A.

Ronald Pies
SUNY Upstate Medical University, Syracuse, New York, and Tufts University School of Medicine, Boston, Massachusetts, U.S.A.

INTRODUCTION

Clinicians and researchers working with elderly patients face a paradox. We know that depressive symptoms and disorders are a source of great emotional and physical suffering in the elderly, yet the origins of late-life depression are not well understood. Moreover, as Blazer and Hybels (1) put it, "Older adults appear to be at greater biologic vulnerability to depression, yet community surveys in Western societies have repeatedly documented a lower frequency of late-life depressive symptoms ... [and] disorders...compared to midlife." Indeed, prevalence figures vary from study to study, depending on criteria for "depression" and the population studied. In general, community studies have shown that about 25% of elderly persons report having depressive symptoms, but only about 5% meet full criteria for major depression. In settings that care for more compromised elders, such as medical hospitals and long-term care facilities, the rates of depression are higher (2).

To complicate matters further, the relationship between biologic and psychosocial factors in late-life depression is dauntingly complex. As Blazer and Hybels note, "psychological dimensions have biological mechanisms and biological models imply input from the environment" (1). Indeed, there is a subtle "bidirectionality" that seems to govern the relationship between biologic and psychologic factors in late-life depression, so that causal mechanisms are difficult to tease out. This bidirectional relationship—which itself may be an oversimplification—is the focus of the present chapter. In particular, we discuss how four common types of medical illness in the elderly influence, and are influenced by, affective symptoms and syndromes.

This necessarily involves a discussion of so-called comorbidity between "psychiatric" and "medical" disorders. Yet this dichotomy risks perpetuating an unfounded Cartesian dualism, which artificially separates mind and body. It might be more accurate to say that this chapter describes how those pathologic signs and symptoms that are often treated by internists, cardiologists, or oncologists interact in complex ways with those treated by psychiatrists.

While many kinds of medical and neurologic disorders might have served as the focus of our chapter, we have selected four that are commonly seen in consultation-liaison and geriatric psychiatry settings, and which appear to have important connections to affective syndromes—cardiac disease, chronic obstructive pulmonary disease (COPD), diabetes mellitus, and cancer. Owing to space limitations, our focus is on unipolar (not bipolar) depressive symptoms and disorders. The important issue of bipolar disorder and medical comorbidity is comprehensively reviewed by Newcomer (3). Finally, we will discuss how specific pharmacologic interventions for depressed elderly patients may complicate underlying medical conditions.

EPIDEMIOLOGY OF MEDICAL-AFFECTIVE COMORBIDITY: AN OVERVIEW

There is good evidence that medical comorbidities are common among outpatients with major depression, in both primary care and specialty settings. For example, in the STAR*D study (4), the prevalence of significant medical comorbidity in this mixed-age population was nearly 53%. The prevalence of medical comorbidities in depressed, elderly populations is not precisely known. However, in a recent study of elderly patients hospitalized for treatment of major depression ($N = 195$), nearly three-fourths had at least one comorbid medical condition requiring first-line treatment, nearly half had two, and one-fourth had three or more (5). Similarly, in a study of 1801 elderly primary care patients, Noel et al. (6) found high rates of medical illness in a cohort with major depression or dysthymic disorder. Chronic lung disease was found in 23.3% of the sample, diabetes in 23.2%, cancer (excluding skin cancer) in 10.9%, and heart disease in 27.6%. Study participants had an average of 3.8 medical diagnoses, suggesting that the problem of medical comorbidity is substantial in elderly patients with depression. Notably, severity of depression made larger independent contributions to three of the four general health indicators (mental functional status, disability, and quality of life) than did severity of medical comorbidities.

The issue of medical-depressive comorbidity may also be investigated by examining the prevalence of depression in populations defined as "medically ill." There is substantial evidence that depression is often not recognized in primary practice, and that few depressed older adults receive adequate treatment in primary care settings (7,8). However, diagnosing depression, and delineating its boundaries, is by no means straightforward in older and medically ill cohorts. For example, in a study of 49 patients hospitalized for medical illness, Clarke et al. (9) found that all participants described being "depressed, down, or sad." The authors concluded, "Demoralization, which involves feelings of being unable to cope, helplessness, hopelessness and diminished personal esteem, characterizes much of the depression seen in hospitalized medically ill patients." Aside from "boundary issues" (e.g., major depression vs. demoralization), numerous medical illnesses can directly produce signs and symptoms that overlap significantly with those of DSM-IV depressive disorders, such as major depression and dysthymia. This may complicate diagnosis of depression, as well as determination of its prevalence among the medically ill. For example, as will be discussed below, there is some risk of overdiagnosing depression in patients with congestive heart failure whose anergia is a direct manifestation of their cardiac illness or in patients who become demoralized, though not depressed, as a result of their numerous medical setbacks (10).

Notwithstanding these nosologic and diagnostic complexities, some studies convincingly point to high rates of depressive symptoms among numerous medically ill (but not necessarily elderly) cohorts. Our focus in this chapter, however, is on patients with cardiovascular and chronic lung disease ("cardiopulmonary disease"), cancer, and diabetes.

Among patients with ischemic heart disease ("coronary artery disease," in the older literature), a recent review (11) cited rates of depression ranging from 18% to 65%, depending on presence or absence of recent myocardial infarction (MI), and whether major or minor depression was considered. However, a contemporaneous study puts the figure at the lower end of this range (12). With respect to chronic lung disease, the prevalence of depressive symptoms has been difficult to establish. However, one recent study (13) found that in patients with severe COPD, the prevalence of depression was 25.0% compared with 17.5% in controls and 19.6% in patients with mild to moderate COPD.

Among patients with cancer, depressive symptoms may occur in up to 58% of patients, and depressive disorders in up to 38% of patients (14). However, there is wide variability in prevalence rates, owing to varying study methods, measures of depression, and type of cancer (14), as discussed below.

Finally, several recent studies find that the risk of depression in diabetic cohorts is approximately twice that of nondiabetic comparison groups (15,16). Again, prevalence rates vary considerably, depending on the population studied and the methodology used, as detailed below.

With respect to the four comorbid medical conditions discussed, it is difficult to find reliable data on prevalence of depression exclusively in patients older than age 65 years.

THE ARROW OF CAUSALITY: A BIOPSYCHOSOCIAL MODEL

Blazer and Hybels suggest that a biopsychosocial model of the etiology of depression is "especially applicable to the elderly, primarily because it reminds us that the origins of late-life depression are multiple and range across all three domains" 91). Yet, these authors caution "even so, this model can be misleading, given the tight connection between the domains." Moreover, Ghaemi (17) has cautioned that a reflexive use of the biopsychosocial model can lead to inappropriately eclectic treatment of psychiatric disorders. Given these conundrums, the determination of "what caused what?" in elderly patients with comorbid depression and medical illness is extremely complex. Nevertheless, based on the available evidence, we have attempted to depict a plausible set of interactions in Figure 1.

There is little doubt that a "primary" or underlying medical illness can have profound effects not only on mood, but also on neuroendocrine and immune function, self-care, and degree of social interaction. Yet, this causal relationship (primary disease—alterations in mood, physiology, etc.) may well be mediated by the patient's premorbid personality, ego defenses, and characteristic coping style (1). There is some evidence of this from the psychosomatic medicine literature. Drossman et al. (18), for example, studied the health outcome of women with gastrointestinal disorders who used varying "coping strategies" to deal with their illness. Variables such as daily pain, number of visits to physicians, days spent in bed, and psychologic distress were studied in relation to adaptive or maladaptive coping styles. The authors found that patients who had "a profoundly pessimistic view of [their] illness"—e.g., a "catastrophizing" coping style—were likely to have a poorer outcome, even after controlling for other factors. Interestingly, a history of physical abuse appeared to magnify the effect of such "catastrophizing." Similarly, Gross (19) studied the effect of (presurgery) coping strategies on relief of pain, following laminectomy. At 6-week follow-up, patients scoring high on a measure of "self-reliance" rated their pain as significantly less than did those having lower

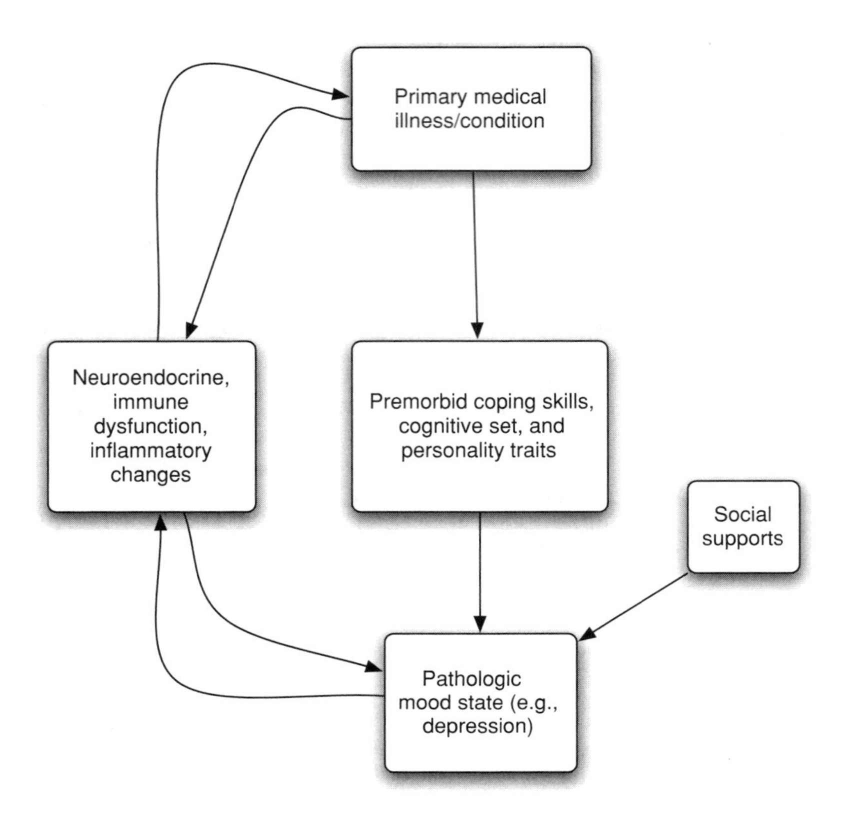

FIGURE 1 Biopsychosocial interactions in Disease States

self-reliance scores. This effect was found after controlling for the patient's presurgical medical status and level of pain. Taken together, these studies suggest that the overall health outcome of "primary" pathophysiologic processes (gastrointestinal disease, postsurgical pain, etc.) may be mediated or mitigated by habitual ego defenses and coping styles.

Our diagram suggests that once a pathologic mood state arises in the course of a primary medical illness, it may in turn set off a variety of pathophysiologic events that can exacerbate the underlying medical condition. This, in turn, may lead to a reactive worsening of the patient's mood, in what amounts to a "vicious circle" or aversive cascade of synergistic events. To appreciate these complex interactions, consider an elderly patient who experiences a cerebrovascular accident. It is well established that as many as 39% of patients with acute stroke may become depressed within the first few weeks of the event, but the etiology of poststroke depression (PSD) is not clear (20). PSD may be the result of direct insult to biogenic amine tracts in the brain, psychologic reaction to loss of function, neuroendocrine disturbance, or some combination of these factors. Indeed, neuroendocrine disturbance is common in the immediate poststroke period, including elevation of serum cortisol (21). Elevations of serum cortisol are also commonly seen in many patients with major depression, particularly in those with "psychotic depression" (22). Pathologically elevated levels of corticosteroids are known to have wide-ranging effects on a variety of bodily functions, including adverse effects on glucose, electrolytes, enzyme activity, and brain function (23).

While the temporal sequence and causal connections are not clearly understood in PSD, one may hypothesize that elevated cortisol levels in already depressed poststroke patients may "feed back" upon the brain in ways that may adversely affect both brain function and structure, with a consequent worsening of the patient's mood and cognitive function (24). Thus, as suggested in our diagram, pathophysiologic alterations of neuroendocrine function may reinforce depressive mood states, and vice versa. We believe that this paradigm may aid our general understanding of medical-affective comorbidity across a variety of disease states in the elderly. We acknowledge, however, that this is still a heuristic hypothesis, and greatly in need of further study. More specific etiopathologic relationships will be discussed for each of the four major disease groups reviewed.

Cardiopulmonary Disease and Depression in the Elderly

One recent study finds that approximately 20% of patients with ischemic heart disease (IHD) suffer from comorbid depression (12). It is not surprising that a diagnosis of IHD, and its accompanying limitations, can provoke feelings of sadness and loss for many patients. While IHD may sometimes precipitate depression, analysis of putatively "reactive" post-MI depression reveals that the mood episodes often begin before the acute cardiac event (25). However, despite increasing evidence that depression significantly impairs cardiovascular outcome, some cardiologists remain somewhat skeptical of this link (26), perhaps reasoning that depression is an "understandable," time-limited response to illness.

In fact, meta-analyses of prospective data suggest that depression is an independent predictor of IHD in otherwise healthy individuals, even after controlling for risk factors such as smoking. The increased risk is approximately 60%, and is greater for those with clinical depression as opposed to depressive symptoms (27,28).

The impact of even mild depression on those with existing IHD may be still greater, with significantly increased cardiac morbidity and mortality (29,30). A meta-analysis found that, after adjusting for other risk factors, depression doubled mortality risk in patients with IHD over two years (31). Major depression has been found to have a similar adverse impact on cardiac prognosis as left ventricular dysfunction and a past history of MI (11). Depression appears to worsen prognosis for those with stable IHD, after acute MI or coronary artery bypass surgery (12). Older studies (before 1992) suggested that depression was associated with a three-fold increase in cardiac mortality risk (30).

Depression may contribute to IHD and its consequences via both direct physiologic effects and indirect effects on cardiac risk factors. Thus, depression is associated with *autonomic imbalance*, including elevated sympathetic and/or diminished parasympathetic tone. The resulting reduction in heart rate variability (HRV), in turn, may increase mortality in IHD patients, perhaps by precipitating ventricular arrhythmias in response to ventricular premature contractions (32,33).

Depression-related immune dysfunction may worsen IHD via inflammatory cytokine (e.g., interleukin-6, tumor necrosis factor alpha) activation of vulnerable coronary plaque, with subsequent thrombus formation. However, this link may be bidirectional, with IHD-related immune abnormalities also contributing to depression (34).

Enhanced platelet aggregation ("stickiness"), associated with increased levels of platelet factor 4 and β-thromboglobulin, is characteristic of depression, and may also contribute to and worsen IHD (35). Somatic-vegetative depressive symptoms, but not anxiety or anger, were recently found to contribute to subclinical atherosclerosis, as measured by an increase in mean carotid intima-media thickness over a 3-year period (36).

The depression-to-IHD link may be strengthened by the patient's inability to modify IHD risk factors, such as smoking, physical inactivity, and poor diet. This adverse interaction may be exacerbated by nonadherence to medications and medical recommendations. Social isolation, psychosocial stress, and low levels of perceived support are related to both depression and IHD, and could mediate bidirectional effects on these conditions (12,31), particularly in elderly populations.

Antidepressant treatment of depression in patients with IHD seems warranted to improve quality of life, level of functioning, adherence to medical recommendations, and perhaps cardiac outcome itself. However, there has been long-standing concern about the safety of antidepressants in this population [summarized by Harnett (10)], particularly among elderly patients. Tricyclic antidepressants (TCAs), while possibly more efficacious than selective serotonin re-uptake inhibitors (SSRIs) in severe depression, are associated with orthostatic hypotension, cardiac conduction delay, and anticholinergic effects (Table 1). TCAs may be particularly arrhythmogenic in the face of myocardial ischemia, sometimes leading to sudden death.

Several recent studies have examined the treatment of depression in patients with ischemic heart disease. The Sertraline Antidepressant Heart Attack Randomized Trial (SADHART) (37), designed primarily to evaluate antidepressant safety, was a randomized, double-blind, placebo-controlled trial that included 369 patients who received a diagnosis of major depression after hospitalization for an acute coronary syndrome (ACS), e.g., acute MI or unstable angina. Though cardiac testing precluded antidepressant use for approximately one month after the ACS, sertraline was otherwise found to be safe, with 20% fewer associated severe cardiac events than with placebo. Although this difference was not statistically significant, the study was most likely underpowered to show statistically significant safety benefit.

Antidepressant efficacy was notable in the subgroup with Hamilton Depression Rating Scale score greater than 18, depressive onset before the ACS, or past history of major depression. More than half of depressive episodes associated with the ACS had their onset long before the acute cardiac event (and this is likely an underestimate, since patients on an antidepressant at the time of their ACS were excluded from the study). In contrast, depression following ACS was highly placebo responsive (25).

The Enhancing Recovery in Coronary Heart Disease Patients (ENRICHD) study (38) was the first multicenter clinical trial in behavioral medicine sponsored by the National Heart, Lung and Blood Institute. Six months of cognitive behavioral therapy (CBT) was compared to "usual care" in 2481 post-MI patients with depression and/or low-perceived social support. At six months, CBT was superior to usual care. At 29 months, both groups were equally improved and CBT conferred no benefit on cardiac morbidity (i.e., recurrent MI) or mortality.

TABLE 1 Medication Side Effects and Complications

	Medical condition and medication-related issues/complications			
Class of agent	Cardiac/Ischemic heart disease	Diabetes	COPD/pulmonary disease	Cancer
Antidepressants				
SSRI/SNRI	SSRIs usually first-line agents; venlafaxine may ↑ BP at high doses	SSRIs may have hypoglycemic effects; venlafaxine has little effect on glucose levels	SSRIs may improve respiratory function	SSRIs are first-line agents for comorbid cancer & depression; mirtazepine, venlafaxine may be helpful; hyponatremia may occur with any SSRI
Tricyclics	TCAs may worsen conduction disorder, increase risk of arrhythmia during ischemia, worsen orthostasis in CHF	Generally avoid because of hyperglycemic effects	Anticholinergic effects may dry airways; respiratory function usually not affected but some reports suggest respiratory depression possible	Avoid anticholinergic effects (constipation, urinary retention) in cancer patients with xerostomia, stomatitis, status post gastrointestinal, genitourinary surgery
Bupropion	Generally safe; rare hypertension, arrhythmia	Little effect on glucose levels	Generally well tolerated in smokers w/COPD	Preliminary data suggests efficacy, safety
Mood Stabilizers				
Lithium	Occasional sinus node dysfunction w/preexisting cardiac disease	Some patients may show Li-related glucose dysregulation, perhaps due to weight gain	Does not compromise small airways, respiratory drive at therapeutic blood levels	May ameliorate chronic leukopenia following chemotherapy or radiotherapy

(*Continued*)

TABLE 1 Medication Side Effects and Complications (*Continued*)

Class of agent	Medical condition and medication-related issues/complications: Cardiac/coronary artery disease	Diabetes	COPD/pulmonary disease	Cancer
Divalproex	Usually no cardiac problems	Indirect effects on glucose via weight gain	No major effect on COPD	Risk of thrombocytopenia; rare blood dyscrasia; antineoplastic effect
Carbamazepine	May cause conduction abnormalities	Usually no major effects on glucose	No major effect on COPD	May cause leukopenia; many drug interactions; generally not recommended
Lamotrigine	Usually no cardiac problems	Usually no major effects on glucose	No major effect on COPD	Limited data in cancer patients but may have role as adjunctive analgesic
Antipsychotics				
Neuroleptics (typical APs)	Orthostatic hypotension related to α-1 blockade; QTc ++ prolonged w/thioridazine and others	Typical antipsychotics associated with risk of glucose elevation intermediate between risperidone, olanzapine	Rare reports of respiratory distress, arrest; overdose may cause respiratory suppression	Prolactin $\uparrow$ is theoretical concern, but no definitive link between APs and cancer risk. Risks are dry mouth, EPS, constipation, hypotension
Atypical APs	Orthostatic hypotension with quetiapine, risperidone, olanzapine; less w/aripiprazole, ziprasidone; moderate QTc prolongation w/ziprasidone	Glucose elevation: Clozapine > olanzapine >> quetiapine > risperidone > ziprasidone > aripiprazole; Monitor BMI, glucose	Rare reports of acute respiratory failure associated with quetiapine, olanzapine, in COPD patients; respiratory depression w/combination of clozapine and benzodiazepine	Agranulocytosis risk with clozapine; prolactin $\uparrow$ w/risperidone; some atypicals may aid sleep, appetite, weight in cachectic cancer patients; risks = dry mouth, constipation, hypotension

Abbreviations: AP, antipsychotic; ++, marked; CHF, congestive heart failure; BMI, body mass index; EPS, extrapyramidal side effects; SNRI, Serotonin norepinephrine reuptake inhibitor.
Source: From Ref. 90.

A secondary analysis of ENRICHD reviewed antidepressant use in a subgroup of the 1834 depressed patients (39). The therapy patients were referred for possible medication, preferably sertraline, if severely depressed or failing to respond to CBT. Antidepressant use was more common in the CBT group (21% received SSRIs) than in the usual care group (14.6% received SSRIs). At 29 months, there was a remarkable 43% lower risk of death or recurrent MI in the SSRI group and a 28% lower risk in those receiving non-SSRI antidepressants.

The Canadian Cardiac Randomized Evaluation of Antidepressant and Psychotherapy Efficacy (CREATE) trial (40) studied the role of 12 weeks of interpersonal psychotherapy (IPT) and the SSRI citalopram in 284 depressed IHD patients who were not immediately post-MI. The four treatment possibilities were (i) IPT + citalopram, (ii) IPT + placebo, (iii) clinical management + citalopram, and (iv) clinical management + placebo. Patients were more depressed than in SADHART or ENRICHD (24-item Hamilton Depression Rating Scale score of 20 or higher). Citalopram was superior to placebo, and IPT was not better than clinical management in alleviating depression. As with SADHART, response was greater in those with recurrent depression.

It is uncertain if the potential benefits of SSRIs on IHD-related morbidity and mortality stem from amelioration of underlying depression or from pharmacologic effects on IHD pathophysiology. Sertraline decreased platelet activation in the SADHART study (41). Paroxetine, but not nortriptyline, reduced β-thromboglobulin and platelet factor 4 in a small study (42). The "antiplatelet" effects of SSRIs have also been suggested in large, retrospective databases noting increased risk of upper gastrointestinal bleeding (43). HRV is lessened by TCAs and is either increased or unaffected by SSRIs (32). Additionally, successful CBT in IHD patients with depression was associated with improved HRV (32)—perhaps affirming the "mind-body" connections depicted in Figure 1. Other interventions that might simultaneously ameliorate depression and IHD include cardiac rehabilitation (11), exercise (44), and omega-3 fatty acids (45).

Heart failure (HF), affecting five million elderly people in the United States, is the fastest growing form of cardiovascular disease in the past 10 years. (HF is now preferred to "congestive heart failure," because not all patients have volume overload.) Prevalence of depression in HF (21.5%) (46) is similar to that in IHD, but increases with increasing heart failure severity. Depression is associated with increased HF-related morbidity, mortality, and health care costs (46).

While a complete discussion of depression and comorbid COPD is beyond the scope of this chapter, a recent comprehensive review (47) strongly suggests a bidirectional relationship. On one hand, depression increases morbidity and reduces quality of life and adherence to planned care in patients with COPD. On the other hand, COPD may lead to depression as a patient's reaction to illness-related loss, as an effect secondary to medications such as corticosteroids, or by directly affecting the brain. Specifically, chronic hypoxemia and derangement of the cerebral microvasculature may be involved in the increased susceptibility to comorbid late-onset depression often seen in patients with COPD. The relationship between COPD and depression is further mediated by tobacco use. Young and depressed adults are more likely to smoke, which in turn increases late-life COPD risk. Additionally, in those with a history of depression, smoking cessation is less successful and can precipitate acute depression (47).

Diabetes Mellitus and Depression in the Elderly

Diabetes mellitus (DM) has recently gained attention in psychiatry because of the metabolic side effects of atypical antipsychotics. Yet from a national and worldwide public health perspective, diabetes is a wide-ranging concern and an emerging epidemic. Seven percent of the U.S. population (20.8 million people) is estimated to have DM, including 6.2 million who may be undiagnosed (48). The worldwide prevalence of DM in 2000 was 2.8% (171 million) and is expected to reach 4.4% in 2030 (366 million) (49).

The concurrence of diabetes and depression has long been noted. Meta-analyses suggest that the presence of diabetes doubles the risk of comorbid depression (15,16). Reported prevalence of depression in diabetes [e.g., 17.6% (16), 25% (50)] is more variable, depending on the population studied and the methodology used. For example, studies utilizing self-report mood scales find higher rates of depression than do those relying upon observed-administered structured interviews.

The sensitivity of diagnostic assessment for depression in patients with diabetes may be enhanced by relying on cognitive rather than somatic symptoms such as appetite, energy, and psychomotor changes that may be directly referable to diabetic illness (51). Depressed patients with diabetes reported a greater number of somatic diabetic symptoms, even after controlling for severity of diabetes (52).

What is the direction of causality in the diabetes–depression relationship? As with IHD, a diagnosis of diabetes, with its attendant limitations in activities of daily living, may precipitate feelings of sadness and loss. However, major depression has increasingly been found to precede the development of type 2 diabetes, rather than simply develop as a consequence (53). A meta-analysis of nine longitudinal studies (54) concluded that depression is an independent risk factor for DM, even after controlling for confounds such as weight, race, and socioeconomic status. Major depression or high depressive symptoms, in a recent large Norwegian study, increased the likelihood of developing type 2 diabetes mellitus by 37%. (55). The causal sequence is less clear with type 1 diabetes, which more often precedes depression diagnosis (53).

Depression may increase the risk of DM through a number of mechanisms (51,56). Mood disorders are associated with activation/dysregulation of counter-regulatory hormone systems including the sympathoadrenal, hypothalamic-pituitary-adrenocortical, and hypothalamic-growth hormone axes. These systems counteract the hypoglycemic effects of insulin by increasing glucose concentration via increased glucose production, enhanced glycogen breakdown, lipolysis, and inhibition of peripheral glucose transport and utilization. Depressed patients have been found, in particular, to exhibit decreased glucose utilization in the left frontal cortical areas (51). Recently, a cohort of young and depressed Finnish men were found to be insulin resistant (57).

Depression may also lead to diabetes via immune system activation. Cytokines are proteins, such as interleukins (ILs), interferons (IFNs), and tumor necrosis factor (TNF), that are released by immune system cells to generate an immune response. Some data suggest that the inflammatory cytokines IL-1 and IL-6, associated with depression, may also be diabetogenic (51).

The nature of the diabetes–depression interrelationship is complex, and probably includes psychosocial as well as physiologic links. Most studies, but not all (58), suggest that diabetes and depression worsen each other's outcome.

Depressive episodes in patients with either type 1- or type 2 diabetes are more recurrent, longer in duration, and more refractory to antidepressant treatment, especially when glycemic control is poor (50,53).

Physical inactivity, a strong risk factor for type 2 diabetes, may also be seen in major depression, and might contribute to the depression–diabetes link in a mutually reinforcing way. For example, compared with nondepressed diabetic patients, depressed diabetic patients exercise less, exhibit poorer self-care, and show decreased adherence to diet and treatment recommendations. Depressed diabetic patients also experience decreased quality of life, increased morbidity and mortality (59), increased hospitalization and health care costs (60), and poorer glycemic control, which itself is associated with diabetic complications (61).

Diabetes-related cerebrovascular disease may further worsen depressive symptomatology via so-called "vascular depression" mechanisms (62). Diabetic peripheral neuropathy pain and depression are also correlated (63). Sociocultural factors such as race (e.g., Native American, African-American), less education, unmarried status, and poor social support are also associated with depression in individuals with diabetes (51).

Given the overlapping pathophysiologies of diabetes and depression, it is not surprising that the treatment of one condition might ameliorate the other—for instance, aggressive antidiabetic treatment (e.g., insulin as opposed to oral hypoglycemics) may improve mood (50). However, amelioration of depression, associated with modest improvements in glycemic control in some studies (50), may vary with the differing metabolic effects of various antidepressants (56). Thus, monoamine oxidase inhibitors have been associated with hypoglycemia [summarized by Harnett (10)], whereas the TCAs nortriptyline (64) and imipramine (65,66) have been associated with hyperglycemia. TCAs could worsen diabetes via noradrenergic enhancement, blockade of M3 (muscarinic) receptors in pancreatic β-cells, or antagonism of 5-HT 2c receptors.

In contrast, SSRIs may modestly reduce hyperglycemia and increase insulin sensitivity (67,68,69), although longer studies are needed to see if such benefits persist. Preliminary evidence suggests that dual-mechanism antidepressants (e.g., venlafaxine, duloxetine) have a neutral effect on glucose homeostasis (56).

A recent major study of subjects with diabetes and depression found significant improvement in levels of glycosylated hemoglobin (Hb A-1-C) with open-label sertraline. In a subsequent 1-year maintenance phase, sertraline significantly delayed depressive recurrence as compared to placebo. Both maintenance groups sustained the lower Hb A-1-C levels during the depression-free interval (until recurrence). However, final Hb A-1-C in the two groups did not differ (68).

Consistent with the pathways shown in Figure 1, CBT may also improve mood and glycemic control in depressed diabetics (50). Psychologic intervention, mostly using variants of cognitive behavioral therapy, has more commonly aimed at improving glycemic control in diabetics without manifesting psychiatric illness. One meta-analysis found improvements in glycemic control and psychologic distress, but not in weight and serum glucose concentrations, in patients with type 2 diabetes (70) who receive psychological interventions. In those with type 1 diabetes, psychologic treatments tend to improve glycemic control in children and adolescents, but not in adults (71).

It is hoped that the elucidation of the diabetes–depression interrelationship will lead to more specific and effective treatment of both conditions.

Cancer and Depression in the Elderly

Of all the medical comorbidities, cancer most merits an "understandable" depressive response in the popular consciousness. Unfortunately, the refrain, "If *you* had cancer, wouldn't *you* be depressed?" leads to under-recognition and lack of treatment of mood disorders in individuals with cancer. Approximately 25% of patients with cancer will need evaluation and treatment of depression in the course of their illness (72). Depression rates vary with type of cancer, with higher rates occurring with pancreatic (73), oropharyngeal, and breast cancers (74), and lower rates with lymphoma, gastric cancer, and leukemia (74). Rates are also affected by diagnostic bias (see discussion below of inclusive vs. exclusive approach), assessment instrument used, type of cancer treatment given, and severity of disease. Depression may persist long after treatment and may be related to the intensity of the initial chemotherapeutic regimen (74).

Depression invariably impacts quality of life and often reduces adherence to care. It may also independently predict mortality in cancer patients, though there have been discrepant reports. A prior diagnosis of depression was associated with enhanced death risk in a tumor registry database of almost 25,000 elderly women with breast cancer. Though the depressed women were less likely to receive optimal treatment, greater mortality also occurred in the women who received "definitive" care (75). A Danish registry of over 20,000 patients with breast cancer found that depression diagnosed after early-stage cancer surgery and before later-stage surgery predicted greater natural-cause mortality (76).

The diagnosis of depression in patients with cancer has been controversial, owing to the overlap of somatic symptoms of depression, such as fatigue and anorexia, with the direct manifestations of the medical illness (77). An " inclusive" approach that includes all depressive symptoms irrespective of origin has increasingly been suggested to enhance diagnostic sensitivity. An "exclusive" approach omits somatic symptoms, such as fatigue and anorexia, and emphasizes cognitive features of depression. This method might enhance diagnostic specificity (lack of false positives), but at the price of diminished sensitivity. Knowledge and experience with specific medical illnesses can also be helpful to the psychiatrist in determining the origin of symptoms.

A study examining four groups (major depression without cancer, normal-comparison, cancer with major depression, and cancer without major depression) found six Hamilton Depression Rating Scale items that optimally diagnosed depression in patients with cancer—late insomnia, agitation, psychic anxiety, diurnal mood variation, depressed mood, and genital symptoms (78).

Cancer-related fatigue is itself a significant problem, experienced by more than 50% of patient with advanced cancer, and is related to both depression and pain (79). Low hemoglobin levels, often leading to fatigue, have also been associated with depression in patients with cancer (80).

While cancer-related pain often contributes to depression, it has also been argued that pain should be controlled before making a psychiatric diagnosis (72). Depression in a patient with cancer might also reflect a substance-induced mood disorder, e.g., secondary to corticosteroids, metoclopramide (Reglan), antiestrogens, exogenously administered cytokines (interferon-α, IL-2), or other chemotherapeutic agents (amphotericin-B, cycloserine, L-asparaginase, procarbazine, vinblastine, vincristine) (74).

The link between depression and cancer may also be explained by immune system activation, with cytokines leading to the syndrome of "sickness behavior" (81,82). This is a departure from the previous notion of depression association with immunosuppression (83). Infections (and cancers and their treatments) cause production of proinflammatory cytokines, which signal the brain to induce symptoms of sickness such as sleepiness, malaise, anhedonia, anorexia, decreased libido, withdrawal from social activities, inability to concentrate, hyperalgesia, and fever. This leads the organism to adjust its priorities so as to facilitate recovery from infection. Thus, sickness behavior, seen in all mammals and birds, may have evolutionary benefit, analogous to a fear response when exposed to a predator.

Cancer patients with depression were found to have significantly higher IL-6 levels than those without depression (84). Increased tumor burden, tissue destruction, chemotherapy, and radiation treatment are all associated with production of inflammatory cytokines, especially IL-1, IL-6, and TNF. These immune stimulators may induce depression/sickness behavior via HPA axis activation, blockade of glucocorticoid receptors (impairing negative feedback to the HPA axis and the inflammatory cytokines), or by induction of an enzyme that degrades L-tryptophan, the primary precursor of serotonin (74).

While there is justification to support the use of antidepressants and psychosocial treatments for depression in patients with cancer, a recent critical review emphasized the dearth of high-quality supportive evidence, especially when the criterion is alleviation of clinical depression, rather than improvement of depressive symptoms (85). Tricyclic antidepressants, SSRIs, mirtazapine, and mianserin have been recommended for depressed patients with cancer (86). Venlafaxine, duloxetine, bupropion, and tricyclics may mitigate neuropathic pain, while fluoxetine, paroxetine, and venlafaxine may reduce hot flashes in patients with cancer (74). Mirtazapine may be more helpful than SSRIs for illness- and treatment-related nausea and cachexia. Stimulants, modafinil, and bupropion help fatigue (87). While SSRIs are often preferred, subtle side effects should be considered, i.e., nausea, hyponatremia with mental status change, and drug interactions. Fluoxetine decreases the metabolism of a wide range of medications (by cytochrome P450 3A4 inhibition), and P450 2D6 inhibitors (e.g., paroxetine) may alter the clinical effect of tamoxifen (88).

In an innovative study, 40 patients with malignant melanoma due to receive high-dose IFN-α therapy were treated with either paroxetine or placebo, two weeks prior to the cancer treatment (89). Major depression developed in 11% of the paroxetine group (2 of 18 subjects) and 45% of the placebo group (9 of 20 subjets) over 12 weeks of IFN-α treatment. Severe depression in one of the subjects receiving paroxetine and seven of the subjects receiving placebo-necessitated discontinuation of the IFN-α treatment. It was not known if decreasing depressive symptoms lessened the effectiveness of IFN-α.

MEDICATION EFFECTS UPON MEDICAL COMORBIDITY

The pharmacologic treatment of mood disorders in the elderly is discussed in chapter 16. Our focus here is on the ways in which medication for mood disorders (mainly antidepressants and mood stabilizers) may affect the four main disease classes we have examined. In brief, the main concerns with these agents in depressed elderly patients with comorbid medical illness include the following:

- Anticholinergic side effects (dry mouth, constipation, etc.) with low-potency antipsychotics
- Hypotension and dizziness
- Cardiac conduction abnormalities and dysrhythmias
- Respiratory suppression
- Deleterious effects on neuroendocrine function
- Blood dyscrasias
- Drug drug interactions
- GI side effects of serotonergic agents can be obscured by comorbid medical illness
- Falls, ataxia with SSRIs, lithium, anticonvulsants

More detailed information is summarized in Table 1.

CONCLUSION

The Cartesian duality of "mind" and "body" has become increasingly untenable in the modern practice of medicine. In this chapter, we have outlined the complex, bidirectional relationship between depression and several highly prevalent medical illnesses in elderly populations (1). We have noted that depression-related immune dysfunction may worsen IHD via inflammatory mechanisms, even as IHD contributes to the patient's depression. We have reviewed data showing that depression may increase the risk of DM through a number of mechanisms (51,56) even as diabetes-related cerebrovascular disease may worsen depressive symptomatology. We have noted that a prior diagnosis of depression may be associated with increased risk of death among elderly women with breast cancer (75), while cancer-related pain often contributes to depression (72). Mood problems may also arise in these medically ill elderly patients as a result of medication-related side effects or drug interactions. As research sheds light on the molecular, neuroendocrine, and psychosocial bases for these complex interactions, our treatment of depressed, medically ill patients should be greatly enhanced.

ACKNOWLEDGMENT

The authors wish to thank Sandra A. Jacobson, MD, for her helpful comments on a portion of this chapter. We also appreciate the editing assistance of Margaret Trainor, Terri Niland, and Chantelle Marshall.

REFERENCES

1. Blazer DG, Hybels CF. Origins of depression in later life. Psychol Med 2005; 35(9):1241–1252.
2. Raj A. Depression in the elderly: Tailoring medical therapy to their special needs. Postgrad Med 2004; 115(6):26–42.
3. Newcomer JW. Medical risk in patients with bipolar disorder and schizophrenia. J Clin Psychiatry 2006; 67(suppl 9):25–30.
4. Yates WR, Mitchell J, Rush AJ, et al. Clinical features of depressed outpatients with and without co-occurring general medical conditions in STAR*D. Gen Hospital Psychiatry 2004; 26(6):421–429.

5. Proctor EK, Morrow-Howell NL, Dore P, et al. Comorbid medical conditions among depressed elderly patients discharged home after acute psychiatric care. Am J Geriatr Psychiatry 2003; 11(3):329–338.
6. Noel PH, Williams JW, Unutzer J, et al. Depression and comorbid illness in elderly primary care patients: Impact on multiple domains of health status and well-being. Ann Fam Med 2004; 2(6):555–562.
7. Unutzer J, Katon W, Sullivan M, et al. Treating depressed older adults in primary care: Narrowing the gap between efficacy and effectiveness. Milbank Q 1999; 77(2):225–256.
8. Unutzer J, Katon W, Callahan CM, et al. Collaborative care management of late-life depression in the primary care setting: A randomized controlled trial. JAMA 2002; 288(22):2836–2845.
9. Clarke DM, Cook KE, Coleman KJ, et al. A qualitative examination of the experience of "depression" in hospitalized medically ill patients. Psychopathology 2006; 39(6):303–312.
10. Harnett DS. The difficult-to-treat psychiatric patient with co-morbid medical illness. In: Dewan MJ, Pies R, eds . The Difficult-to-Treat Psychiatric Patient. Washington, D.C.: American Psychiatric Press, 2001:325–357.
11. Zellweger MJ, Osterwalder RH, Langewitz W, et al. Coronary artery disease and depression. Eur Heart J 2004; 25(1):3–9.
12. Lett HS, Blumenthal JA, Babyak MA, et al. Depression as a risk factor for coronary artery disease: Evidence, mechanisms, and treatment. Psychosom Med 2004; 66(3):305–315.
13. van Manen JG, Bindels PJ, Dekker FW, et al. Risk of depression in patients with chronic obstructive pulmonary disease and its determinants. Thorax 2002; 57(5):412–416.
14. Massie MJ. Prevalence of depression in patients with cancer. J Natl Cancer Instit Monogr 2004; 32:57–71.
15. Anderson RJ, Freedland KE, Clouse RE, et al. The prevalence of comorbid depression in adults with diabetes: A meta-analysis. Diabetes Care 2001; 24(6):1069–1078.
16. Ali S, Stone MA, Peters JL, et al. The prevalence of co-morbid depression in adults with type 2 diabetes: A systematic review and meta-analysis. Diabet Med 2006; 23(11):1165–1173.
17. Ghaemi SN. Paradigms of psychiatry: Eclecticism and its discontents. Curr Opin Psychiatry 2006; 19(6):619–624.
18. Drossman DA, Leserman J, Li Z, et al. Effects of coping on health outcome among women with gastrointestinal disorders. Psychosom Med 2000; 62(3):309–317.
19. Gross AR. The effect of coping strategies on the relief of pain following surgical intervention for lower back pain. Psychosom Med 1986; 48(3–4):229–241.
20. Chemerinski E, Robinson RG. The neuropsychiatry of stroke. Psychosomatics 2000; 41(1):5–14.
21. Johansson A, Ahren B, Nasman B, et al. Cortisol axis abnormalities early after stroke—Relationships to cytokines and leptin. J Intern Med 2000; 247(2):179–87.
22. Schatzberg AF, Posener JA, DeBattista C, et al. Neuropsychological deficits in psychotic versus nonpsychotic major depression and no mental illness. Am J Psychiatry 2000; 157(7):1095–1100.
23. Starkman MN. Psychiatric manifestations of hyperadrenocorticism and hypoadrenocorticism (Cushing's and Addison's Disease). In: Wolkowitz OM, Rothschild AJ, eds. Psychoneuroendocrinology. Washington, D.C.: American Psychiatric Press, 2003:165–188.
24. Rothschild AJ. The hypothalamic-pituitary-adrenal axis and psychiatric illness. In: Wolkowitz OM, Rothschild AJ, eds. Psychoneuroendocrinology. Washington, D.C.: American Psychiatric Press, 2003:139–163.
25. Glassman AH, Bigger JT, Gaffney M, et al. Onset of major depression associated with acute coronary syndrome: Relationship of onset, major depression disorder history, and episode severity to sertraline benefit. Arch Gen Psychiatry 2006; 63(3):283–288.
26. Frasure-Smith N, Lesperance F. Reflections on depression as a cardiac risk factor. Psychosom Med 2005; 67(suppl 1):S19–S25.
27. Rugulies R. Depression as a predictor for the development of coronary heart disease: A review and meta-analysis. Am J Prev Med 2002; 23(1):51–61.
28. Wulsin TR, Singal BM. Do depressive symptoms increase the risk for the onset of coronary disease? A systematic quantitative review. Psychosom Med 2003; 65(2):201–210.

29. Lesperance F, Frasure-Smith N, Talajic M, et al. Five-year risk of cardiac mortality in relation to initial severity and one-year changes in depression symptoms after myocardial infarction. Circulation 2002; 105(9):1049–1053.
30. van Melle J, de Jong P, Spijkerman TA, et al. Prognostic association of depression following myocardial infarction with mortality and cardiovascular events: A meta-analysis. Psychosom Med 2004; 66(6):814–822.
31. Barth J, Schumacher M, Herman-Langen C. Depression as a risk factor for mortality in patients with coronary heart disease. Psychosom Med 2004; 66(6):802–813.
32. Carney RM, Freedland KE, Veith RC. Depression, the autonomic nervous system, and coronary heart disease. Psychosom Med 2005; 67(suppl 1):S29–S33.
33. Carney RM, Howells WB, Blumenthal JA, et al. Heart rate turbulence, depression and survival after acute myocardial infarction. Psychosom Med 2007; 69(1):4–9.
34. Kop WJ, Gottidiener JS. The role of immune system parameters in the relationship between depression and coronary artery disease. Psychosom Med 2005; 67(suppl 1):S37–S41.
35. Bruce EC, Musselman DL. Depression, alterations in platelet function and ischemic heart disease. Psychosom Med 2005; 67(suppl 1):S34–S36.
36. Stewart JC, Janicki DL, Muldoon MF, et al. Negative emotions and 3-year progression of subclinical atherosclerosis. Arch Gen Psychiatry 2007; 64(2):225–233.
37. Glassman AH, O'Connor CM, Califf RM, et al. Sertraline treatment of major depression in patients with acute MI or angina. JAMA 2002; 288(14):701–709.
38. Berkman LF, Blumenthal J, Burg M, et al. Effects of treating depression and low perceived social support on clinical events after myocardial infarction: The Enhancing Recovery in Coronary Heart Disease Patients (ENRICHD) Randomized Trial. JAMA 2003; 289(23):3106–3116.
39. Taylor CB, Youngblood ME, Catellier D, et al. Effects of antidepressant medication on morbidity and mortality in depressed patients after myocardial infarction. Arch Gen Psychiatry 2005; 62(7):792–798.
40. Lesperance F, Frasure-Smith N, Koszycki D, et al. Effects of citalopram and interpersonal psychotherapy on depression in patients with coronary artery disease: The Canadian Cardiac Randomized Evaluation of Antidepressant and Psychotherapy Efficacy (CREATE) Trial. JAMA 2007; 297(4):367–379.
41. Serebruany VL, Glassman AH, Malinin AJ, et al. Platelet/endothelial biomarkers in depressed patients treated with selective serotonin reuptake inhibitor sertraline after acute coronary events: The Sertraline AntiDepressant Heart Attack Randomized Trial (SADHART) Platelet Substudy. Circulation 2003; 108(8):939–944.
42. Pollock BG, Laghrissi-Thade F, Wagner WR. Evaluation of platelet activation in depressed patients with ischemic heart disease after paroxetine or nortriptyline treatment. J Clin Psychopharmacol 2000; 20(2):137–140.
43. van Walraven C, Mamdani MM, Wells PS, et al. Inhibition of serotonin reuptake by antidepressants and upper gastrointestinal bleeding in elderly patients: Retrospective cohort study. BMJ 2001; 323(7314):655–658.
44. Lett HS, Davidson J, Blumenthal JA. Nonpharmacologic treatments for depression in patients with coronary heart disease. Psychosom Med 2005; 67(suppl 1):S58–S62.
45. Parker G, Gibson NA, Bratchie H, et al. Omega-3 fatty acids and mood disorders. Am J Psychiatry 2006; 163(6):969–978.
46. Rutledge T, Reis VA, Linke SE, et al. Depression in heart failure. A meta-analytic review of prevalence, intervention effects, and associations with clinical outcomes. J Am Coll Cardiol 2006; 48(8):1527–1537.
47. Norwood R, Balkissoon R. Current perspectives on management of co-morbid depression in COPD. COPD 2005; 2(1):185–193.
48. National Institute of Diabetes and Digestive and Kidney Diseases. National Diabetes Statistics fact sheet, 2005. Bethesda, MD: National Diabetes Information Clearinghouse. Online at http://diabetes.niddk.nih.gov/dm/pubs/statistics/index.htm#7 (accessed July 2, 2007).

49. Wild S, Roglic G, Green A, et al. Global prevalence of diabetes: Estimates for the year 2000 and projections for 2030. Diabetes Care 2004; 27(5):1047–1053.
50. Lustman PJ, Clouse RE. Depression in diabetic patients: The relationship between mood and glycemic control. J Diabetes Complications 2005; 19(2):113–122.
51. Musselman DL, Betan E, Larsen H, et al. Relationship of depression to diabetes types 1 and 2: Epidemiology, biology and treatment. Biol Psychiatry 2003; 54(3):317–329.
52. Ludman EJ, Katon W, Russo J, et al. Depression and diabetes burden. Gen Hosp Psychiatry 2004; 26(6):430–436.
53. Talbot F, Nouwen A. A review of the relationship between depression and diabetes in adults. Is there a link? Diabetes Care 2000; 23(10):1556–1562.
54. Knol MJ, Twisk JW, Beekman AT, et al. Depression as a risk factor for the onset of type 2 diabetes mellitus. A meta-analysis. Diabetologia 2006; 49(5):837–845.
55. Engum A. The role of depression and anxiety in onset of diabetes in a large population-based study. J Psychosom Res 2007; 62(1):31–38.
56. McIntyre RS, Soczynska JK, Konarski JZ, et al. The effect of antidepressants on glucose homeostasis and insulin sensitivity: Synthesis and mechanisms. Expert Opin Drug Saf 2006; 5(1):157–168.
57. Timonen M, Rajala U, Jokelainen J, et al. Depressive symptoms and insulin resistance in young adult males: Results from the Northern Finland 1966 birth cohort. Mol Psychiatry 2006; 11(10):929–933.
58. Engum A, Mykletun A, Midthjell K, et al. Depression and diabetes: A large population-based study of sociodemographic, lifestyle, and clinical factors with depression in type 1 and type 2 diabetes. Diabetes Care 2005; 28(8):1904–1909.
59. Fenton WS, Stover ES. Mood disorders: Cardiovascular and diabetes comorbidity. Curr Opin Psychiatry 2006; 19(4):421–427.
60. Simon GE, Katon WJ, Lin EH, et al. Diabetes complications and depression as predictors of the health care costs. Gen Hosp Psychiatry 2005; 27(5):344–351.
61. Lustman PJ, Anderson RJ, Freedland KE, et al. Depression and poor glycemic control. A meta-analytic review of literature. Diabetes Care 2000; 23(7):934–942.
62. Jacobson AM, Samson JA, Weinger K, et al. Diabetes, the brain and behavior: Is there a biological mechanism underlying the association between diabetes and depression? Int Rev Neurobiol 2002; 51:455–479.
63. Vileikyte L, Leventhal H, Gonzales JS, et al. Diabetic peripheral neuropathy and depressive symptoms: The association revisited. Diabetes Care 2005; 28(10):2378–2383.
64. Lustman PJ, Griffith LS, Clouse RE, et al. Effects of nortriptyline on depression and glycemic control in diabetes: Results of a double-blind, placebo-controlled trial. Psychosom Med 1997; 59(3):241–250.
65. Ghaeli P, Shahsavand E, Mesbahi M, et al. Comparing the effects of 8-week treatment with fluoxetine and imipramine on fasting blood glucose of patients with major depressive disorder. J Clin Psychopharmacol 2004; 24(4):386–388.
66. Derijks HJ, de Koning FH, Meyboom RH, et al. Impaired glucose homeostasis after impramine intake in a diabetic patient [Letter to the Editor]. J Clin Psychopharmacol 2005; 25(6):621–623.
67. Lustman PJ, Freedland KE, Griffith LS, et al. Fluoxetine for depression in diabetes. A random double-blind placebo-control trial. Diabetes Care 2000; 23(5):618–623.
68. Lustman PJ, Clouse RE, Nix BD, et al. Sertraline for prevention of depression recurrence in diabetes mellitus. A randomized, double-blind, placebo-controlled trial. Arch Gen Psychiatry 2006; 63(5):521–529.
69. Paile-Hyvarinen M, Wahlbeck K, Eriksson JG. Quality of life and metabolic status in mildly depressed women with type 2 diabetes treated with paroxetine: A single blind randomized placebo-controlled trial. BMC Fam Pract 2003; 4:7.
70. Ismail K, Winkley K, Rabe-Hesketh S. Systematic review and meta-analysis of randomized controlled trials of psychological interventions to improve glycaemic control in patients with type 2 diabetes. Lancet 2004; 363(9521):1589–1597.

71. Winkley K, Ismail K, Landau S, et al. Psychological interventions to improve glycaemic control in patients with type 1 diabetes: Systemic review and meta-analysis of randomized controlled trials. BMJ 2006; 333(7558):65–68.
72. Miller K, Massie MJ. Depression and anxiety. Cancer J 2006; 12(5):388–397.
73. Boyd AD, Riba M. Depression and pancreatic cancer. J Natl Compr Cancer Netw 2007; 5(1):113–116.
74. Raison CL, Miller AH. Depression in cancer: New developments regarding diagnosis and treatment. Biol Psychiatry 2003; 54(3):283–294.
75. Goodwin JS, Zhang DD, Ostir GV. Effect of depression on diagnosis, treatment, and survival of older women with breast cancer. J Am Geriatr Soc 2004; 52(1):106–111.
76. Hjerl K, Anderson EW, Keiding N, et al. Depression as a prognostic factor for breast cancer mortality. Psychosomatics 2003; 44(1):24–30.
77. Harnett DS. Psychopharmacologic treatment of depression in the medical setting. In: Hall RCW, ed. Recent Advances in Psychiatric Medicine. Longwood, FL: Ryandic Publishing, 1989:91–105.
78. Guo Y, Musselman DL, Manatunga AK, et al. The diagnosis of major depression in patients with cancer: A comparative approach. Psychosomatics 2006; 47(5):376–384.
79. Rao A, Cohen HJ. Symptoms management in the elderly cancer patients: Fatigue, pain, and depression. J Natl Cancer Instit Monogr 2004; 32:150–157.
80. Skarstein J, Bjelland I, Dahl AA, et al. Is there an association between hemoglobin, depression, and anxiety in cancer patients? J Psychosom Res 2005; 58(6):477–483.
81. Dantzer R. Cytokine, sickness behavior and depression. Neurol Clin 2006; 24(3):441–460.
82. Dantzer R, Kelley KW. Twenty years of research on cytokine-induced sickness behavior. Brain Behav Immun 2007; 21(2):153–160.
83. Raison CL, Capuron L, Miller AH. Cytokines sing the blues: Inflammation and the pathogenesis of depression. Trends Immunol 2006; 27(1):24–31.
84. Jehn CF, Kuehnhardt D, Bartholomae A, et al. Biomarkers of depression in cancer patients. Cancer 2006; 107:2723–2729.
85. Williams S, Dale J. The effectiveness of treatment for depression/depressive symptoms in adults with cancer: A systematic review. Br J Cancer 2006; 94(3):372–390.
86. Evans DL, Charney DS, Lewis L, et al. Mood disorders in the medically ill: Scientific review and recommendations. Biol Psychiatry 2005; 58(3):175–189.
87. Moss EL, Simpson JS, Pellitier G, et al. An open-label study of the effects of bupropion SR on fatigue, depression and quality of life of mixed-site cancer patients and their partners. Psychooncology 2006; 15(3):259–267.
88. Jin Y, Desta Z, Stearns V, et al. CYP2D6 genotype, antidepressant use, and tamoxifen metabolism during adjuvant breast cancer treatment. J Natl Cancer Instit 2005; 97:30–39.
89. Musselman DL, Lawson DH, Gumnick JF, et al. Paroxetine for the prevention of depression induced by high-dose interferon alpha. N Engl J Med 2001; 344:961–966.
90. Jacobson SA, Pies RW, Katz IR. Clinical Manual of Geriatric Psychopharmacology. Washington, D. C.: American Psychiatric Press, 2007.

12 Substance Use Disorders and Late-Life Depression

E. Nalan Ward

West End Clinic, Outpatient Addiction Services, Department of Psychiatry, Massachusetts General Hospital, and Department of Psychiatry, Harvard Medical School, Boston, Massachusetts, U.S.A.

INTRODUCTION

By 2030, it is projected that 21% of the American population will be older than 65 years (1). In 2000, the number of the elderly in need of substance-abuse treatment was about 1.7 million. This number will double to 4.4 million by 2020 (2).

Historically, alcohol has been the most commonly reported primary substance of use among the elderly. Interestingly, between 1995 and 2002 the number of treatment admissions among older adults who report alcohol as their primary substance declined from 86.5% to 77.5%. During this same time period, there was an increase in geriatric inpatient admissions for a primary diagnosis of substance use disorders amounting to a 106% increase for men and a 119% increase for women (3).

Among the elderly with depression, the rates of substance use disorders are higher than among the general elderly population. The prevalence of substance use disorder among elderly patients with major depression has been estimated between 15% and 20% in various psychiatric settings such as outpatient, inpatient, and specialty geriatric clinics (4–7). Even a past history of major depressive disorder seems to predict higher rates of alcohol use disorders.

The majority of the elderly do not receive the substance abuse and mental health treatment that they need. Screening early intervention and preventive services are very limited from both a substance abuse and mental health perspective. Given the rapidly growing numbers of the elderly and the already limited access to mental health care, the future is certain to present a challenge in addressing the needs of elderly depressed adults with co-occurring substance use disorders.

EPIDEMIOLOGY

Alcohol Use

The National Institute for Alcohol Abuse and Alcoholism (NIAAA) recommends, "no more than one drink a day" for individuals older than 65 years (8). The Center for Substance Abuse Treatment (CSAT) Treatment Improvement Protocol (TIP 26) on Substance Abuse Among Older Adults, recommends (9)

1. no more than one drink per day for men,
2. maximum of two drinks on any drinking occasion (New Year's Eve, weddings), and
3. somewhat lower limits for women.

According to the 2006 National Survey on Drug Use and Health (NSDUH) the prevalence of any alcohol use was 48.0% among 60- to 64-year-old people (10). Of those, 35.2% were current alcohol users, meaning they reported having at least one alcoholic drink within the last month. Binge alcohol users were reported to be about 10.1%, and 2.7% were heavy alcohol users.

Among adults aged 65 years and older, the estimated prevalence of alcohol use in 2006 was 38.4%. Of those, 30.8% were current alcohol users (nonbinge or heavy use), 6.0% were binge alcohol users (nonheavy use), and 1.6% were heavy alcohol users (10).

Illicit Drug Use

According to the NSDUH, adults aged 50 to 59 years showed an increased rate of current illicit drug use between 2002 and 2005 No further change was reported in 2006 (10). The reported increase may partially reflect the aging of the baby boomer cohort, whose lifetime rates of illicit drug use are higher than those of preceding cohorts. Specifically, among 60- to 64-year-old people, 2.1% used illicit drugs in the past month whereas the percentage fell to 0.7% for persons aged 65 years or older. Marijuana was the most commonly used illicit drug (1.1%), followed by prescription-type drugs used nonmedically (0.7%) and cocaine (0.2%). According to a 2005 Drug and Alcohol Services Information Services Report (DASIS) from the Substance Abuse and Mental Health Services Administration (SAMHSA), opiates were the most commonly reported primary nonalcohol drug of abuse, for all drug abuse inpatient admissions aged 50 years and older (3). Between 1995 and 2005, primary opiate admissions increased from 6.6% to 10.5% of admissions aged 65 years or older. This comes as no surprise given the increased prevalence of prescription opioid abuse in adult population.

COMORBIDITY

In the elderly population, comorbidity rates for mental health disorders and substance abuse vary, ranging from 7% to 38% of those with psychiatric illness and 21% to 66% of those with substance abuse. Among the elderly, alcohol abuse and depression are the most commonly comorbid pair. Prigerson et al. (6) reported the rate of co-occurring mental health and substance abuse disorders as 13.5% between age 55 and 64 years and 7.3% among those aged 65 to 74 years in an outpatient setting. The observed comorbidity rates tend to be even higher in psychiatric inpatient settings. In one study, one-third of the elderly inpatients were diagnosed with co-occurring psychiatric and substance use disorders (5). In particular, the substance use disorder tends to be alcohol abuse and the psychiatric diagnosis is usually is depression.

Psychiatric comorbidity rates are high among patients with diagnosed substance use disorders such as older veterans with alcohol dependence, older adults attending alcohol dependence rehabilitation programs, and hospitalized elders with prescription drug dependence. In such instances, a mood disorder seems to be the predominant psychiatric comorbidity (11,12). This pattern is also illustrated in a study of Italian primary care practice users of benzodiazepines between the ages of 65 and 84 years. Of the 1156 subjects, 36.5% were found to have a depressive disorder (13).

Comorbidity of substance use and mood disorders seems to be associated with poor outcomes, increased health care cost, increased mortality and suicidal ideation (14,15).

CLINICAL PRESENTATION AND DIAGNOSIS

Depression can predispose to substance abuse and substance abuse can lead to clinical depression. In most cases where an individual has been abusing substances for a long time, it can be difficult to tease out which came first. Often, a patient does not acknowledge the presence of substance abuse even while seeking treatment for a mood disorder, as demonstrated in the following vignette:

Alcohol Use Disorders and Depression in Elderly

> Mrs. V, a 72-year-old retired woman, was first admitted to inpatient medical care for broken ribs and pneumonia. Within six months after her discharge, she was admitted for the second time after falling at home. Both times, she was brought into hospital by her adult son who found her on the floor intoxicated. Since her husband's death two years earlier, Mrs. V had been suffering from clinical depression. Her treatment included visits to a psychotherapist and prescription of an *antidepressant* by her primary care physician. Her son was upset over her drinking. He complained of finding her drunk on many occasions at her home, and he noted the presence of hidden, empty bottles. Despite this evidence of alcohol use and its untoward consequences, however, she denied having any problems with drinking and expressed interest only in being treated for depression.

The medical team therefore sought consultation from the addiction services team.

In practice, every elderly depressed patient should be screened for substance use disorders. Obtaining a history of the presence or absence of past substance use disorders in relation to depressive disorder can guide clinicians toward a more successful treatment outcome. In the elderly, diagnosis of substance use disorders can be challenging because the DSM-IV-TR criteria do not apply as clearly as they do to younger patients. The Consensus Panel on Substance Abuse Among Older Adults (TIP 26) has emphasized, for example, that DSM-IV-TR criteria may not be adequate to diagnose older adults with alcohol problems (10).

Physiologic Dependence

As adults age, vulnerability to some of alcohol's negative consequences may increase (16). The decreased physiologic volume of distribution results in a higher blood alcohol level for a given amount of intake. Decreased hepatic metabolism can contribute to the higher blood level as well. Many older adults, especially those who begin their drinking later in life, show increased sensitivity to alcohol's intoxicating effects with less development of tolerance. Even in the absence of signs of physiologic dependence, however, the consequences of alcohol use can be quite severe (17).

Substances Taken in Larger Amounts than Intended

Cognitive impairment, whether as a result of alcohol consumption or an independent disorder, can impair an individual's self-monitoring capacity. As a result, the individual is not fully aware of the amount of alcohol used. He or she may drink more than intended and may fail to report with accuracy the amount of use (9).

Giving up Important Social, Occupational Activities

Assessing the severity of the effects of alcohol use on the basis of interference with social, work, or family responsibilities is more complicated in elderly retired patients whose schedules may be less busy with activities and responsibilities (9).

Due to the limitations of DSM-IV-TR alcohol use disorders criteria for elderly patients, The Consensus Panel on Substance Abuse among Older Adults (TIP 26) recommends use of the terms *at-risk* and *problem drinkers*. This model is preferred over the use of DSM-IV-TR diagnostic categories by some substance abuse specialists because it provides more flexibility in capturing drinking patterns of the elderly. An at-risk drinker is one whose pattern of alcohol use, although not yet causing problems, may bring about adverse consequences e.g., imprudent operation of a motor vehicle after drinking at a party. Problem drinking signifies a more hazardous level of consumption.

For those who treat persons with late-life depression, diagnosing comorbid substance use disorders can be challenging due to impaired cognition, judgment, and altered mood.

A thorough alcohol use history should be obtained from the patient, family members, or from other health care providers. The age of onset of problem drinking becomes important in the differential diagnostic process. Elderly patients who had an early onset of alcoholism, typically present with a long history of pathologic alcohol use beginning in their 20s or 30s, with multiple consequences of drinking in different aspects of their lives such as alcohol-related medical illness (e.g., pancreatitits, cirrhosis); legal problems; loss of job, marriage, and relationships; financial loss; history of detoxification; outpatient treatment, rehabilitation, and residential programs. Behavioral and personality problems, history of familial alcoholism, and recurrent clinical depression are common. Elderly patients with early-onset alcoholism also often present with a history of cognitive decline, disinhibition, poor judgment and memory loss as a result of the cumulative effects of chronic alcohol use. Depressed patients with longstanding, prior comorbid, severe alcoholism may have a relatively poor prognosis (18).

On the other hand, those with late-onset alcoholism present with onset of drinking after the age of 55 or 60 years, usually in response to losses, life changes, or the death of a loved one. They tend to have fewer complications from chronic drinking. Comorbid depression is again common among these patients, but it seems to be related to a loss or a life change. The depression among late-onset drinkers is thought to be more amenable to treatment. Approximately one-third of older adults with a drinking problem tend to be late-onset problem drinkers (19). These patients demonstrate less cognitive decline and loss compared to early-onset alcoholics. These patients have fewer alcohol-related chronic illnesses, such as cirrhosis, but medically will be as much affected by alcohol as early-onset alcoholics (e.g., Diabetes mellitus, drug–alcohol interactions, and falls) (9).

In the general adult population, depression is more common among women and alcoholism is seen predominantly in males. Gender differences in drinking patterns and the prevalence of depression tend to diminish over time among the elderly as women live longer than men and late-onset alcoholism affects more women than men (9).

A topic of special interest in the elderly population is the interface of pain and drinking problems. A 2005 study by Brennan et al. (20) demonstrated that older adults with problem drinking tend to use alcohol more to manage their pain than their peers without problem drinking. Also, this group with problem drinking reported more severe pain and more disruption of daily activities due to pain compared to older nonproblem drinkers. The authors emphasized the need to screen and monitor drinking behaviors of older patients presenting with pain, especially those with preexisting alcohol problems (20).

Drug-Use Disorders and Depression in the Elderly

The elderly adults use a higher number of prescribed- and over-the-counter medications than any other age group (21). Prescription drug misuse and abuse are not uncommon among the elderly. Misuse of drugs in the elderly patients includes such behaviors as using more or less than the prescribed dose, use for contraindicated purposes, mixing medications inappropriately with one another or with alcohol, skipping doses, or hoarding drugs (22). The diagnostic ambiguity of comorbid substance abuse and depression is illustrated in the following vignette:

> Mr. G, a 68-year-old male patient with a history of recurrent major depressive disorder, opioid and sedative hypnotic dependence in partial remission, Cluster B personality disorder traits, Hepatitis C, and liver cirrhosis, was followed by a team consisting of a primary care physician, a psychiatrist, and a neurologist. He was treated with an antidepressant and a low-dose antipsychotic. Typically, he presented with drug seeking behavior. He insisted that the only medication that helped him was lorazepam and his clinicians suspected that he used this and/or other prescription drugs illicitly. Occasionally, he appeared disinhibited and easily *agitated*. When he was asked to reflect on his behavior, Mr. G invariably attributed his presentation to being depressed, feeling down, and being on the wrong medications. His primary care physician and his neurologist cautioned him repeatedly that he should stay away from benzodiazepines and narcotic painkillers, because they would only complicate his already compromised health. Nonetheless, falls and amnesia continued and laboratory testing showed the presence of diazepam in his blood at the time of one of his emergency department visits for confusion.

Benzodiazepines and Sedative-Hypnotics

Although geriatric specialists advise limiting the use of this group of medications in the elderly, many older patients are still prescribed benzodiazepines on a daily basis for at least one year or at doses considered to be high (14,23,24). Patients with a prior history of illicit or prescription drug abuse and depressive disorders have been reported to be at higher risk for misusing prescribed benzodiazepines A group at special risk for benzodiazepine abuse is those patients with opioid dependence who are maintained on methadone therapy (25). Not much is known about the aging patients on methadone maintenance, but it is suggested that they be monitored vigilantly for benzodiazepine misuse, abuse, or dependence. Chronic use of psychoactive substances in the elderly is associated with multiple complications related to aging. The older body's ability to metabolize and eliminate drugs is diminished, resulting in greater drug accumulation, increased neurotoxicity and consequently impaired psychomotor performance, gait problems, falls, confusion, mood lability, and amnesia.

Chronic prescription of benzodiazepines and/or opioids can lead to physiologic dependence with tolerance and withdrawal. The elderly depressed patients can develop iatrogenic dependence without realizing it. A study from Mayo Clinic showed that one-third of the elderly patients who were admitted to the hospital due to prescription drug dependence had a mood disorder (26), Chronic users of benzodiazepines, according to available studies tend to be older, female, and with psychologic distress, dysphoria, and depression (26,27). An expert consensus panel (TIP 26) recommended that sedative-hypnotics be prescribed for only 7 to 10 days at a time to older adults, with frequent monitoring of use in patients treated longer than 2 to 3 weeks, and that benzodizapines used to treat anxiety disorders not be prescribed longer than four months (9).

Opioids and Cocaine

According to the 2005 Healthcare Cost and Utilization Project Data on community hospital inpatient stays, opioids were the most frequently named drugs cited for a drug abuse hospitalization in older patients (12.2% of the elderly drug abuse stays). Most abused opioids were misused legal prescription medications. Cocaine abuse was responsible for 4.3% of these drug abuse stays for patients 65 and above (28). The remaining 83.2% of drug abuse hospitalizations for those 65 years and older were for drug abuse classified as "other"(usually 2 or more drugs).

SCREENING TOOLS AND OTHER DIAGNOSTIC INSTRUMENTS

As the elderly proportion of the U. S. population increases, health care providers should become more vigilant in screening older adults for substance use as well as psychiatric disorders. Because most elderly patients never consult a mental health specialist, this screening may need to take place in primary care or community settings. Studies have indicated, however, that primary care screening of substance abuse disorders may be implemented ineffectively. In one study, for example, 263 elderly patients with a history of substance abuse were screened by medical staff and only 3 of 88 problem users of benzodiazepines, 29 of 76 smokers, and 33 of 99 problem drinkers were correctly identified (29). Another study revealed a higher rate of screening for problem alcohol use among internists than among geriatricians (30).

Perhaps the failure to recognize substance abuse disorders in primary care settings can be understood in part as a consequence of the challenging nature of the task. Elderly patients with substance use problems have a tendency to hide their behaviors and minimize their reported substance use. Depressed patients who show poor self-care and social isolation may be at particular risk for comorbid substance abuse. The clinician should therefore look for evidence of intoxication such as shuffling gait, slurred speech, unexplained falls and bruises, cognitive decline, amnesia, or new seizure activity. Liver function test abnormalities and anemia are common laboratory findings in persons with substance use disorders, and confirmation of substance abuse in some cases may be obtained through the presence of unprescribed intoxicants on a urine- or blood toxicology screen.

The clinician's approach to an elderly depressed patient who may be abusing substances should be nonjudgmental, motivational, and supportive. Clinicians should ask a standard series of questions to understand the quantity and the frequency of alcohol use.

1. "Do you drink alcohol?"
2. "On average, how many days a week do you drink?"
3. "On a day when you drink alcohol, how many drinks do you have?"
4. "What is the maximum number of drinks you consumed on any given occasion in the past month?"

Eight or more drinks per week or two or more occasions of binge drinking during the past month are indicative of alcohol-use problems (31).

The CAGE Questionnaire and the Michigan Alcoholism Screening Test-Geriatric Version (MAST-G) are two well-known, alcohol-screening instruments that have been validated for use with older adults (32,33). A more recent study has suggested that the Alcohol Use Disorders Identification Test—AUDIT and AUDIT-5—are both appropriate screening instruments for detecting problem drinking in older adults with mental illness (34). The sensitivity, specificity, and positive predictive value of AUDIT and AUDIT-5 were superior to CAGE.

Although abuse of legal and illegal drugs other than alcohol is a growing problem for the elderly, there are no validated screening or assessment instruments available. In addition, effective screening and identification of substance use disorders among groups such as depressed patients with physical disabilities, chronic pain, or elderly depressed minorities are understudied areas.

NEUROPSYCHOLOGICAL TESTING AND NEUROIMAGING

Of the 20 million alcoholics in the United States, up to 2 million alcoholics will develop permanent and debilitating conditions that require lifetime custodial care (35). Examples of such conditions include alcohol-induced persisting amnestic disorder (also called Wernicke-Korsakoff syndrome) and dementia, which seriously affects many mental functions in addition to memory (e.g., language, reasoning, and problem-solving abilities).

Heavy drinking promotes shrinkage of brain tissue and leads to neurodegenerative changes and cognitive decline over time. Some of the effects of heavy alcohol use on brain function are similar to those observed with Alzheimer disease. Alcohol-related changes may be reversible compared to normal aging or Alzheimer disease. Atrophy can decrease and cognitive performance may improve after abstinence from alcohol (36).

Comorbid psychiatric conditions such as depression, anxiety, schizophrenia, and use of other drugs can interact to aggravate alcoholism's effects on the brain and behavior (37). In the case of elderly depressed patients with comorbid alcohol or drug abuse, the cognitive presentation can be very confusing. Patients may seem unresponsive to traditional treatment modalities. Addressing substance use disorders may help improve the cognitive function or may stop progression of cognitive decline in such patients.

Magnetic resonance imaging studies show brain shrinkage in chronic alcoholics. This is most marked in the frontal regions and especially in older alcoholics (38). Other areas vulnerable to shrinkage are the limbic system, thalamus, hypothalamus, right hemisphere, and cerebellum (39).

For purposes of differential diagnosis, there might be benefits in obtaining neuropsychological testing along with imaging in such cases to measure executive functions controlled by frontal lobes, such as problem solving abilities, reasoning, and the ability to inhibit irrelevant responses and to measure spatial cognition controlled by right hemisphere (35).

The Center for Substance Abuse Treatment (CSAT) Treatment Improvement Protocol for Older Adults (TIP 26) recommends using an Orientation/Memory/Concentration Test or the Mini Mental Status Examination to screen for cognitive dysfunction in older substance abusers. Visuospatial performance tends to be significantly abnormal among patients with heavy drinking, so the Panel

TABLE 1 Intervention with Older Adults with Alcohol Use.

Preventive education for abstinent, low-risk drinkers
Brief, preventive intervention with at-risk drinkers
Alcoholism treatment for abusing/dependent (heavy) drinkers

recommends using the "draw-a-clock-test" to assess visuospatial functioning and the Neurobehavioral Cognitive Status Examination (NCSE) to assess for abstract thinking and visual memory (9).

TREATMENT

The treatment of co-occurring substance use and mental health problems among older adults is an understudied area, but existing studies support the effectiveness of concurrent treatment of substance abuse and depression in reducing alcohol use and improving depressive symptoms.

The Center for Substance Abuse Treatment's Treatment Improvement Protocol on Older Adults (TIP 26) has recommended several approaches for the effective treatment of elderly patients with substance abuse problems. These include brief interventions, cognitive behavioral approaches, group-based approaches, individual counseling, medical/psychiatric approaches, marital and family involvement/family therapy, case management/community–linked services, and outreach (9).

Once an elderly is screened and identified as having a substance use problem, the least intensive treatment options should be utilized first. A common sequence is to try brief intervention initially, and follow-up with motivational interviewing. Brief intervention, a nonconfrontational approach that relies upon tools from motivational psychology and behavioral self-control training, has been shown to reduce alcohol use in older adults (40–42). The studies have shown that older adults can be engaged in brief intervention, that this technique is acceptable in this population, and that there is a substantial reduction in drinking and in alcohol-related harm and health care utilization among at-risk drinkers receiving the interventions compared with a control group.

For elderly depressed patients who are at-risk drinkers, an older-adult–specific brief intervention should be conducted. During the intervention, the patient should get nonconfrontational feedback on screening questions, followed by some information on drinking patterns in elderly patients with depression. Some time should be spent on reasons for drinking. It is very important for the provider to understand the role of alcohol in relation to depression. The psychological as well as medical consequences of drinking should be discussed. This intervention may be a good opportunity for the clinician to introduce the concepts of self-medicating and mood-altering effects of hazardous drinking. Reasons to cut down normal drinking limits in elderly and cutting down strategies need to be discussed. An agreement outlining a drinking plan should be written and signed by the patient and the clinician. The agreement should be reviewed during the follow-up visit. Once patient is engaged in this paradigm, the clinician should periodically monitor the patient's drinking pattern along with mood changes (Table 1).

A more intensive intervention, a confrontation during which family members give feedback, is usually conducted by an addiction specialized counselor. The intervention includes the patient, family, and friends. When family is present, no more than one or two close relatives should be involved. During intervention, clinicians should be mindful about monitoring feelings of shame and embarrassment, especially with a depressed elderly patient (9).

For depressed patients who are more severe problem drinkers, or who fail to respond to interventions, motivational interviewing should be considered.

Motivational interviewing techniques use the concept of stages of change. The specific stages are precontemplation (unreadiness to consider change), contemplation (readiness to consider change), action, and maintenance. In this model, the differences in readiness to change are acknowledged. The clinician is understanding and respectful of the patient's perspective and his or her ambivalance about the need to change. The clinician helps the patient identify the negative consequences of continued drinking and supports an effort to develop greater insight and behavioral changes. Motivational counseling has been proven to be effective with older adults (43).

When elderly patients do not respond to less intensive approaches such as brief intervention, intervention, and motivational interviewing, clinicians should consider referral to specialized substance abuse or dual diagnosis programs. Inpatient detoxification or dual diagnosis admission may be required for those who are in high risk of serious withdrawal symptoms, suicidal, with untreated depression, unstable medical condition, mixed addictions, and who are unstable psychosocially (44).

TREATMENT OF COMORBID SUBSTANCE ABUSE AND DEPRESSION IN ELDERLY

According to SAMHSA's recent review, methods for the evaluation and treatment of co-occurring substance use and mental health problems among older adults remain understudied. Depression and alcohol use are the most commonly cited co-occurring disorders in older adults. Co-occuring mental health and substance use disorders are associated with poor health outcome, greater inpatient and outpatient service utilization, and increased suicidal ideation and attempts, compared to either disorder alone (45).

A study by Oslin et al. (46) highlighted the importance of identifying and treating comorbid depression and substance abuse. In their study cohort, approximately 80% of moderate- and high alcohol consuming patients reduced their drinking by more than 90% while receiving treatment for depression. Reducing alcohol use, in this study, was associated with a modest benefit on depression outcomes, compared to older adults who continued to drink. Reduced alcohol use and diminished relapses during treatment of depression were also associated with reduced depression in another randomized clinical trial that compared treatment of elderly depressed alcohol-dependent adults with sertraline and psychosocial support with or without adjunctive naltrexone (47). Interestingly, the presence of naltrexone in this particular study conferred no additional benefit in treating alcohol dependence. These findings are consistent with a recommendation from SAMHSA's Older Americans Substance Abuse and Mental Health Technical Assistance Center (TAC) that concurrent treatment of substance abuse and depression in elderly may be effective both in reducing alcohol use and improving depressive symptoms (45).

PREVENTION/EARLY INTERVENTION

Data on the prevention and early intervention of co-occurring disorders in older adults are limited. There are no standard prevention programs for older adults. Prevention (and early intervention) strategies to treat co-occurring substance abuse and mental health problems in older adults should include programs that combine medication with psychotherapy for depression and integrated service delivery approaches.

The Primary Care Research in Substance Abuse and Mental Health for Elderly (PRISM-E) study compared treatment engagement of older primary care patients (age 65 years and older) receiving care through two distinct services models, including integrated substance abuse and mental health treatment and enhanced referral to a specialty mental health clinic. In the integrated model, substance abuse and mental health services were colocated in the primary care setting. In the specialty clinic model, treatment was offered at a separate location. The authors concluded older patients preferred the integrated primary care site and engaged more in treatment in this model. The integrated model was superior in engaging patients with at-risk alcohol use, suicidal ideation and increased distress, and severe depression (48).

CONCLUSION

Alcohol and drug abuse continue to be public health problems among the rapidly growing elderly population. In the elderly, alcohol abuse and depression are very commonly present together. There are many barriers to screening and early detection of these comorbid conditions. Comorbidity of substance use and mood disorders seems to be associated with poor outcomes, increased health care cost, increased mortality, and suicidal ideation. Available studies indicate the importance of screening for, and addressing, these conditions in primary care settings.

REFERENCES

1. U.S. Census Bureau. U.S. Interim Projections by Age, Sex, Race, and Hispanic Origin: Table 2a. Projected Population of the United States, by Age and Sex: 2000 to 2050. www.census.gov/ipc/www/usinterimproj
2. Gfroerer J, Penne M, Pemberton M, et al. Substance abuse treatment need among older adults in 2020: The impact of the aging baby-boom cohort. Drug Alcohol Depend 2003; 69(2):127–135.
3. Substance Abuse and Mental Health Services Administration, Office of Applied Studies. (November 8, 2007). The DASIS Report: Older Adults in Substance Abuse Treatment: 2005. Rockville, MD. http://www.oas.samhsa.gov/
4. Regier DA, Farmer ME, Rae DS, et al. Comorbidity of mental disorders with alcohol and other drug abuse: Results from the Epidemiologic Catchment Area (ECA) study. J Am Med Assoc 1990; 264(19):2511–2518.
5. Devanand DP. Comorbid psychiatric disorders in late life depression. Biological Psychiatry 2002; 52(3):236–242.
6. Prigerson HG, Desai RA, Rosenheck RA. Older adult patients with both psychiatric and substance abuse disorders: Prevalence and health service use. Psychiatr Q 2001 Spring; 72(1):1–18.
7. Speer DC, Bates K. Comorbid mental and substance disorders among older psychiatric patients. J Am Geriatr Soc 1992; 40:886–890.

8. National Institute on Alcohol Abuse and Alcoholism. Alcohol Alert No. 40: Alcohol and Aging. Bethesda, MD: The Institute, 1998.
9. Treatment Improvement Protocol (TIP) #26. Substance Abuse Among Older Adults. U.S. Department of Health and Human Services. Public Health Service, Substance Abuse and Mental Health Services Administration, Center for Substance Abuse Treatment. Rockville, MD: 1998. http://www.ncbi.nlm.nih.gov
10. Substance Abuse and Mental Health Services Administration. Results from the 2006 National Survey on Drug Use and Health: National Findings (Office of Applied Studies, NSDUH Series H-32, DHHS Publication No. SMA 07–4293). Rockville, MD: 2007 http://www.oas.samhsa.gov/
11. Blixen CE, McDougall GJ, Suen L. Dual diagnosis in elders discharged from a psychiatric hospital. Int J Geriatr Psychiatry 1997; 12(3):307–313.
12. Brennan PL, Nichols KA, Moos RH. Long-term use of VA mental health services by older patients with substance use disorders. Psychiatric Services 2002; 53(7):836–841.
13. Blow FC, Cook CA, Booth BM, et al. Age-related psychiatric comorbidities and level of functioning in alcoholic veterans seeking outpatient treatment. Hosp Community Psychiatry 1992; 43(10):990–995.
14. Balestrieri M, Marcon G, Samani F, et al. Mental disorders associated with benzodiazepine use among older primary care attenders-a regional survey. Soc Psychiatry Psychiatr Epidemiol 2005; 40(4):308–315.
15. Bartels SJ, Coakley E, Oxman TE, et al. Suicidal and death ideation in older primary care patients with depression, anxiety and at-risk alcohol use. Am J Geriatr Psychiatry 2002; 10(4):417–427.
16. NIAAA Research Monograph No. 33. Alcohol Problems and Aging. NIH Pub. No. 98–4163. Bethesda, MD: NIAAA, 1998.
17. Dufour M, Fuller RK. Alcohol in the elderly. Annu Rev Med 1995; 46:123–132.
18. Cook B, Winokur G, Garvey M, et al. Depression and previous alcoholism in the elderly. Br J Psychiatry 1991; 158:72–75.
19. Liberto JG, Oslin DW, Puskin PE. Alcoholism in older persons: A review of the literature. Hos Community Psychiatry 1992; 43(10):975–984.
20. Brennan PL, Schutte KK, Moos RH. Pain and use of alcohol to manage pain: Prevelance and 3 year outcomes among older problem and nonproblem drinkers. Addiction 2005; 100:777–786.
21. Larsen PD, Martin JL. Polypharmacy and elderly patients. AORNJ 1999; 69(3):619–628.
22. Ellor JR, Kurz DJ. Misuse and abuse of prescription and nonprescription drugs by the elderly. Nurs Clin North Am 1982; 17:319–330.
23. Shorr RI, Bauwens SF, Landefeld CS. Failure to limit quantities of benzodiazepine hypnotic drugs for outpatients: Placing the elderly at risk. Am J Med 1990; 89:725–732.
24. Mellinger GD, Balter MG, Uhlenhuth EH. Prevalence and corraletes of the long term use of anxiolytics. JAMA 1984; 251:375–379.
25. Salzman C. Benzodiazepine dependence, toxicity, and abuse: A task force report of the American Psychiatric Association. Washington, D.C.: American Psychiatric Press, 1990.
26. Finlayson RE. Misuse of prescription drugs. Int J Addict 1995; 30(13 &14):1871–1901.
27. Sheahan SL, Hendricks J, Coons SJ. Drug misuse among the elderly: A covert problem. Health Values 1989; 13(3):22–29.
28. Kassed CA (Thomson Healthcare), Levit KR (Thomson Healthcare), Hambrick MM (AHRQ). Hospitalizations Related to Drug Abuse, 2005. HCUP Statistical Brief #39. October 2007. Agency for Healthcare Research and Quality, Rockville, MD. http://www.hcup-us.ahrq.gov/reports/statbriefs/sb39.pdf.
29. McInnes E, Powell J. Drug and alcohol referrals: Are elderly substance abuse diagnosis and referral are being missed? BMJ 1994; 308:444–446.
30. Reid MC, Tinetti ME, Brown CJ, et al. Physician awereness of alcohol use disorders among older patients. J Gen Intern Med 1998; 13:729–734.
31. AMSHA—Get Connected! Linking Older Americans With Medication, Alcohol, and Mental Health Resources. DHHS Pub. No. (SMA) 03–3824. Rockville, MD: Center for

Substance Abuse Treatment, Substance Abuse and Mental Health Services Administration, 2003.
32. Ewing JA. Detcting Alcoholism: The CAGE Questionnaire. JAMA 1984; 252:1905–1907.
33. Blow FC, Brower KJ, Schulenberg JE, et al. The Michigan Alcoholism Screening Test-geriatric version (MAST-G): A new elderly-specific screening instrument. Alcohol Clin Exp Res 1992; 16:372.
34. Philpot M, Pearson N, Petratau V, et al. Screening for problem drinking in older people referred to a mental health service: A comparison of CAGE and AUDIT. Aging Ment Health 2003; 7(3):171–175.
35. Rourke SB, Loberg T. The neurobiological correlates of alcoholism. In: Nixon SJ, ed. Neuropsychological Assessment of Neuropsychiatric Disorders, 2nd ed. New York, NY: Oxford University Press, 1996:423–485.
36. Oscar-Berman M, Marinkovic K. Alcoholism and the Brain: An overview. Alcohol Res Health 2003; 27(2):125–133.
37. Petrakis IL, Gonzalez G, Rosenheck R, et al. Comorbidity of alcoholism and psychiatric disorders. Alcohol Res Health 2002; 26:81–89.
38. Pfefferbaum A, Sullivan EV, Mathalon DH, et al. Frontal lobe volume loss observed with magnetic resonance imaging in older chronic alcoholics. Alcohol Clin Exp Res 1997; 21;521–529.
39. Gambert S, Albrecht III C. The Elderly. In: Gitlow S, ed. Substance Use Disorders: A Practical Guide. Philadelphia, PA: Lippincott, Williams and Wilkins, 2006:1038–1048.
40. Blow FC, Barry KL. Older patients with at-risk and problem drinking patterns: New developments in brief interventions. J Geriatr Psychiatry Neurol 2000; 13(3):115–123.
41. Barry KL, Oslin DW, Blow FC. Alcohol Problems in Older Adults: Prevention and Management. New York, NY: Springer Publishing Co, 2001.
42. Fleming MF. Identification and treatment of alcohol use disorders in older adults. In: Gurnack AM, Atkinson R, eds. Treating Alcohol and Drug Abuse in the Elderly. New York, NY: Springer Publishing Co, 2002:85–108.
43. Miller WR, Rollnick S. Motivational Interviewing. New York, NY: Guilford Press, 1991.
44. ASAM Patient Placement Criteria for the Treatment of Substance-Related Disorders, 2nd ed. Washington, D.C.: American Society of Addiction Medicine, 1996.
45. Substance Abuse and Mental Health Services Administration. Older Americans Substance Abuse and Mental Health Technical Assistance Center. Evidence-Based Practices for Preventing Substance Abuse and Mental Health Problems in Older Adults. Rockville, MD: 2005.
46. Oslin DW, Katz IR, Edell WS, et al. Effects of alcohol consumption on the treatment of depression among elderly patients. Am J Geriatr Psychiatry 2000; 8(3):215–220.
47. Oslin DW. Treatment of late-life depression complicated by alcohol dependence. Am J Geriatr Psychiatry 2005; 13(6):491–500.
48. Bartels SJ, Coakley E, Zubritsky C, et al. Improving access to geriatric mental health services: A randomized trial comparing treatment engagement with integrated versus enhanced referral care for depression, anxiety, and at-risk alcohol use. Am J Psychiatry 2004; 161(8):1455–1462.

13 Barriers to Psychiatric Treatment for the Geriatric Patient: Cultural Issues

Yolonda Colemon
Albert Einstein College of Medicine, Yonkers, New York, U.S.A.

Iqbal Ahmed
Professor of Psychiatry, John A. Burns School of Medicine, University of Hawaii, Honolulu, Hawaii, U.S.A.

INTRODUCTION

The population is becoming more diverse and the number of ethnic elderly persons is growing dramatically. It has been essential that primary care and mental health providers are aware of how cultural and ethnic issues relate to the mental health of these patients. The global population of elders is expected to double from 500 million in 1990 to one billion in 2025 (1). With this expansion, the number of ethnic minority elderly will also increase, shifting the demographic of countries like the United States at marked rates. It is predicted that non-Caucasian individuals will account for 20% of the U.S. elderly by the year 2050 (2), with those older than 85 years becoming the fastest growing segment of the population as a whole (3). As these numbers have increased, we have realized that there is a paucity of knowledge about how these significant populations are impacted by mental health issues, such as mood disorders and suicide. Ethnic minority elders who are new to the country, having spent most of their productive years elsewhere, are at greater risk for depression when they move into communities without peers or ethnic community supports, such as churches. Issues such as minority status, discrimination, and socioeconomic status may be additional risk factors for depression and other psychiatric problems. The goal of this chapter is to examine how affective change is viewed by patients and physicians from different cultures, how suicide is viewed by different cultures, and the attitudes toward Western medicine and talk therapy that may be encountered in members of ethnic minorities.

In most literature, culture, ethnicity, and race are used interchangeably, but it is important to understand the differences between these terms as they relate to transcultural psychiatry. Culture is a system of values, beliefs, and learned behaviors shared across a group of people that can evolve over time and with each generation (4). Ethnicity is a group identification based on a common cultural heritage, including beliefs, customs, place of origin, religion, diet, language, dress, self-concept, and normative expectations. Race is a number of broad divisions of the human species into groups, based on a common geographic origin, certain shared physical characteristics, and a characteristic distribution of gene frequencies (5).

GENERAL ISSUES

Culture is a learned phenomenon and shapes the way an individual perceives the social and natural world. Culture can include both subjective and objective components of human behavior (6). Culture can influence and shape the recognition and expression of psychiatric illness. It influences the meaning of symptoms and the appropriateness of behavior as viewed by society. It can affect the dialogue and interaction between patient and physician. Culture can influence illness and health seeking behavior in one of the following four ways:

1. It defines what is "normal" compared to abnormal in symptoms and functioning.
2. It provides people with ideas about causality.
3. It determines who the patient is as well as the health care decision-making hierarchy.
4. It defines the steps that are taken in seeking health care (7).

Cultural factors can affect both the psychotherapeutic and pharmacologic treatment of psychiatric disorders in the elderly.

Psychotherapy

A critical issue in conducting psychotherapy with ethnic elders is to determine their degree of assimilation, and to clarify to what extent the four items above are relevant. Sue and Sue (8) have identified several generic themes that should guide counseling of minority persons (*i*) Culture-bound values (e.g., communication patterns, degree of individual centeredness, verbally expressive, open, or analytical, i.e., believing in cause and effect); the degree to which distinctions are made between mental and physical illness. (*ii*) Class-bound values, time orientation such as a focus on immediate, short-term goals. (*iii*) Language (*iv*) The stage of racial or cultural identity development that influences social interactions and self-view.

Sakauye (9) has identified a variety of factors that may arise in the therapeutic session. There may be issues related to authority figures. Patients may be overly deferential, inhibited, or ashamed of revealing personal feelings, or they may be hostile and suspicious. There is usually a need for bilingual therapists. Established immigrants may have more social and health-related issues. However, even among established elderly immigrants, they may say that they cannot fully express their emotional state in English and that they can only express the true meaning when they revert to their language of origin (10). Finally, therapists must insure that patients do not take refuge in cultural differences in order to explain away all emotional reactions and behaviors.

Transference issues are more complex when working with different cultural groups. Therapists often find that their elderly patients may experience transference at different generational levels; sometimes the therapist is the parent, sometimes the sibling or spouse, and at other times the therapist may be a child or even grandchild. In some ethnic groups with broader family relationships, transference towards the therapist may include aunts and uncles, cousins, and other kin.

It is important to heed Sue and Sue's admonition that the reason minority group individuals underutilize and prematurely terminate therapy is often because of the services themselves. Such services are typically antagonistic or inappropriate to belief systems and life experiences of culturally different clients.

Pharmacotherapy

Various racial/ethnic groups appear to respond differently to medication treatments. There are probably a number of variables responsible for this. Among the variables are variations in physicians prescribing practices, different patterns of illness behavior, different pharmacokinetics among the groups that are determined by genetics or other cultural factors, different dietary practices, and different culturally determined attitudes toward medication consumption (11). Dietary consumption of certain vegetables and fruits such as corn, star fruit, hebals such as St. John's wort, which may vary among different groups, affects cytochrome P450 enzymes such as 3A4 leading to alteration of levels of most antidepressants. Ethnicity and race can have "biologic effects" on mechanisms of drug response. These effects are on pharmacodynamics and pharmacokinetics of medications, including psychotropics (12). Drug interactions are affected through the differences in the frequencies of specific cytochrome P450 enzyme polymorphisms among the different ethnic groups, and the resultant effects on the pharmacokinetics of the medications. For example, while most Caucasians are rapid metabolizers, about 7% may be poor metabolizers of drugs metabolized by CYP 450 2D6, Asians and African-Americans are intermediate metabolizers. Mexicans tend to have a more rapid metabolism, while rates of ultrarapid metabolism of 20% to 30% have been noted among Arabs and Ethiopians, far more than the 1% to 5% rate among Europeans. Drugs such as paroxetine, sertraline, fluoxetine, and venlafaxine are metabolized by CYP 450 2D6. On the other hand, approximately 20% of Asians and African-Americans are poor metabolizers of drugs metabolized by CYP 2C19. These drugs include antidepressants citalopram, escitalopram, and clomipramine.

Culture has "nonbiologic effects" on medication response primarily through effects on factors such as patient compliance, placebo effects of medications, and drug interactions (interaction of dietary habits and alternative treatments such as herbal remedies, etc.). These factors in turn may be affected by patient factors, physician factors, and interactional factors (13).

This chapter will focus on the main ethnic minority groups in the United States, and their cultural beliefs regarding depression.

SPECIFIC ETHNIC MINORITY GROUPS

African-Americans

The number of African-Americans in this United States has grown, but the number of whites outnumbers that of African-Americans by almost 2:1. By 2005, the number of African-Americans in this country was 39.7 million, making them the second largest population group behind Hispanic-Americans (14). The percentage of whites in the U.S. population older than 65 years is 14% compared to 8% of African-Americans (15). African-Americans make up a diverse group, most are descendents of slaves from West African countries, but others immigrated from the Caribbean, Central and South America, or South or East Africa.

Although African-Americans are a diverse ethnic group, the same socioeconomic issues challenge many. Nearly 25% of all African-Americans had incomes more than $50,000 in 1997. The median income of an African-American married couple at that time was 87% of the median income of their white counterparts. In 1999, approximately 22% of African-American families were living below poverty level. 79% of those older than 25 years were high school graduates in 2000 and 17% had a bachelors' degree or higher (16).

The rates of depression among African-Americans and whites are similar, but the suicide rates in the two groups differ. According to the CDC's report on suicide injury in 2005 (17), the age-adjusted suicide rate per 100,000 for white men aged 65 to 85+ years (32.7) was more than three times that of African-American men (10.25) of the same age group. Older White women (4.8) were more than three times higher than older African-American women (1.44). Further, African-American elders have less suicidal ideation and tend to have passive as opposed to active suicidal ideation (18,19). Attitudes toward depression differ greatly from those of whites. African-Americans, along with Asians and Hispanics, were less likely to believe that depression is due to biologic changes and were more likely to believe that nonpharmacologic treatments, such as counseling or prayer, were more effective than medications (20). Cooper and colleagues (21) conducted a national telephone survey of primary care patients that had been identified as having depressed mood or anhedonia within the past month. Their finding showed that African-Americans were twice as likely as whites to find the use of antidepressant medication unacceptable. African-Americans elders were found to use antidepressant medications at half the frequency of whites (22). It may be important to explore attitudes towards various treatment modalities with African-American patients before making recommendations and to keep an open dialogue about such issues to improve the rate of treatment adherence.

Ethnic differences also have been reported in regard to psychopharmacology (i.e., drug metabolism) and prescription patterns of antidepressants. African-Americans may develop higher plasma concentrations of antidepressants, which may lead to faster response rates (23). Some studies have shown that antidepressants, particularly selective serotonin reuptake inhibitors, are less likely to be prescribed for African-American elders (24). Despite the availability of depression treatment, many people do not seek help for their symptoms, but in the case of African-Americans, help is not always offered. Recent studies show that depression is less likely to be detected in African-American by their primary care physicians (25,26). African-Americans are also less likely to receive mental health services from any source when compared to whites (27,28), and are more likely to delay treatment (29). Distrust of the medical profession may affect the treatment of African-Americans. There are historical events, most notably the 1932 U.S. Public Health Service Tuskegee Syphilis Study, that highlight racial discrimination against African-Americans in medical research (30,31). Such events have led to a lack of participation in research studies and low rates of trust in medical professionals (32,33). African-Americans are less likely to report symptoms to their physician or other practitioners (nurses, social worker, clergy, etc.), therefore, practitioners should actively elicit reports of mood and feelings from this group and be ready to treat or refer for appropriate behavioral health treatment (34).

Asian-Americans and Pacific Islanders

The term Asian-American Pacific Islanders (AAPI) describes a diverse ethnic and cultural group of individuals, including 28 Asian groups and 15 Pacific Islanders groups (35). There are 32 primary languages and a variety of dialects within each language. According to the 2000 Census data, this is one of the fastest growing populations in the United States increasing to 10.2 million people at last count. More than 800,000 of the U.S. AAPI population are older thanthe age of 65 years (36).

The migration history to the United States varies by group and has been affected by the political climate of the native country. Chinese-Americans were among the first group to arrive in large groups more than 150 years ago. Many Japanese-Americans began to migrate to the U.S. mainland and Hawaii before 1945. The Immigration Act of 1965 brought large number of Chinese, Filipinos, and

Koreans to the United States. In 1975, after the ending of the Vietnam War, a large number of Southeast Asians began to arrive. The first wave after 1975 were mostly educated Vietnamese, but a second wave of Southeast-Asians came to the United States after 1978 to escape persecution. This group included Vietnamese, Chinese-Vietnamese, Cambodians, Lao, Hmong, and Mien. In 1960, most Asians were descended from Chinese and Japanese immigrants, but now more than half are foreign-born (37).

It is important to remember that the length of time in the United States influences the level of acculturation within the family. Families may range from a "traditional family" that holds to traditional values and has very little contact with mainstream American to the "Americanized family" that speaks only English and seems not to maintain traditional values (37). In most traditional Asian families, there is a high value placed on community and a mutual dependence between parents and children. The expectation is that the parents care for the children when they are young and the children care for the parents when they become elderly. In most traditional Asian households, the elders are expected to maintain full authority and financial control over their children, no matter how old the children become or where they live. In most cases, it is the eldest male (grandfather, father, or eldest son) who has been charged with making decisions for the family. Mental health providers need to be aware of this hierarchy when treating Asian family members that uphold these traditions. These values are different from the traditional American family model. Providers may find that elders that migrate later in life may have a more difficult time adapting to a new country and life cycle. Many come to the United States to be with the younger family members and this may disrupt their normal life cycles. This disruption can put these elders at risk for mental health difficulties, but few may actually seek help because of the stigmatization of mental illness, language barriers, social isolation, and limited access to services (38). Families try hard to protect loved ones from what is perceived as an embarrassing situation, therefore delaying mental health treatment until the point where the illness is severe and requires hospitalization. Even then, patients tend to terminate treatment prematurely (39). A large number of AAPI may seek treatment through providers of complementary or alternative medicine (CAM) or prefer a traditional healer to a Western doctor. Asians will often use CAM when pain is the main complaint, a frequent occurrence in a population characterized by a high level of somatization (40).

There are lower rates of major depression in Asians than in other ethnic groups. The 12-month prevalence is 3.4% compared to 5.28% in the general U.S. population. The lifetime prevalence of depression in Asians is 6.9% compared to 13.23% in the United States (41,42). The prevalence rates may be an underestimation because of the stigma of mental illness in this population.

On the other hand, the rates of suicide appear to be higher among Asians compared to other ethnic minority groups. A study of rates of suicide using the 1990 census found that Asian-American elderly had 50% the suicide rate of Caucasian-American elderly. Among the ethnic minorities, however, Asian-American elderly had the highest rates of completed suicide (43). The highest rate within the older Chinese age groups for both men and women runs contrary to Hispanic and African-American groups where rates decrease with age (44). As a group, for all women residing in the United States, East Asian women have the highest proportional rate of suicide over the age of 65 (45). Not only are Asian-American elderly at risk for suicide, they have a higher proportion of death and suicidal ideation as compared to other minority elder groups. In one study, using the Paykel suicide questionnaire to probe thoughts about death, suicide, or attempts at suicide, Asian-American elderly had the highest proportion of death ideation (37.8%) or suicidal ideation (11.8%) in comparison to African-American, Hispanic and Caucasian groups (46). Taken together, these studies reveal that Asian-American elderly are at higher risk for suicide than other ethnic minority elder groups. A possible reason for the higher rates of suicide among elderly Chinese- and Japanese-Americans that has been proposed it that it is due to their children's acculturation, with its subsequent cultural conflict between generations (47).

In addition to the issue of stigma, depression may also go underreported due to high incidence of somatization instead of psychologic complaints (48). Unexplained symptoms that have been worked up and treated in other settings and remain unresolved may be considered "red flags" for further probing. It is important to become aware of idioms of distress used in the patient's cultural and ethnic group. The challenges in diagnosis and treatment are illustrated in a study by Yeung et al. (49), who investigated the illness beliefs of depressed Chinese-American patients, and found that 76% complained of somatic symptoms, 14% reported psychologic symptoms including irritability, rumination, and poor memory. No patients spontaneously reported depressed moods. Seventy-two percent of the patients did not know the name of their illness or did not consider it a diagnosable medical problem. Only 10% labeled their problems psychiatric. Help was sought from general hospitals (69%), lay help (62%), alternative treatments (55%), spiritual treatment (14%), self-administered alternative treatments (10.5%), and mental health practitioners (3.5%). The authors concluded that many Chinese-Americans do not consider depressed mood a symptom to report to their physicians, and many are unfamiliar with depression as a treatable psychiatric disorder.

Hispanic-Americans

Hispanic-Americans are the largest minority population in the United States (50) and one of the fastest growing. In the year 1990, 5.1% of Hispanics were 65 years and older. This number is expected to be 14.1% in the year 2020 (51). The United States has the fifth largest Spanish speaking population in the world, exceeded only by Mexico, Columbia, Spain, and Argentina. The terms Hispanic and Latino are often used interchangeably. Hispanic signifies Spanish origin or language, and Latino refers to those of Latin-American descent (i.e., descendents of Cuba, Mexico, Puerto Rico, South or Central America).

Hispanics in the United States make up a diverse group of people with various backgrounds and cultural experiences, so it is important to note that there may be differences among the subgroups of this population. Approximately 48% of elderly Hispanics are Mexican, 15% Cuban, 12% Puerto Rican, and 25% from other Hispanic groups (52). These subgroups may differ with respect to their life experiences, natural histories, and risk for psychiatric disorders, especially as it pertains to their experiences with war and trauma. Hispanics are a heterogeneous group that includes Native American, African-American, white, or some mixture of these three. They are younger, poorer, less educated, and more likely to be foreign born than whites in the United States. 40% of all Hispanics are foreign born. They are more likely to live with family, and less likely to have insurance or speak English. There are varying dialects within the Spanish language. Some elderly Hispanics did not speak Spanish at all, but other native languages, such as Mexicans who only speak Nahuatl. Approximately 45% of Hispanics have limited English proficiency (53).

As the Hispanic population continues to grow, it is important that physicians and other practitioners understand how depressive symptoms can manifest in this population. Preoccupation with somatic complaints in Hispanics with depression has been well documented in the literature (54–56). Somatic symptoms are a culturally sanctioned justification for seeking treatment, because it would be stigmatizing to express psychologic distress explicitly. This is particularly true of elderly Hispanic women (57). Hispanics tend to present more to the primary care provider for assistance with mental health problems, rather than seek out a behavioral health provider (58), but rates of depression treatment are lower in Hispanics than in whites (59).

Three universal themes throughout the Hispanic community have been identified as protective factors against suicide and depression. *Familismo* is the concept of emphasizing close relationships with extended family. Family is viewed by many Hispanics as the cornerstone of one's existence. Loyalty, reciprocity, and solidarity are all greatly valued. *Fatilismo* is the expectation of adversity, and the idea that outcomes in one's life may be decided by fate, luck, or a higher power (60). *Religion* is also protective and serves as a source of support and coping for elderly Hispanics (61,62). It has been hypothesized that if there is a belief in an afterlife, then suffering in this life can be easier to endure (63). Certain subgroups may be more at risk for mental illness than others. American-Puerto Ricans have greater mental health concerns and lifetime depression rates that are more than double those for Mexican-Americans and Cuban-Americans. They were also twice as likely as whites to have depression in a given year (64,65).

Native Americans and Alaska Natives

The Native Americans and Alaska Natives constitute 1.5% of the total U.S. population. This population rose by 1% from 2004 to 2005 to 4.5 million people (50). The indigenous population of North America is referred to by various terms, including Native American, Alaska Native, American-Indians, Native American-Indians, Indians, Natives, and First Nations. Most live in the western states of California, Arizona, New Mexico, South Dakota, Alaska, and Montana. This is a diverse population with multiple subgroups that originate from different regions of the country. Indigenous groups that shared environments tended to develop similar skills, beliefs, and customs. There are more than 560 federally recognized tribes, each with unique culture and history. 62% live in urban, suburban, or rural nonreservation areas (66). Although most Native Americans do not live on reservations, most maintain close family and political associations with reservations or trust land communities. Native Americans and Alaska Natives are generally a younger population when compared with whites because of higher mortality rates, lower education, and lower average incomes. There is also limited access to mental health services.

The prevalences of any mood disorder (15.3%), major depressive disorder (12.4%), and dysthymic disorder (3%) were significantly greater in Native Americans than in African-Americans. Rates of major depression and dysthymic disorder also were significantly different from whites. During 2001 to 2002, 5.3% of the U.S. population had experienced major depressive disorder in the previous year and 13.2% of people had experienced it during their lifetimes. Those at greatest risk were women, Native Americans, people aged between 45 and 64 years, those who were widowed, separated, or divorced, and those with lower incomes (42). Being Asian-, Hispanic-, or African-American decreased risk.

Psychologic distress among American-Indian and Alaska Native (AIAN) individuals can be understood in the context of the multigenerational trauma that Native people have experienced (67). The trauma dates back to colonial and military subrogation that contributed to the loss of connection to tribal lands, separation of family members, and the disappearance of tribal land. This trauma may be associated with high rates of suicide among American-Indian and Alaskan Natives in addition to the alcohol and drug use, and interpersonal violence.

Often AIANs have great mistrust of formal health care systems. Many contemporary Indian/Native communities have long-standing traditional healing and support for personal and family development. Usually family leaders arrange access to this healing. American-Indians commonly use native healers. The medicinal use of plants and roots is common in some Indian communities. Several targeted studies suggest that American-Indians and Alaska Natives use alternative therapies at rates that are equal to or greater than the rates for Caucasians (68).

CONCLUSIONS

Multiple practical and cultural barriers to care exist for ethnic minorities with depression. These include limited knowledge about available services, services which may not be sensitive to cultural needs, lack of financial resources and access to transportation, cultural stereotypes and norms, including a strong belief and preference for family care. Effective culturally appropriate prevention and treatment strategies must be developed which incorporate services geared to meet specific needs of ethnic minority elders, including services in their native language and incorporation of various traditional cultural values, such as respect for elders and cooperation. In addition, interventions to explore in the future include providing social support for families, information regarding diagnosis of depression, availability of community resources, initiatives to develop depression screening, both in primary care and community. As the ethnic minority elderly population increases in the 21st century, increasing the availability of culturally competent formal services will be another needed intervention.

In the meantime, understanding the particular dilemmas, that ethnic minority elderly face, will enable clinicians to better serve this population. Awareness of individuals' particular sociocultural background, acculturation stressors, cultural beliefs about mental illness and treatment, cultural practices, differences in diet, ethnobiological differences in pharmacogenomics, and role of the family will enable clinicians to better engage with their ethnic minority elderly patients and their families. The knowledge that mental health issues are prevalent and yet underrecognized for this population must prompt us to renew our efforts to reach out to this underserved population at risk.

REFERENCES

1. Desjarlais R, Eisenberg L, Good B, et al. World Mental Health Problems and Priorities in Low Income Countries. Oxford, UK: Oxford University Press, 1995.
2. Mintzer J, Hendrie H, Faison W. Geriatrics: Minority and cultural issues. In: Sadock BJ, Sadock V, Kaplan HI, eds. Kaplin and Sadock's Comprehensive Textbook of Psychiatry, 8th ed. Baltimore, MD: Lippincott Williams & Wilkins, 2004.

3. Baker FM, Lightfoot OB, Psychiatric care of ethnic elders. In: Gaw AC, ed. Culture, Ethnicity, and Mental Illness. Washington, D.C.: American Psychiatric Press, 1993.
4. Matsumoto D, Culture and Psychology. San Francisco, CA: Brooks/Cole, 1996.
5. Gaw AC. Concise Guide to Cross-Cultural Psychiatry. Washington, D.C.: American Psychiatric Publishing, Inc., 2001.
6. Lim R, ed. Clinical Manual of Cultural Psychiatry. Washington, D.C.: American Psychiatric Press, 2006.
7. Ferran E, Tracy LC, Gany FM, et al. Culture and multicultural competence. In: Kramer EJ, Ivey SL, eds. Immigrant Women's Health: Problems and Solutions. San Francisco, CA: Jossey-Bass, 1999.
8. Sue DW, Sue D. Counseling the Culturally Different: Theory and Practice, 2nd ed. New York, NY: Wiley, 1990.
9. Sakauye K. Ethnocultural aspects of aging in mental health. In: Sadavoy J, Jarvik LF, Grossberg GT, Meyers BS, eds. Comprehensive Textbook of Geriatric Psychiatry, 3rd ed. New York, NY: WW Norton, 2004.
10. Sadavoy J, Lazarus LW. Individual therapy. In: Sadavoy J, Jarvik LF, Grossberg GT, Meyers BS, eds. Comprehensive Textbook of Geriatric Psychiatry, 3rd ed. New York, NY: WW Nrton, 2004.
11. Turner SM, Cooley-Quille MR. Socioecological and sociocultural variables in psychopharmacological research: Methodological considerations. Psychopharmacol Bull 1996; 30:183–192.
12. Smith MW. Ethnopsychopharmacology. In: Lim RF, ed. Clinical Manual of Cultural Psychiatry. Washington, D.C.: American Psychiatric Press, Inc., 2006.
13. Ahmed I. Psychological aspects of giving and receiving medications. In: Tseng WS, Streltzer J, eds. Culture and Psychotherapy: A Guide to Clinical Practice. Washington, D.C.: American Psychiatric Press, Inc., 2000.
14. U.S. Census Bureau, U.S. Census Press Release. Nation's population one-third minority. U.S. Department of Commerce, Public Information Office. Released May 10, 2006. Retrieved from http://www.census.gov/Press-Release/www/releases/archives/population/006808.html on May 10, 2008.
15. McKinnon J. The Black population in the United States: March 2002. U.S. Washington, D.C.: Census Bureau, Current Population Reports, Series P20–541. 2003.
16. U.S. Census Bureau: Online. Available: 2001 Statistical abstract of the United States. Retrieved from http://www.census.gov/prod/2002pubs/01statab/pop.pdf on October 26, 2006.
17. Centers for Disease Control and Prevention, United States. Suicide injury deaths and rates per 100000. All races, both sexes, aged 65 to 85+, 2005. Retrieved from http://webappa.cdc.gov/sasweb/ncipc/mortrate10_sy.html on May 10, 2008.
18. Gallo JJ, Cooper-Patrick L, Lesikar S. Depressive symptoms of Whites and African Americans aged 60 years and older. J Gerontol B Psychol Sci Soc Sci 1998; 53:277–286.
19. Lish JD, Zimmerman M, Farber NJ, et al. Suicide screening in a primary care setting at a Veterans Affairs Medical Center. Psychosomatics 1996; 37:413–424.
20. Givens JJ, Houston TK, Van Voorhees BW, et al. Ethnicity and preferences for depression treatment. Gen Hosp Psychiatry 2007; 29:182–191.
21. Cooper LA, Gonzales JJ, Gallo JJ, et al. The acceptability of treatment for depression among African American, Hispanic, and White primary care patients. Med Care 2003; 41:479–489.
22. Grunebaum MF, Oquendo MA, Manly JJ. Depressive symptoms and antidepressants use in a random community sample of ethnically diverse, urban elderly persons. J Affect Disord 2008; 105:273–277.
23. Lin KM, Poland RE, Nakasaki G, eds. Psychopharmacology and Psychobiology of Ethnicity. Washington, D.C.: American Psychiatric Press, 1993.
24. Blazer DG, Hybels CF, Simonsick EM, et al. Marked differences in antidepressant use by race in an elderly community sample: 1986–1996. Am J Psychiatry 2000; 157:1089–1094.
25. Borowsky SJ, Rubenstein LV, Meredith LS, et al. Who is at risk of nondetection of mental health problems in primary care? J Gen Internal Med 2000; 15:381–388.

26. Gallo JJ, Bogner HR, Morales KH, et al. Patient ethnicity and the identification and active management of depression in late life. Arch Internal Med 2005; 165:1962–1968.
27. Kessler RC, Demler O, Frank RG, et al. Prevalence and treatment of mental disorders, 1990 to 2003. N Engl J Med 2005; 352:2515–2523.
28. Miranda J, Cooper LA. Disparities in care for depression among primary care patients. J Gen Internal Med 2004; 19:120–125.
29. Wang PS, Berglund P, Olfson M, et al. Failure and delay in initial treatment contact after first onsent of mental disorders in the National Comorbidity Survey Replication. Arch Gen Psychiatry 2005; 62:603–613.
30. Fairchild AL, Bayer R. Uses and abuses of Tuskegee. Science 1999; 284:9199–9921.
31. Gamble VN. Under the shadow of Tuskegee: African Americans and health care. Am J Public Health 1997; 87:1773–1778.
32. Boulware LE, Cooper LA, Ratner LE, et al. Race and trust in the health care system. Public Health Reports 2003; 118:358–365.
33. Shavers VL, Lynch CF, Burmeister LF. Racial differences in factors that influence the willingness to participate in medical research studies. Ann Epidemiol 2002; 12:248–256.
34. Probst JC, Laditka SB, Moore CG, et al. Race and ethnicity differences in reporting of depressive symptoms. Adm Policy Ment Health 2007; 34:519–529.
35. Ponce N. (1990). Asian and Pacific Islander health data: quality issues and policy recommendations. In Policy Papers, San Francisco, Calif: Asian American Health Forum, Inc.; 1990.
36. He W, Sengupta M, Velkolf VA, et al. Census Bureau. Current population reports, p23–209. +65 in the United States: 2005. Washington, DC: U.S. Government Printing Office, 2005.
37. Lee E. Working with Asian Americans: A guide for clinicians. In: Lee E, ed. New York, NY: The Guilford Press, 1997.
38. Kao RS, Lam ML. Asian American elderly. In: Lee E, ed. Working with Asian Americans: A Guide for Clinicians. New York, NY: The Guilford Press, 1997.
39. Sue D, Sue S. Cultural factors in the clinical assessment of Asian Americans. J Consult Clin Psychol 1987; 55:479–487.
40. Najm W, Reinsch S, Hoehler F, et al. Use of complementary and alternative medicine among the ethnic elderly. Altern Ther Health Med 2003; 9:50–57.
41. Takeuchi D, Chung RCY, Lin KM, et al. Lifetime and twelve-month prevalence rates of major depressive episodes and dysthymia among Chinese Americans in Los Angeles. Am J Psychiatry 1998; 155:1407–1414.
42. Hasin DS, Goodwin RD, Stinson FS, et al. Epidemiology of major depressive disorders: Results frrm the national epidemiologic survey on alcoholism and related conditions. Arch Gen Psychiatry 2005; 62:1097–1106.
43. Baker FM. Suicide among ethnic minority elderly: A statistical and psychosocial perspective. J Geriatr Psychiatry 1994; 27:241–264.
44. Shiang J, Blinn R, Bongar B, et al. Suicide in San Francisco, CA: A comparison of Caucasian and Asian groups, 1987–1994. Suicide Life Threat Behav 1997; 27:80–91.
45. McKenzie K, Serfaty M, Crawford M. Suicide in ethnic minority groups. Br J Psychiatry 2003; 183:100–101.
46. Bartels SJ, Oakley E, Oxman TE, et al. Suicide and death ideation in older primary care patients with depression, anxiety, and at-risk alcohol use. Am J Geriatr Psychiatry 2002; 10:417–427.
47. Diego AT, Yamamoto J, Nguyen LH, et al. Suicide in the elderly: Profiles of Asians and whites. Asian Am Pac Isl J Health 1994; 2:49–57.
48. Chen JP, Chen H, Chung H. Depressive disorders in Asian American adults. Western J Med 2002; 176:239–244.
49. Yeung A, Chang D, Gresham R, et al. Illness beliefs of depressed Chinese American patients in primary care. J Nerv Ment Dis 2004; 192:324–327.
50. U.S. Census Bureau. Press Release, May 10, 2006 (a). Nation's population one-third minority: Online. Retrieved from http://www.census.gov/Press-Release/www/release/archives/population/006808.html on October 26, 2006.

51. U.S. Bureau of the Census, Cheeseman Day J. Population projections of the United States, by age, sex, race and Hispanic origin: 1993–2050. Current Population Reports, U.S. Government Printing Office, 1993:25–1104.
52. U.S. Bureau of the Census. (1993). U.S. Population Estimates, by Age, Sex, Race, and Hispanic Origin: 1980–1991, Current Population Reports, P23-1095, (November 1992), Washington, DC, U.S. Government Printing Office.
53. Kochlar R, Suro R, Tafoya S. The new Latino south: The context and consequences of rapid population growth. Pew Hispanic Center. July 26, 2005; 12. Retrieved at: www.pewhispanic.org
54. Escobar JI. Transcultural aspects of dissociative and somatoform disorders. Psychiatr Clin North Am 1995; 18:555–569.
55. Canino IA, Rubio-Stipec M, Canino G, et al. Functional somatic symptoms: A cross-ethnic comparison. Am J Orthopsychiatry 1992; 8:605–612.
56. Escobar JI, Randolph ET, Hill M. Symptoms of schizophrenia in Hispanic and Anglo veterans. Cult Med Psychiatry 1986; 10:259–276.
57. Angel R, Guarnaccia PJ. Mind, body, and culture: Somatization among Hispanics. Soc Sci Med 1989; 28:1229–1238.
58. Vega WA, Kolody B, Aguilar-Gaxiola S, et al. Gaps in service utilization by Mexican Americans with mental health problems. Am J Psychiatry 1999; 156:928–934.
59. Unützer J, Katon W, Callahan CM, et al. Depression treatment in a sample of 1801 depressed older adults in primary care. J Am Geriatric Soc 2003; 51:505–514.
60. Hoppe SK, Martin HW. Patterns of suicide among Mexican Americans and Anglos, 1960–1980. Soc Psychiatry 1986; 21:83–88.
61. Beyene Y, Becker G, Mayen N. Perception of aging and sense of well-being among Latino elderly. J Cross Cultural Gerontol 2002; 17:155–172.
62. Weisman A, Rosales G, Kymalainen J, et al. Ethnicity, family cohesion, religiosity and general emotional distress in patients with schizophrenia and their relatives. J Nerv Ment Dis 2005; 193:359–368.
63. Hovey JD. Religion and suicidal ideation in a sample of Latin American immigrants. Psychol Rep 1999; 85:171–177.
64. Oquendo MA, Ellis SP, Greenwald S, et al. Ethnic and sex differences in suicide rates relative to major depression in the United States. Am J Psychiatry 2001; 158:1652–1658.
65. Moscicki EK, Rae DS, Regier DA, et al. The hispanic health and nutrition survey: Depression among Mexican Americans, Cuban Americans and Puerto Ricans. In: Garcia M, Arana J, eds. Research Agenda for Hispanics. Chicago, IL: University of Illinois Press, 1987.
66. U.S. Census Bureau. American Indian and Alaska Natives (AIAN) aata and links. 2006 (b). Online. Retrieved: http://factfinder.census.gov/home/aian/index.html.
67. Duran E, Duran B. Native American Postcolonial Psychology. Albany, NY: State University of New York Press, 1995.
68. Fleming CM. American Indian and Alaska native patients. In: Lim R, ed. Clinical Manual of Cultural Psychiatry. Washington, D.C.: APPI Press, 2006.

14 Bereavement in Later Life

Christine Moutier
Department of Psychiatry, University of California, San Diego, California, U.S.A.

Sidney Zisook
Department of Psychiatry, University of California, San Diego, and Psychiatry Service, Veterans Affairs San Diego Healthcare System, San Diego, California, U.S.A.

A man's dying is more the survivors' affair than his own.
– Thomas Mann (1875–1955)

INTRODUCTION

Physicians across almost all specialties are faced with the clinical dilemma of distinguishing between normal grief due to the loss of a loved one and syndromes that warrant clinical treatment such as major depressive disorder. When presented with a bereaved patient, the clinician faces a number of questions: Is the patient experiencing normal grief or a pathologic depression? Should these symptoms be treated, or left to resolve on their own in what many believe to be a restorative process? And, if intervention is appropriate, which therapeutic domain maximizes the probability of a successful outcome? These issues, perplexing in any clinical encounter, pose an additional set of challenges when the patient is elderly as the loss may be accompanied by a host of factors associated with aging, such as poor health, impaired cognitive abilities, declining income, decreasing independence, and the loss of social and occupational roles to name a few.

This chapter will serve to elucidate the diagnostic differences between normal grief, complicated grief, and depressive disorders, as well as other medical and psychiatric complications of grief. More subtle subsyndromal depressive states are discussed and recommendations for treatment options for complicated grief, bereavement-related depression are presented.

BEREAVEMENT

Bereavement is the state of profound loss due to the death of a loved one. The grief that accompanies this loss is characterized by a multidimensional experience encompassing intense emotions, physical symptoms, transient cognitive changes, functional role impairment, and alterations in the way the bereaved views themselves and the world around them. Bereavement is best viewed as a process rather than a state. Many investigators (1–3) have described the grief process in terms of stages bereaved individuals pass through, as they accept and adjust to the loss of a loved one. These stages are typically described as an initial period of disbelief and denial, followed by a time of intense emotional discomfort as the reality of the loss registers with the bereaved. This second, intermediate stage may include crying spells and a myriad of feelings, including anguish, guilt, anxiety, fear, and apathy. The bereaved may become socially withdrawn in an attempt to avoid interactions that may arouse painful memories. Somatic disturbances may appear in the form of gastrointestinal complaints, problems with sleep and appetite, chest pain, heart palpitations, dyspnea, dizziness, tremulousness, and other distressing symptoms. The grief process culminates in a period of reorganization and recovery as the bereaved comes to terms with the loss.

These stages, although potentially useful in delineating the journey from numbness to acute anguish to reconciliation and, ultimately, the ability to accept and cope with the loss, are best viewed as highly variable from person to person (4) and fluid even within the individual. Although some investigators have attempted to validate the "stage theory" of grief and bereavement, (5) others emphasize the uniqueness of each person's grief and the difficulties inherent in expecting a uniform process (6,7).

An alternate model of grief postulates several relatively independent tasks that challenge many, if not most, bereaved individuals (*i*) working through the intensely painful, emotional, and cognitive responses that accompany the loss of a loved one and accepting positive feelings that also permeate the grief process; (*ii*) finding healthy and adaptive ways of modulating the intense emotional pain and limiting maladaptive coping; (*iii*) maintaining a psychologically and symbolically acceptable continuing relationship with the deceased loved one while coming to grips with the reality of the death; (*iv*) adjusting to a world in which the deceased is missing in a very real and concrete way while maintaining old roles and developing the capacity to master new ones as necessary; (*v*) maintaining key relationships with friends and relatives and becoming available to form new intimate relationships as appropriate; and (*vi*) achieving a healthy and integrated self-concept and stable worldview.

Shear distinguishes the period of *acute* grief, when painful emotions and a preoccupation with images, thoughts, and memories of the deceased often dominate the life of the bereaved from a later form of grief, *integrated* or *abiding* grief, in which the deceased is easily called to mind, often with associated sadness and longing (8). However, different from its acute form, this second form of grief does not persistently preoccupy the mind or disrupt other activities. The bereaved do not forget the people they lost, stop missing their loved ones, or fully relinquish their sadness. The loss becomes integrated into autobiographic memory and thoughts and memories of the deceased are no longer preoccupying or disabling. There may be periods when grief intensity surges; for example, during special times like holidays, birthdays, or anniversaries, or at the time of another loss or during a particularly stressful period. For this reason, many clinicians and researchers consider grief to be life-long process following the death of someone very close.

COMPLICATED GRIEF

Because grief is, by its very definition, a pervasive state of extreme emotional anguish, clinicians cannot easily determine when a bereavement reaction is overly intense or unusually prolonged. Yet, it is clear that for some bereaved persons, grief takes on its own life, and the period of acute, painful, and preoccupying grief does not abate into its integrated or abiding form. "Complicated grief," also called traumatic, hypertrophic, or chronic grief, is characterized by intense and persistent grief generally involving the following: recurrent, intense pangs of grief; persistent yearning, pining, and longing for the deceased; recurrent intrusive images of the person dying; and a distressing admixture of avoidance and preoccupation with reminders of the loss. Positive memories are often blocked or excessively sad, or they are experienced in prolonged states of reverie that interfere with daily activities (9–11). Complicated grief has been associated with concomitant (12) and subsequent physical and mental morbidity, including increases in suicidality (10).

If recently bereaved individuals meet criteria for traumatic grief by six months, then by 13 months they are at increased risk for changes in smoking, eating, depression, and high blood pressure. By 25 months, such individuals express suicidal ideation more often and demonstrate an increased risk to develop heart trouble and new cases of cancer (12).

At least three treatment studies have suggested that the syndrome of complicated grief responds to treatment. In the first open study of individuals with what was then called traumatic bereavement, improvement in grief intensity and associated depressive symptoms was reported with a combination of interpersonal psychotherapy and paroxetine (13). In the second study, a randomized controlled clinical trial, a specific form of psychotherapy, "complicated grief treatment", was found to produce more robust and rapid improvement in complicated grief symptoms (51% much or very much improved) than interpersonal psychotherapy (28%) (14). The third study, a small case report series, suggested the effectiveness of treatment with citalopram monotherapy (15).

A prolonged duration of the bereavement process is not sufficient to determine whether or not an individual suffers from complicated, chronic, pathologic grief. Rather, the clinician should consider the nature of the grief experience and its impact on the bereaved, in addition to its duration, when evaluating an individual who has suffered a loss. Is the grief overwhelming, accompanied by dysphoria, and characterized by an unyielding preoccupation with and idealization of the deceased? Is the intensity of the sorrow unmitigated by time? Investigators have not reached a consensus regarding how long grief lasts before it should be deemed chronic; however, persistent and pervasive grief lasting more than six months and characterized by the features just described requires clinical attention (9,16,17). Careful consideration should be given to whether the grief process has been impeded by another psychiatric disorder, such as major depression, anxiety disorder, or posttraumatic stress disorder (PTSD) (18). Clinicians should determine whether criteria for one or more of these syndromes are met and target treatment accordingly. Risk factors for chronic grief are loss of a child (19), a dependent relationship with the deceased (20), or an unnatural death (21). The condition is frequently reported in young and middle-aged adults, most often in women and adolescents. Prognosis for this condition is guarded and treatment may be protracted and difficult.

MEDICAL AND PSYCHIATRIC MORBIDITY

Medical Morbidity and Mortality

Prebereavement health problems constitute the greatest risk factor for declining health after bereavement. Given the higher incidence of medical morbidity in the older population, it is not surprising that the elderly evince a particular vulnerability to such complications after the loss of a spouse. Thompson et al. (22) suggested that this group (especially older women) suffers an exacerbation in existing conditions and develops new illnesses in the months immediately following the bereavement, although other studies suggest these effects are transient and disappear by 30 months follow-up (23). One explanation for this phenomenon lies in the increased caretaking burden wives assume as they care for their dying husbands (24,25) while neglecting their own health.

Two comprehensive reviews of the mortality of bereavement concluded that the vast majority of studies support an excess mortality rate in bereaved versus nonbereaved individuals (26,27). Since most studies focus on the effects of spousal bereavement, the findings pose particular relevance to the elderly population as the likelihood of becoming widowed between the ages of 65 and 74 years is 8.8% for men and 29.4% for women. The risk of widowhood increases dramatically after the age of 74 years to 21.6% for men and 59.2% for women (28). Several large studies demonstrate higher mortality rates for individuals who have lost spouses than for their married counterparts (29–37). Interestingly, the group at greatest risk of dying (relative to their peers) following spousal bereavement is younger widows (30,31,38), although one study (39) demonstrated that the oldest old persons might be at relatively higher risk compared to controls. Widowers appear to be at greatest risk within the first six to twelve months of bereavement (30,37,40,41); this period of risk may be delayed one or two years in widows (29,30). Other risk factors include Caucasian race (42), moving into a chronic care facility (30), social isolation and lack of social support (30,39,43), living alone or not remarrying (for widowers) (30), sudden deaths for widowers or widows under the age of 50 years, and death from a chronic illness for widowers between 50 and 64 years (27). Parents who lose children under the age of 18 years have also been found to have excess mortality risk by natural causes as well as suicide (44,45). One study of survivors of Israeli soldiers suggested that divorced or widowed mothers who lose a son in war are at higher risk for increased mortality (33).

No consistent pattern emerges for the cause of excess mortality during bereavement (27). Some of the most compelling data implicate death from suicide (31,46,47,48). Other investigators suggest that accidents (30,38,49) and heart disease (50) may be significant contributors to higher mortality rates in bereaved individuals; but cancer, liver cirrhosis, diabetes, and infectious diseases may also contribute.

Major Depression

Clinicians often equate grief with depression when, in fact, they are two distinct phenomena with overlapping features. Bereaved individuals often manifest symptoms of grief that are commonly associated with major depression: crying, insomnia, dysphoria, anorexia, restlessness, fatigue, poor memory, loss of interest, and difficulty in concentrating (23,51–56). Indeed, as a symptom, depression is considered a fundamental aspect of normal grief and bereavement. Clayton (52,57) reported that more than half of all widowed persons experience crying spells, sleep disturbances, low mood, loss of appetite, fatigue, and/or poor memory at some point during the first year of bereavement. Others (55,58) have reported that widows and widowers experience a far greater number of depressive symptoms than do married individuals. Specifically, one-third of all widows and widowers expressed feelings of loneliness, feeling blue, insomnia, diminished interests, thoughts of death or dying, and hopelessness for as long as two years following the death of their spouses.

Differentiating Bereavement and Depression

According to the DSM-IV TR, a diagnosis of major depression applies when either depressed mood or loss of interest in normal activities is present most of the time for at least two weeks. In addition, several other symptoms must coexist during the same period; the syndrome must create either marked distress or psychosocial impairment, and it must not be causally related to medications, drugs, or general medical illness. However, when the syndrome occurs in the context of bereavement, DSM-IV TR conventions dictate a diagnosis of "bereavement" if any or all symptoms of a depressive episode occur within two months of the loss (59). The only exception to this mandate occurs when certain markers of depression severity (e.g., psychomotor retardation, morbid feelings of worthlessness, or suicidal ideation) are present. After the first two months have elapsed, the diagnosis of major depression is relatively straightforward; symptoms that emerge during the first two months pose a more complex diagnostic dilemma. Such episodes are common, occurring in 29% to 58% of widows and widowers one month after their spouse's death (53,60,61), can be disabling, and are often chronic (55).

Bereavement as an Exclusion Criterion for Major Depression

Interestingly, major depression is the only Axis I disorder whose condition is negated by bereavement. If, for example, a person develops a panic disorder, no one would repudiate the diagnosis if the individual also happened to be bereaved. In addition, no other stressors aside from bereavement nullify the diagnosis of major depression. As an illustration, consider an individual, recently divorced, disabled, or impoverished, who manifests symptoms of depression. An astute clinician would recognize the stressor as precipitant to a major depression in a vulnerable person, not simply dismiss the depressive symptoms as a product of the situation (62).

The validity of the bereavement exclusion criteria and the notion that major depression is a disorder that, short of severity markers cannot be diagnosed within the 2-month period following loss of a loved one, currently holds a fair amount of controversy. In a recent review examining antecedent, concurrent and predictive validators, bereavement-related depression occurring within the first two months following the death of a loved one was found to be similar to standard major depression. The conclusion from this study was that the published literature supports the similarity of bereavement-related depression (within the 2-month time period) to standard major depression (63). This finding calls into question the validity of bereavement as an exclusion criterion for diagnosing major depression during the first two months following the death of a loved one.

Bereavement-Related Depression in the Elderly

In the late 1970s, the National Institute on Aging established bereavement and aging as priorities and funded three controlled, prospective, longitudinal studies that looked at depression and its risk factors after late-life bereavement (58). Investigations followed that examined depressive reactions in late-life bereavement (51,53,64–67). In general, these studies reveal that there are more similarities than differences between the depressive reactions experienced by older versus younger individuals. As in younger individuals, the risk for depressive symptoms and syndromes in late life is substantial (23,51,53,68) and remain greater than the risk for married controls for at least two years beyond the death of a loved one (53,55).

On the other hand, several investigators have found that the frequency and intensity of depressive symptoms and syndromes after late-life bereavement may be less than in younger individuals (65,6969–71). Zisook and Shuchter (55) found that risk for major depressive syndrome in older widows and widowers is less than in their younger counterparts only for the first year; by the end of the second year of bereavement the frequency of major depressive syndrome in widows and widowers older than 65 years is identical to the frequency in those younger than 65 years. Therefore, it may not be that older widows and widowers are less distressed or depressed than younger ones, but rather that it takes somewhat longer for the full impact of bereavement to be experienced.

There are more similarities than differences between bereavement-related depression in late life and other forms of major depression. Gallagher-Thompson et al. (72) and Breckenridge et al. (68) emphasized that the depressions experienced by late-life widows and widowers tend to be milder than other major depressive syndromes and that self-depreciation rarely is observed in bereavement reactions. Similarly, Bruce et al. (51) found bereavement increased the risk for dysphoria and major depressive syndrome and that, except for fewer reports of guilt or worthlessness, the major depressive syndrome experienced by widows and widowers roughly parallels other major depressive syndromes in terms of symptomatology. One sleep study found abnormal sleep architecture in depressed elderly widows, further supporting the similarities between a major depressive syndrome associated with loss and a nonbereavement-related depression (73).

Risk Factors for Major Depression Among the Bereaved

Not all bereaved individuals experience a major depressive syndrome after their loss; individuals undergoing a severe life stressor often display amazing adaptive capacities (74–76). But because risk for developing a major depressive syndrome after bereavement is substantial and the morbidity of untreated depression so great, it is important to identify risk factors. In general, no consistent findings on risk factors that relate to gender emerge. Some studies found that older widows are at higher risk (23,51) and other studies reported that older widowers are most vulnerable (77), but most studies have not found substantial differences between bereaved men and women (52,78,79). Loss of a spouse may pose a greater risk than most other types of losses (66). Poor prior physical and mental health (65,80) and prebereavement depression (66) or dysphoria (51) are additional risk factors. A particularly traumatic loss, such as a suicide, may be especially likely to result in persistent depressive syndromes (61). The protective role of social supports in attenuating the risks for depression associated with late-life bereavement appears to be especially important (64,66,80,81). Other investigators have identified early intense reactions soon after the loss (20,79,82,83) and early depressive reactions (61,79,81) as powerful predictors of later depression. Additional risk factors include financial problems, global stress (66), recent disability (64), and subsequent losses in widowers (84). Using a stepwise, logistic regression procedure, Zisook and Shuchter (55) identified a 6-variable model that correctly classified 91% of widows and widowers in terms of major depressive syndrome two years after loss. The six variables are (*i*) presence of a major depressive syndrome soon after the loss, (*ii*) intense symptoms of depression soon after the death, (*iii*) family history of major depression, (*iv*) increased alcohol consumption soon after the loss, (*v*) poor physical health around the time of the death, and (*vi*) a sudden and unexpected death.

Subsyndromal Depression

When evaluating clinically relevant manifestations of bereavement-related depression, one must include the minor and subsyndromal depressions, in addition to the more familiar major depression, in the equation (85). As defined in the DSM-IV (86) appendix, minor depressive episodes differ from major depressive episodes primarily in the number of depressive symptoms—fewer than five. Subsyndromal depression has been defined in many ways: Judd's definition requires two or more depressive symptoms, lasting for two weeks or more, in the absence of a minor or major depression. He found that subsyndromal syndromes often correlate with marked disability and precede a full major depressive syndrome (87). Indeed, these attenuated forms of depression occur more frequently than do major depressive syndromes. Such subsyndromal depressions may be quite common in elderly persons and may be associated with substantial suffering and morbidity (88–90). Unfortunately, despite its prevalence in this vulnerable population, the condition often goes unrecognized (91,92). For a more detailed general discussion of the nonmajor depressive syndromes, see Chapter 2 in this book. During the first two years of spousal bereavement, minor and subsyndromal depressions may be the prodromes of major depression, may represent residual symptoms and/or syndromes as a major depression is improving or even reflect the aftermath of a partially remitted major depression. It is also possible that these depressions constitute independent mood disturbances or forms of attenuated depression important in their own right. Often, widows and widowers shift back and forth between phases of no depression, subsyndromal depression, minor depression, and major depression. An individual who experiences a major depressive episode six to eight weeks after his or her spouse dies can expect to spend roughly 38% of the next two years in a major depressive state, 38% with either minor or subsyndromal depression, and only 24% depression free. These percentages are similar to rates reported for nonbereaved depressed populations (93). And these minor and subsyndromal manifestations of depression are not innocuous. Widows and widowers with minor and subsyndromal manifestations of depression experience psychosocial morbidity roughly midway between those with no depression and those with major depression (85).

Substance Abuse

Individuals who have lost a spouse are at high risk for increased substance use including alcohol and tobacco (94–96) and drugs (primarily sedatives and hypnotics) (97). Clayton (57) found a higher incidence of alcohol use in a sample of older widows and widowers compared to married controls. Many studies suggest that such increases occur in people with preexisting alcohol problems. Valanis et al. (98), for example, noted no new cases of heavy or problem drinking in widowed individuals. Similarly, Zisook et al. (99) measured changes in alcohol consumption in middle-aged and elderly widowed individuals (mean age = 61 years) and found that approximately equal numbers increased (30%) and decreased (26%) the number of days per month they drank. However, when looking at the quantity of alcohol consumed, Zisook reported more widows and widowers increased (34%) than decreased (10%) their quantity of alcohol consumption. Risk factors for increased drinking included the amount of drinking prior to bereavement, being male, a history of depression, dissatisfaction with social and emotional supports, and experiencing a depressive episode soon after the death.

Anxiety Disorders

Parkes (100) found that an array of symptoms typically associated with anxiety often accompany grief. Restlessness, tension, insomnia, headaches, and irritability may characterize the first year of spousal bereavement. Parkes further noted that panic attacks often punctuate the first several months of bereavement. Clayton (101,102) suggested an increased prevalence of anxiety symptoms in widows than in their married counterparts. Widows reported an increased frequency of anxiety attacks, insomnia, weight loss, fatigue, decreased concentration, poor memory, shortness of breath, palpitations, and blurred vision. Maddison and Viola (97) similarly reported increased nervousness, panic feelings, fears, insomnia, and trembling in widows one year after losing their husbands. Jacobs et al. (103) found that more than 40% of bereaved spouses reported at least one type of anxiety disorder based on the modified *Structured Clinical Interview for DSM-III*. There were higher than expected rates for panic and for generalized anxiety disorders during the first year, for agoraphobia in the first six months, and for social phobia in the latter six months.

According to Zisook et al. (104,105), older widows and widowers used more over-the-counter "nerve pills," as well as more prescribed antianxiety medications and hypnotics. This group also demonstrated higher risk rates of several anxiety symptoms during the first seven months of spousal bereavement, elevated scores on Hopkins Symptom Checklist scales of anxiety, somatization, interpersonal sensitivity, and obsessions compared to community norms. Individuals at greatest risk for continued high-anxiety seven months after bereavement tended to be female, younger, and of lower socioeconomic status. Additional risk factors included lack of environmental support, presence of unresolved grief, and increased depression and anxiety symptom intensity soon after the loss. The risks for panic and generalized anxiety disorders were highest among those who had a previous history of anxiety disorders.

Related to the syndrome of complicated grief described above, several investigators have reported that bereavement, especially after a violent and untimely death, may precipitate an actual episode of PTSD (3,104). Indeed, in the first published epidemiologic study of PTSD using DSM-IV criteria, Breslau et al. reported that the sudden and unexpected death of a loved one accounted for more PTSD than any other stressor (106). Rynearson (21,107–110) and Parkes (111) have compared the reactions to such traumatic losses as suicide, homicide, or other forms of unnatural death to PTSD. Rynearson noted that people bereaved by a homicide event report symptoms typically associated with a posttraumatic stress syndrome: intrusive, vivid, and repetitive images of the death; impaired cognitive processes; nightmares, heightened arousal; hypervigilance; and avoidance. Zisook et al. reported that almost 10% of recently bereaved widows and widowers experienced PTSD, even after an expected death following a chronic illness (112). According to Middleton et al. (113), grief complicated by PTSD can be differentiated from other bereavement reactions by hyperarousal, avoidance, nightmares, and intrusive, recurrent, or traumatic images that often reflect the scene of the death. A paucity of data exists on whether or when bereavement is likely to lead to PTSD in the elderly and more work is warranted in this area.

TREATMENT OF BEREAVEMENT-RELATED DEPRESSION SYNDROMES

To Treat or not to Treat?

Just as a clinician would treat any other Axis I disorder that emerges in the context of bereavement, so too should one assess the need for treatment when symptoms of depression occur after the loss of a loved one. Even subsyndromal depressive syndromes occurring in the context of bereavement can be chronic, associated with poor functioning, and replete with risk factors for major depressive episodes, raising questions of whether and how these minor variants of depression should be treated (92).

Although there are overwhelming data to support treating major depressive episodes, less is known about the risk-to-benefit ratios of treating minor and subsyndromal depression. What is known is that minor depressions are associated with significant morbidity (114) and respond to antidepressant medications (115). Therefore, minor episodes of depression should be treated if they significantly interfere with function, impede the normal flow of grief, or persist without showing signs of spontaneously abating. Whether to treat subsyndromal symptoms is even more controversial, as subsyndromal symptoms of depression also are associated with biopsychosocial morbidity (87) but fail to demonstrate a clear response to treatment. Subsyndromal symptoms warrant treatment only when they clearly are an early manifestation of a more robust major depressive episode (i.e., prodromal symptoms) or represent residual symptoms after partial remission from a major depressive episode. In the latter situation, ample data suggests that such residual symptoms correlate with prolonged functional impairment and are strong predictors of imminent recurrent full-blown episodes (93).

Major depressive disorders, even when the episode's onset falls near the time of death of a loved one, have been associated with chronicity, recurrence, impaired interpersonal and occupational functioning, feelings of worthlessness, suicidal ideation, medical morbidity, and poor overall adjustment to widowhood. Such depressive episodes add to the already substantial pain, suffering, and poor functioning associated with bereavement, and also have biologic underpinnings similar to other nonbereavement major depressions. They predict prolonged biopsychosocial impairment (92). Thus, they appear to be at last as clinically significant as other major depressive episodes not associated with bereavement and, just as any major depressive episode is worthy of treatment, so too are those syndromes associated with bereavement.

There are increasing but still too limited data on the efficacy of psychopharmacology, psychotherapy, or both for the treatment of major depression associated with bereavement in the elderly. However, there is little reason to think such depressive episodes will not respond to adequate treatment, as most studies consistently support the effectiveness of the treatment studied. Psychopharmacologic trials suggest that such interventions are safe and effective and that treatment of depression does not interfere with grief. Indeed, studies suggest that depression interferes with grief and that the treatment of depression facilitates the work of grief. However, they also found that grief resolution requires more than short-term medication treatment (13,91). Alternative or augmenting treatment options include a wide range of psychotherapies. Both cognitive and interpersonal therapies, for example, have been found effective for the acute treatment of mild- to moderate major depressive episodes. A more thorough discussion of the two most common treatment modalities, psychopharmacologic intervention, and psychotherapy, follows:

Psychopharmacologic Intervention

Unfortunately, the place of antidepressant medications in the treatment of bereavement-associated depression remains largely uncharted by controlled data. In general, these depressions are underdiagnosed and undertreated, and even recognized psychopharmacology experts have traditionally recommended caution (116,117). Two open studies with tricyclic antidepressants support the safety and efficacy of these medications for bereavement-related major depressive syndromes (118,119), while noting that residual grief symptoms remained even after six to eight weeks of antidepressant therapy. An open-label study suggested that bupropion-sustained release effectively reduces both depressive symptoms and grief intensity in widows and widowers meeting criteria for major depressive syndromes within two months of their loss, technically considered to have the Axis V code of bereavement rather than Major Depression (120). Perhaps early treatment for those depressive syndromes seen within months of the death of a loved one helps prevent some of the prolonged suffering, morbidity, and even mortality associated with bereavement.

In the only randomized, placebo-controlled study on bereavement-related major depression, Reynolds and colleagues (121) found that nortriptyline was more effective than placebo in achieving remission of major depressive episodes, that interpersonal therapy was not more effective than placebo, and that the combination of medication and psychotherapy was more effective than either treatment alone. Thus, the available data overwhelmingly support the acute pharmacologic treatment of bereavement-related depression, perhaps as early as six to eight weeks after the loss, and certainly anytime thereafter.

There is no reason to think that any one class of medications is more effective than others for the treatment of bereavement-related depression. As with treating other, nonbereavement-related depressions, selection should be based on past- or family history of response or, to a lesser extent, on clinical subtype. In the absence of information on past history or specific subtypes known to be preferentially responsive to a particular class of medications, side effects and toxicity guide the choice of medications. Of course, the issues surrounding the pharmacologic treatment of older, nonbereaved individuals also apply when treating older, depressed patients who have lost a loved one. Clinicians should consider prescribing lower doses of antidepressant medications in this population than in their younger counterparts. Concerns surrounding polypharmacy are relevant in this group as the elderly often take multiple medications for various ailments. Special attention should be paid to adherence issues, as older individuals may suffer from visual or hearing losses and not perceive instructions well, or they may have problems with memory and easily forget when and how much medication should be taken. Clinicians should, whenever possible, involve family members or other caregivers when treating older, bereaved individuals.

Psychotherapy

There is a paucity of data evaluating the efficacy of psychotherapy for the treatment of bereavement-related depression, and only one small psychotherapy study specifically focused on treating depression in the elderly. In that study, a small case report series, results suggested the potential effectiveness of interpersonal psychotherapy for bereavement-related depression following loss of a spouse in late life (122). We have advocated a psychotherapeutic approach that addresses both grief and depression, and includes the following components (123):

(a) Establish a supportive relationship with the bereaved individual and possibly their family.
(b) Obtain a detailed assessment of the bereaved individual's relationship to the deceased as it began and evolved over time, the events, and associated feelings surrounding the death, the impact of the loss, social support, other stressors, and background and family issues.
(c) Probe the psychologic, behavioral, and cognitive responses to the death.
(d) Assess coping strategies, encouraging flexibility, and "healthy" responses while discouraging less healthy coping strategies (e.g., alcohol or drugs).
(e) Accept the person's pain and anguish without offering platitudes or empty reassurance.
(f) Help the person accept their own idiosyncratic responses without feeling guilty for not grieving the way they think they should or others tell them are "normal."
(g) Help facilitate acceptance of the loss, as the person is ready, while simultaneously fostering the development of adaptive symbolic and psychologic ties to the deceased.
(h) Explore ongoing relationships with key friends and relatives.
(i) Attend to psychologic, social, and medical needs as necessary.
(j) Some individuals may need help attending to requirements of everyday life, such as paying bills, housekeeping, or child care; others may need help with grief-specific tasks necessitated by the loss, such as funeral arrangements and tracking important papers and documents.
(k) Consider referral to social services or grief support services.
(l) For unflappable avoidance or numbness, consider evocative techniques such as guided imagery, visiting the grave, or writing letters.
(m) For pervasive preoccupation with painful images, consider treatment aimed at anxiety reduction and distraction.
(n) Help the bereaved person understand that grief is a life-long process, but recognize that people learn to go on.
(o) Treatment goals must take into account that depression is often chronic, recurrent, and pleiomorphic in its manifestations over time.
(p) Understand that grief work is exhausting and demanding, often for the therapist as well as the patient.

An Integrative Model for Treatment

Most bereaved individuals do not require professional help. Their arduous journey through the grief process will ultimately culminate in an acceptable level of adjustment to a life without their loved one. Some, however, will find themselves facing a potentially serious psychiatric disorder in the midst of trying to cope with their loss. When confronted with such an individual, the clinician must decide whether and which interventions—psychotherapeutic, psychopharmacologic, or a combination of the two—are appropriate. The major factors that determine when and how to treat are past history; time since death; and the intensity, duration, and pervasiveness of the depressive syndrome.

Past History

The more vulnerable the person is, the sooner (after the loss) active treatment should begin. The risk of developing a major depressive syndrome more than doubles if the person has had only one episode of major depression before the death of a spouse; if a person has had two or more previous episodes, the risk is more than six-fold greater than if the person was never before depressed (85). Thus, for a patient with a history of recurrent major depressive episodes, treatment should begin by the time the death of a loved one is considered imminent. Such a person is vulnerable to an exacerbation or relapse of the depressive illness after the death, and prevention is warranted. If first seen after the death, a bereaved person with a history of recurrent depression should be either observed closely or started on prophylactic treatment. The decisions regarding which treatment or combination of treatments are best for each unique person are based on the patient's preferences; the severity, duration, proximity, and treatment-response of previous depressions; the likelihood of the patient promptly initiating treatment should depression develop; the intensity of grief and depressive symptoms at the time of the initial evaluation; and the general medical health of the patient. In other words, the risk factors previously described help to guide treatment.

Time Since Death

Compared with the past history and the nature of the depressions, time since death is a relatively minor factor. The question is not so much how long to wait before treating, but rather under what circumstances one should wait. If there is no past or family history of major depression and the syndrome is relatively mild in terms of severity, reactivity, and impairment, treatment may be delayed for at least the first two months, if not longer. The clinician may then initiate treatment with educational-supportive psychotherapy, using the same general guidelines as one would for nonbereavement depressions. If the depression does not fully respond to psychotherapeutic interventions, antidepressant medications should be given. Aggressive treatment of minor or subsyndromal depressive syndromes during the first few months of bereavement is rarely necessary. However, the farther the patient is from loss, the more therapeutic intervention may be warranted, even in these subthreshold variants. The more vulnerable the person is in terms of past or family history, and the more intense or autonomous the symptoms are, the earlier in the course of bereavement intervention is justified. Suicidal or melancholic symptoms, for example, require prompt intervention regardless of the proximity to bereavement (or any other psychosocial stressor, for that matter).

Nature of Symptoms

As in all other depressions, the decision of when and how to treat is dependent on the intensity, autonomy, duration, and pervasiveness of the syndrome. The more severe and autonomous the depression is, the more likely it is that somatic treatment is necessary. Even in the absence of previous episodes or immediately after the death of a loved one, if depressive symptoms are severe, present in the absence of grief triggers, and associated with suicidal ideation or melancholic features, aggressive pharmacologic treatment should prevail. Conversely, if the depressive symptoms and the impairment are mild, seem most pronounced around reminders of the deceased, and are not associated with significant impairment, suicidal thoughts, or melancholic features, education and support may be all that is necessary. If the bereaved person does not have close friends or a supportive social milieu, a support group might be helpful for this type of mild depression. For depression between these two extremes, combinations of somatic and psychotherapeutic interventions are indicated.

No single form of psychotherapy or antidepressant medication is currently designated the "best" treatment for bereavement-related depression, and few studies exist which focus on the treatment of older, bereaved individuals. Cognitive-behavioral and interpersonal therapy have both proved effective for treating depression; indeed, there are no strong data demonstrating that either of these forms of therapy is superior to the other. Similarly, all classes of antidepressant medications are about equally effective, but differences in their side-effect profiles usually dictate which medication is best suited for an individual patient. It is important to address the individual's specific needs and resources, as well as the availability of various treatment modalities, in choosing the best approach. A paradigm that includes education, supportive psychotherapy, and medication management maximizes the probability of successful treatment (123,124).

CONCLUSIONS

Grief and depression are by no means identical and constitute two separate, albeit intertwined, phenomena. Despite—or perhaps because of—the pain, disability, and life disruption associated with bereavement, many individuals experience enormous growth and development throughout the grief process. Although the shattering impact of losing a loved one should never be minimized, many individuals emerge from the experience with a renewed sense of who they are and with an expanded repertoire of competencies. However, a substantial minority of bereaved individuals may find their loss precipitating the onset, persistence, or exacerbation of a psychiatric disorder. In such cases, the problem should not be rationalized or minimized. Psychiatric disturbances that emerge in the context of bereavement, including depressive syndromes, warrant full clinical attention. Sadness, unhappiness, loneliness, and other dysphoric experiences commonly characterize "normal" grief, but major depression does not. Bereavement-related depressions respond just as well to treatment as do other nonbereavement-related depressions. More studies are needed in the area of late-life bereavement; a particular dearth of literature exists in the area of treatment strategies geared toward this population. An integrative approach combining patient support, family education, psychotherapy, and pharmacologic therapy is ideal.

REFERENCES

1. Bowlby J. Attachment and Loss. Loss: Sadness and Depression, Vol. 3. New York, NY: Basic Books, 1980/1981.
2. DeVaul RA, Zisook S, Faschingbauer TR. Clinical aspects of grief and bereavement. Prim Care 1979; 6:391–402.
3. Horowitz MJ. Stress Response Syndromes. Northvale, NJ: Aronson, 1986.

4. Shuchter S, Zisook S. The course of normal grief. In: Stroebe MS, Stroebe W, Hansson RO, eds. Handbook of Bereavement: Theory, Research and Intervention. Cambridge, UK: Cambridge University Press, 1993:23–43.
5. Maciejewski PK, Zhang B, Block SD, et al. An empirical examination of the stage theory of grief. JAMA 2007; 297:716–723.
6. Bonanno GA, Boemer K. The stage theory of grief. JAMA 2007; 297:2693.
7. Silver RC, Wortman CB. The stage theory of grief. JAMA 2007; 297:2692.
8. Shear K, Shair H. Attachment, loss, and complicated grief. Dev Psychobiol 2005; 47:253–267.
9. Horowitz MJ, Siegel B, Holen A, et al. Diagnostic criteria for complicated grief disorder. Am J Psychiatry 1997; 154:904–910.
10. Prigerson HG, Bridges J, Maciejewski PK, et al. Influence of traumatic grief on suicidal ideation among young adults. Am J Psychiatry 1999; 156:1994–1995.
11. Shear MK, Frank E, Foa E, et al. Traumatic grief treatment: A pilot study. Am J Psychiatry 2001; 158:1506–1508.
12. Prigerson HG, Bierhals AJ, Kasi SV, et al. Traumatic grief as a risk factor for mental and physical morbidity. Am J Psychiatry 1997; 154:616–623.
13. Zygmont M, Prigerson HG, Houck PR, et al. A post hoc comparison of paroxetine and nortriptyline for symptoms of traumatic grief. J Clin Psychiatry 1998; 59:241–245.
14. Shear K, Frank E, Houck PR, et al. Treatment of complicated grief: A randomized controlled trial. JAMA 2005; 293:2601–2608.
15. Simon NM, Thompson EH, Pollack MH, et al. Complicated grief: A case series using escitalopram. Am J Psychiatry 2007; 164:1760–1761.
16. Lichtenthal WG, Cruess DG, Prigerson HG. A case for establishing complicated grief as a distinct mental disorder in DSM-V. Clin Psychol Rev 2004; 24:637–662.
17. Prigerson HG, Shear MK, Jacobs SC, et al. Consensus criteria for traumatic grief. A preliminary empirical test. Br J Clin Pharmacol 1999; 174:67–73.
18. Simon NM, Shear KM, Thompson EH, et al. The prevalence and correlates of psychiatric comorbidity in individuals with complicated grief. Compr Psychiatry 2007; 48:395–399. Epub 2007 Jul 5.
19. Raphael B. The Anatomy of Bereavement. New York, NY: Basic Books, 1983.
20. Parkes CM, Weiss RS. Recovery from Bereavement. New York, NY: Basic Books, 1983.
21. Rynearson EK. Psychological adjustments to unnatural dying. In: Zisook S, ed. Biopsychosocial Aspects of Bereavement. Washington, D. C.: American Psychiatric Association, 1987.
22. Thompson LW, Breckenridge JW, Gallagher D, et al. Effects of bereavement on self-perceptions of physical health in elderly widows and widowers. J Gerontol B Psychol Sci Soc Sci 1984; 39:309–314.
23. Gallagher-Thompson DE, Breckenridge J, Thompson LW, et al. Effects of bereavement on indicators of mental health in elderly widows and widowers. J Gerontol 1983; 38:565–571.
24. Hutchin S. The distress of care giving, 146th Annual Meeting of the American Psychiatric Association. San Francisco, CA: 1993.
25. Moss MS, Moss SZ, Rusbinstein R, et al. Impact of elderly mother's death on middle age daughters. Int J Aging Hum Dev 1993; 37:1–22.
26. Stroebe M, Schut H, Stroebe W. Health outcomes of bereavement. Lancet. 2007; 370:1960–1973.
27. Stroebe MS, Stroebe W. The mortality of bereavement: A review. In: Stroebe MS, Stroebe W, Hansson R, eds. Handbook of Bereavement: Theory, Research and Intervention. Cambridge, UK:Cambridge University Press, 1993.
28. He W, Sengupta M, Velkoff VA, et al. 65+ in the United States: 2005. U. S. Census Bureau, Current Population Reports. Washington, D. C.: U. S. Government Printing Office, 2005:23–209.
29. Cox PR, Ford JR. The mortality of widows shortly after widowhood. Lancet 1964; 1:163–164.

30. Helsing KJ, Szklo M. Mortality after bereavement. Am J Epidemiol 1981; 114:41–52.
31. Kaprio J, Kaoskenvuo M, Rita H. Mortality after bereavement: A perspective study of 95647 widowed persons. Am J Public Health 1987; 77:283–287.
32. Kraus AS, Lilienfeld AM. Some epidemiological aspects of the high mortality rate in the young widowed group. J Chronic Dis 1959; 10:207–217.
33. Levav I, Friedlander Y, Kark J, et al. An epidemiologic study of mortality among bereaved patients. N Engl J Med 1988; 319:457–461.
34. Li G. The interaction effect of bereavement and sex on the risk of suicide in the elderly: An historical cohort study. Soc Sci Med 1995; 40:825–828.
35. Lillard LA, Waite LJ. Till death do us part—Marital disruption and mortality. Am J Sociol 1995; 100:1131–1156.
36. Manor O, Eisenbach Z. Mortality after spousal loss: Are there socio-demographic differences? Soc Sci Med 2003; 56:405–413.
37. Rees W, Lutkins S. Mortality of bereavement. BMJ 1967; 4:13–16.
38. Mellstrom D, Nilsson A, Oden A, et al. Mortality among the widowed in Sweden. Scand J Soc Med 1982; 10:33–41.
39. Bowling A, Charlton J. Risk factors for mortality after bereavement: A logistic regression analysis. J R Coll Gen Pract 1987; 37:551–554.
40. Erlangsen A, Jeune B, Bille-Brahe U, et al. Loss of partner and suicide risks among the oldest old: A population-based registry study. Age Ageing 2004; 33:378–383.
41. Young M, Benjamin B, Wallis C. Mortality of widowers. Lancet 1963; 2:454–456.
42. Elwert F, Christakis N. Widowhood and race. Am Sociol Rev 2006; 71:16–41.
43. Gallagher-Thompson DE, Futerman A, Farberow N, et al. The impact of spousal bereavement on older widows and widowers. In: Stroebe MS, Stroebe W, Hansson RO, eds. Handbook of Bereavement: Theory, Research and Intervention. Cambridge, UK: Cambridge University Press, 1993:227–239.
44. Li J, Precht DH, Mortensen PB, et al. Mortality in parents after death of a child in Denmark: A nationwide follow-up study. Lancet 2003; 361:363–367.
45. Qin P, Mortensen PB. The impact of parental status on the risk of completed suicide. Arch Gen Psychiatry 2003; 60:797–802.
46. Ajdacic-Gross V, Ring M, Gadoa E, et al. Suicide after bereavement: an overlooked problem. Psychol Med 2008; 38:673–676.
47. Agerbo E. Midlife suicide risk, partner's psychiatric illness, spouse and child bereavement by suicide or other modes of death: A gender specific study. J Epidemiol Community Health 2005; 59:407–412.
48. MacMahon B, Pugh TF. Suicide in the widowed. Am J Epidemiol 1965; 81:23–31.
49. Jones DR. Heart disease mortality following widowhood: Some results form the OPCS logitudinal study. J Psychosom Res 1987; 31:325–333.
50. Jones DR, Goldblatt PO, Leon DA. Bereavement and cancer: Some results using data on deaths of spouses from the Longitudinal Study of the Office of Population Censuses and Surveys. Br Med J 1984; 298:461m–464m.
51. Bruce ML, Kim K, Leaf PJ, et al. Depressive episodes and dysphoria resulting from conjugal bereavement in a prospective community sample. Am J Psychiatry 1990; 145:608–611.
52. Clayton PJ. Bereavement and depression. J Clin Psychiatry 1990; 51:34–40.
53. Harlow SD, Goldberg EL, Comstock GW. A longitudinal study of the prevalence of depressive symptomatology in elderly widowed and married women. Arch Gen Psychiatry 1991; 48:1065–1068.
54. Weller RA, Weller EB, Fristad MA, et al. Depression in recently bereaved prepubertal children. Am J Psychiatry 1991; 148:1536–1540.
55. Zisook S, Schuchter SR. Major depression associated with widowhood. Am J Geriatr Psychiatry 1993; 1:316–326.
56. Zisook S, Shuchter SR, Sledge P. Diagnostic and treatment considerations in depression associated with late-life bereavement. In: Schneider LS, Reynolds CF, Lebowitz BD, et al., eds. Diagnosis and Treatment of Depression in Late Life: Results of the NIH

Consensus Development Conference. Washington, D. C.: American Psychiatric Press, 1991:419–435.
57. Clayton PJ. The sequelae and nonsequelae of conjugal bereavement. Am J Psychiatry 1979; 136:1530–1534.
58. Lund DA, Caserta MS, Dimond MF. The course of spousal bereavement in later life. In: Stroebe MS, Stroebe W, Hansson R, eds. Handbook of Bereavement: Theory, Research and Intervention. Cambridge, UK: Cambridge University Press, 1993:240–254.
59. American Psychiatric Association. Diagnostic and Statistical Manual of Mental Disorders, 3rd ed. Text Revision. Washington, D. C.: American Psychiatric Association, 2000.
60. Clayton PJ, Halikas JA, Maurice WL. The depression of widowhood. Br J Psychiatry 1972; 120:71–77.
61. Gilewski MJ, Farberow NL, Gallagher DE, et al. Interaction of depression and bereavement on mental health in the elderly. Psychol Aging 1991; 6:67–75.
62. Zisook S, Shuchter SR. Bereavement. Current Psychiatric Therapy II 1997; 34:248–252.
63. Zisook S, Shear K, Kendler KS. Validity of the bereavement exclusion criterion for the diagnosis of major depressive episode. World Psychiatry 2007; 6:38–43.
64. Goldberg EL, Comstock GW, Harlow SD. Emotional problems and widowhood. J Gerontol B Psychol Sci Soc Sci 1988; 43:5206–5208.
65. McHorney CA, Mor V. Predictors of bereavement depression and its health services consequences. Med Care 1988; 26:882–893.
66. Norris FH, Murrell SA. Social support, life events, and stress as modifiers of adjustment to bereavement by older adults. Psychol Aging 1990; 5:429–436.
67. Zisook S, Shuchter SR. Early psychological reaction to the stress of widowhood. Psychiatry 1991; 54:320–333.
68. Breckenridge JN, Gallagher D, Thompson LW, et al. Characteristic depressive symptoms of bereaved elders. J Gerontol 1986; 41:163–168.
69. Faletti MV, Gibbs JM, Clark C, et al. Longitudinal course of bereavement in older adults. In: Lund DA, ed. Older Bereaved Spouses: Research with Practical Applications. New York, NY: Taylor & Francis/Hemisphere, 1989:37–51.
70. Mor V. Hospice Care Systems. New York, NY: Springer Press, 1987.
71. VanZandt S, Mou R, Abbott R. Mental and physical health of rural bereaved and nonbereaved elders: A longitudinal study. In: Lund DA, ed. Older Bereaved Spouses: Research with Practical Applications. New York, NY: Hemisphere, 1989:25–35.
72. Gallagher-Thompson DE. Similarities and differences between normal grief and depression in older adults. Essence 1982; 5:127–140.
73. Reynolds CF, Hoch CC, Buysse DJ, et al. Electroencephalographic sleep in spousal bereavement and bereavement-related depression of late life. Biol Psychiatry 1992; 31:69–82.
74. Chentsova-Dutton Y, Zisook S. Adaptation to bereavement. Death Stud 2005; 29:877–903.
75. Pollock GH. The mourning-liberation process in health and disease. Psychiatr Clin North Am 1987; 10:345–354.
76. Silverman PR. Widowhood and prevention intervention. Fam Coord 1972; 21:95–102.
77. Richards JG, McCallum J. Bereavement in the elderly. N Z Med J 1979; 89:201–204.
78. Feinson MC. Aging widows and widowers: Are there mental health differences? Int J Aging Hum Dev 1986; 23:241–255.
79. Zisook S, Shuchter SR. Depression through the first year after the death of a spouse. Am J Psychiatry 1991; 148:1346–1352.
80. Nuss S, Zubenko GS. Correlates of persistent depressive symptoms in widows. Am J Psychiatry 1992; 149:346–351.
81. Dimond M, Lund DA, Caserta MS. The role of social support in the first two years of bereavement in an elderly sample. Gerontologist 1987; 27:599–604.
82. Farberow NL, Gallagher DE, Gilewski MJ, et al. An examination of the early impact of bereavement on psychological distress in survivors of suicide. Gerontologist 1987; 27:592–598.

83. Lund DA, Dimond MF, Caserta MS, et al. Identifying elderly with coping difficulties after two years of bereavement. Omega 1985; 16:213–223.
84. Siegel JM, Kuykendall DH. Loss, widowhood, and psychological distress among the elderly. J Consult Clin Psychol 1990; 58:519–524.
85. Zisook S, Paulus M, Schuchter SR, et al. The many faces of depression following spousal bereavement. J Affect Disord 1997; 45:85–95.
86. American Psychiatric Association. American Psychiatric Association: Diagnostic and Statistical Manual of Mental Disorders, DSM-IV. Washington, D. C.: American Psychiatric Association, 1994.
87. Judd LL, Paulus MP, Wells KB, et al. Socioeconomic burden of subsyndromal depressive symptoms and major depression in a sample of the general population. Am J Psychiatry 1996; 153:1411–1417.
88. Blazer DG. Epidemiology of depressive disorders in late life. In: Schneider LS, Reynolds CF, Lebowitz BD, et al., eds. Diagnosis and Treatment of Depression in Late Life: Results of the NIMH Consensus and Development Conference. Washington, D. C.: American Psychiatric Press, 1994:9–20.
89. Blazer DG, George LK. The epidemiology of depression in an elderly community population. Gerontologist 1987; 27:281–287.
90. Broadhead WE, Blazer DG, George LK, et al. Depression, disability days, and days lost from work in a prospective epidemiologic survey. JAMA 1990; 264:2524–2528.
91. Pasternak RE, Reynolds CF, Miller MD, et al. The symptom profile and two-year course of subsyndromal depression in spousally bereaved elders. Am J Geriatr Psychiatry 1994; 2:210–219.
92. Zisook S, Shuchter SR, Sledge PA, et al. The spectrum of depressive phenomena after spousal bereavement. J Clin Psychiatry 1994; 55:29–36.
93. Judd LL, Akiskal HS, Maser JD, et al. A prospective 12-year study of subsyndromal and syndromal depressive symptoms in unipolar major depressive disorders. Arch Gen Psychiatry 1998; 55:694–700.
94. Blankfield A. Grief and alcohol. Am J Drug Alcohol Abuse 1983; 9:435–446.
95. Klerman GL, Izen J. The effects of bereavement and grief on physical health and general well being. Adv Psychosom Med 1977; 8:63–104.
96. Osterweis M, Solomon F, Green M, eds. Bereavement: Reactions, Consequences, and Care. Washington, D. C.: National Academy Press, 1984.
97. Maddison D, Viola A. The health of widows in the year following bereavement. J Psychosom Res 1968; 12:297–306.
98. Valanis B, Yeaworth RC, Mullis MR. Alcohol use among bereaved and nonbereaved older persons. J Gerontol Nurs 1987; 13:26–32.
99. Zisook S, Shuchter S, Mulvihill M. Alcohol, cigarette and medication during the first year of widowhood. Psychiatr Ann 1990; 20:318–326.
100. Parkes MC. Effects of bereavement on physical and mental health—A study of the medical records of widows. Br Med J 1964; 2:274–279.
101. Clayton PJ. Mortality and morbidity in the first year of widowhood. Arch Gen Psychiatry 1974; 30:747–750.
102. Clayton PJ, Desmarais L, Winokur G. A study of normal bereavement. Am J Psychiatry 1968; 125:168–178.
103. Jacobs SC, Hansen F, Kasl S, et al. Anxiety disorders in acute bereavement: Risk and risk factors. J Clin Psychiatry 1990; 51:267–274.
104. Zisook S, Mulvihill M, Shuchter SR. Widowhood and anxiety. Psychiatr Med 1990; 8:99–116.
105. Zisook S, Shuchter SR, Sledge P, et al. Aging and bereavement. J Geriatr Psychiatry Neurol 1993; 6:137–143.
106. Breslau N, Kessler RC, Chilcoat HD, et al. Trauma and posttraumatic stress disorder in the community: The 1996 Detroit Area Survey of Trauma. Arch Gen Psychiatry 1998; 55:626–632.
107. Rynearson EK. Pathologic grief: The queen's croquet ground. Psychiatr Ann 1990; 20:295–303.

108. Rynearson EK. Psychotherapy of pathologic grief: Revisions and limitations. Psychiatr Clin North Am 1987; 10:487–500.
109. Rynearson EK. Suicide internalized: Existential sequestrum. Am J Psychiatry 1981; 138:84–87.
110. Rynearson EK. Bereavement after homicide: A descriptive study. Am J Psychiatry 1984; 141:1452–1454.
111. Parkes CM. Psychiatric problems following bereavement by murder or manslaughter. Br J Psychiatry 1993; 162:49–54.
112. Zisook S, Chentsova-Dutton Y, Shuchter SR. PTSD following bereavement. Ann Clin Psychiatry 1998; 10:157–163.
113. Middleton W, Raphael B, Martinek N, et al. Pathological grief reactions. In: Stroebe MS, Stroebe W, Hansson RO, eds. Handbook of Bereavement: Theory, Research and Intervention. Cambridge, UK: Cambridge University Press, 1993:44–61.
114. Rollman BL, Reynolds CF. Minor and subsyndromal depression: Functional disability worth treating. J Am Geriatr Soc 1999; 47:757–758.
115. Stewart JW, Quitkin FM, Klein DF. The pharmacotherapy of minor depression. Am J Psychother 1992; 1:23–36.
116. Hollister L. Psychotherapeutic drugs in the dying and bereaved. J Thanatol 1972; 2:623–629.
117. Klein DF, Blank HR. Psychophramacological treatment of bereavement and its complications. In: Kutscher AH, ed. Death and Bereavement. Springfield, IL: Charles C. Thomas, 1969:299–305.
118. Jacobs S, Nelson JC, Zisook S. Treating depressions of bereavement with antidepressants: A pilot study. Psychiatr Clin North Am 1987; 10:501–510.
119. Pasternak RE, Reynolds CF, Schlernitzauer M, et al. Acute open-trial nortriptyline therapy of bereavement-related depression in late life. J Clin Psychiatry 1991; 52:307–310.
120. Zisook S, Shuchter SR, Pedrelli P, et al. Bupropion sustained release for bereavement: Results of an open trial. J Clin Psychiatry 2001; 62:227–230.
121. Reynolds CF, Miller MD, Pasternak RE, et al. Treatment of bereavement-related major depressive episodes in later life: A controlled study of acute and continuation treatment with nortriptyline and interpersonal therapy. Am J Psychiatry 1999; 156:202–208.
122. Miller MD, Frank E, Cornes C, et al. Applying interpersonal psychotherapy to bereavement-related depression following loss of a spouse in late life. J Psychother Pract Res 1994; 3:149–162.
123. Zisook S, Shuchter SR. Treatment of the depressions of bereavement. Am Behav Sci 2001; 44:782–792.
124. Zisook S, Shuchter S. Psychotherapy of the depression in spousal bereavement. Psychother Pract 1996; 2:31–45.

15 Pharmacotherapy of Late-Life Depression: Evidence-Based Recommendations

James M. Ellison

Geriatric Psychiatry Program, McLean Hospital, Belmont, and Department of Psychiatry, Harvard Medical School, Boston, Massachusetts, U.S.A.

E. Yusuf Sivrioglu

Geriatric Psychiatry Unit, Department of Psychiatry, Uludag University Medical Faculty, Bursa, Turkey

Carl Salzman

Department of Psychiatry, Massachusetts Mental Health Center/Beth Israel Deaconess Hospital, and Department of Psychiatry, Harvard Medical School, Boston, Massachusetts, U.S.A.

INTRODUCTION

Antidepressant medications are the most thoroughly researched and most frequently employed modality for treating late-life depression. Though their benefits have repeatedly been shown superior to those of placebo in treating depressed elderly research subjects, many questions about their use in clinical populations remain unresolved. Which of the many available antidepressants should be chosen initially? Are there strong differences between classes or between agents within a class? How should treatment approaches be modified in the care of special populations of depressed elderly such as those with, dementia, psychotic depression, or treatment resistance? How long should the acute and continuation phases of a treatment trial be extended? Under what circumstances and for how long should maintenance treatment be prescribed? And, finally, what gaps are there in our knowledge to guide the design and implementation of more-informative future studies? This chapter will briefly review antidepressants, then address the issues relevant to the special needs of elderly depressed patients by reviewing the available evidence base for treatment decisions regarding the pharmacotherapy of late-life depression.

AGE-ASSOCIATED PHARMACOKINETIC AND PHARMACODYNAMIC CONSIDERATIONS

Age-associated changes in physiology alter drug distribution, decrease metabolism, and reduce excretion, enhancing the effects and side effects of medications. Loss of body water and lean body mass result in relatively lower volumes of distribution and higher plasma levels of drugs, such as lithium, that are distributed primarily in body water. Moreover, an age-associated decrease in plasma albumin, which binds most antidepressants to some degree, results in an increase in the concentration of "free" or "nonbound" medication available for binding at receptor sites. Decreased hepatic demethylation and hydroxylation associated with aging contribute to higher blood levels of many psychotropics that are metabolized in the liver, extending their elimination half-lives. Medications such as divalproex that rely on glucuronidation, which is not altered by aging, are not affected in this way. The elimination of drugs and their metabolites takes place primarily through the kidneys. Between the age of 30 and 80 years, glomerular filtration rate diminishes by approximately 1% per year (1). Reduced renal elimination of active drugs such as lithium or of antidepressants' metabolites (e.g. hydroxydesipramine) can occur as a result of age-associated renal compromise. In contrast, drug absorption can diminish with aging as a result of lower gastric pH, diminished mesenteric blood flow, and reduced intestinal absorption area (2). The overall effect of age-associated pharmacokinetic changes is to increase drug exposure for a given dose by raising peak blood levels and prolonging drug action. These pharmacokinetic effects must be taken into consideration in order to use antidepressants effectively and safely in older patients. Furthermore, drug–drug interactions must be considered because of the greater number of prescribed and over-the-counter medications taken concurrently by the elderly patients.

Higher levels of drug exposure become even more meaningful clinically as a result of the pharmacodynamic changes associated with aging. In the elderly, the effects of anticholinergic medications, for example, can be amplified, resulting in a more deleterious side-effect profile. Similarly, an enhanced response to noradrenergic drugs is observed (3). Response to serotonergic drugs may be altered because of a possible reduction of $5HT_{2A}$ receptors and reuptake sites (4). These pharmacodynamic changes can alter the balance between therapeutic and adverse effects of an antidepressant in older patients.

EVIDENCE BASE AND SUGGESTIONS FOR ACUTE TREATMENT OF LATE-LIFE DEPRESSION

An impressively large literature describes the efficacy, safety, and recommendations for use of antidepressants in the elderly. Several excellent textbooks (5–8) describe their mechanisms of action, benefits and risks, dosing considerations, interactions, and the recommended duration of use. Although a thorough review of each antidepressant falls beyond the scope of this chapter, we will highlight the major distinctions between antidepressant classes, discuss most individual agents, and offer an overview of medications with evidence-based recommendations for use in the elderly.

Our approach to treating late-life depression has evolved from careful review of available published, randomized-controlled trials (RCTs) (9–100) of pharmacotherapy of acute depression in elderly populations as well as from four thoughtful meta-analyses on this topic (101–104) and an expert consensus guideline panel (105) on the treatment of depressive disorders in older patients. More than 90 randomized-controlled trials, summarized in Table 1, were identified by a Medline search and subsequent iterative review of citations within the identified studies.

Heterocyclic antidepressants are the agents with the most extensive evidence base in geriatric cohorts, though newer antidepressants, to a large degree, have superceded at least their initial use. The use of SSRIs in treated late-life depression has been described in more than 40 published controlled studies, whereas only eight describe the use of the newer, dual-action SNRIs in this population. We have identified eight studies for monoamine oxidase inhibitors, three each for bupropion or bupropion and mirtazapine, and none for nefazodone. An additional 19 geriatric depression trials were found for agents not currently available in the United States:

(text continued on page 257)

TABLE 1 Randomized Controlled Trial of Pharmacotherapy of Acute Late Life Depression

Studies	Drugs	*n*	Mean dose or dose range (mg/day)	Age range or mean age	Duration (weeks)	Outcome scales	Results
Allard P (89)	Venlafaxine XR Citalopram	73 75	75–150 20–30	64–89 Mean 73	22	MADRS CGI GDS	Both drugs equally effective in treating depression and in terms of tolerability.
Altamura AC (10)	Fluoxetine Amitriptyline	13 15	20 75	Mean 68.5	5	HAM-D	Shorter latency of action in amitriptyline group. Both drugs are equally effective at the end of the study. Anticholinergic side effects more common in amitriptyline. Significant weight gain observed only in amitriptyline group.
Altamura AC (9)	Amitriptyline Mianserin Trazodone	37 33 36	75 60 150	60–83 Mean 65.83	5	HAM-D	All three drugs were effective at the end of the study. Trazodone showed significantly lower anticholinergic and cardiac side effects when compared to other drugs.
Ather SA (11)	Trazodone Amitriptyline	50 51	100 50	NR	6	HAM-D	Both were drug equally effective at the end of the study. VAS showed an earlier improvement of anxiety with trazodone. Trazodone had fewer anticholinergic side effects than amitriptyline.
Bayer AJ (12)	Trazodone Trazodone-CR	83 83	171.5 150.8	65–90 Mean 78	4	HAM-D CGI	The HAM-D score difference between groups was not significant at the end of the study. Both formulations were equally tolerated.
Bocksberger JP (13)	Moclobemide Fluvoxamine	20 20	433 172	Mean 74.45	4	MADRS CGI	Both group effective in decreasing depression score. Moclobemide showed an earlier effect and was more effective. Tolerability was good for both drugs.

(*Continued*)

TABLE 1 Randomized Controlled Trial of Pharmacotherapy of Acute Late Life Depression (*Continued*)

Studies	Drugs	*n*	Mean dose or dose range (mg/day)	Age range or mean age	Duration (weeks)	Outcome scales	Results
Bondareff W (14)	Sertraline Nortriptyline	105 105	96 78	Mean 67.85	12	HAM-D CGI HAM-A POMS	Efficacy of both drugs was similar at all time points. Secondary measures (memory, cognitive function, quality of life) revealed a significant advantage for sertraline treatment. The safety profiles were similar except that nortriptyline was associated with a significant increase in heart rate.
Bose A (90)	Escitalopram Placebo	132 135	14	Mean 68.3	12	MADRS HAM-D CGI GDS	Efficacy of escitalopram was not significantly different than placebo. Escitalopram was well tolerated.
Branconnier RJ (15)	Bupropion 150 mg Bupropion 450 mg Imipramine Placebo	18 18 18 9	150 450 max. 150 max.	Mean 63.3	5	HAM-D	High and low doses of bupropion and imipramine were equally, and more effective than placebo at the end of the study. At the second week, only bupropion high dose and imipramine groups were more effective than placebo. Side effects observed with both doses of bupropion were not different that placebo. Anticholinergic side effects were significantly higher in imipramine group.
Brion S (59)	Tianeptine 25 mg Tianeptine 37.5 mg Mianserine	100 109 106	25 37.5 30	Mean 78.5	24	MADRS HAM-D	Tianeptine 25 mg and 37.5 mg and mianserine equally effective in treating depression. Impaired vigilance and equilibrium less frequent with Tianeptine 25 mg than with mianserine.
Cassano GB (16)	Paroxetine Fluoxetine	123 119	20–40 20–60	Mean 75.4	52	HAM-D CGI	Both drugs equally effective in treating depression. Efficacy maintained for more than 1 year.

Cohn CK (17)	Sertraline Amitriptyline	161 80	116.2 88.3	65–85 Mean 70.4	8	HAM-D CGI SCL-56 HSC	Two drugs produced similar degree of response to treatment. Anticholinergic side effects were less common and gastrointestinal side effects were more common in sertraline group.
Cohn JB (18)	Nomifensine Imipramine Placebo	21 21 21	152.5 137.5	Mean 66.43	4	HAM-D CGI	Both nomifensine and imipramine were superior to placebo at the end of the study. Compared to imipramine group, fewer patients reported dry mouth, nausea/vomiting, and restlessness/nervousness.
Dalery J (19)	Paroxetine Mianserine	54 62	20 30	60–91 Mean 71.5	24	MADRS AJRS	Both drugs equally effective. Paroxetine more effective in decreasing anxiety score.
De Ronchi D (20)	Fluoxetine Amitriptyline	32 33	20 50–100	Mean 68.8	10	HAM-D MADRS CGI PGI	Both drugs equally effective. CNS adverse effects and weight gain were more frequent with amitriptyline
De Vanna MJ (21)	Moclobemide Mianserin	Total: 80	150–500 50–125	60–80	4	HAM-D	Both drugs were equally effective in treating the depression and both were well tolerated.
Dorman T (22)	Paroxetine Mianserin	30 30	15–30 30–60	>65	6	HAM-D	The ratio of responders was significantly higher in paroxetine group. Mianserin was associated with a greater number of CNS side effects.
Dunner DL (23)	Paroxetine Doxepin	136 135	23.4 105.2	>60 Mean 68	6	HAM-D MADRS HSC CGI	Both drugs were similarly effective in alleviating depression as measured on the HAM-D, MADRS, and HSC. Paroxetine was superior to doxepin on CGI-S, HAM-D retardation factor and depressed mood item. Doxepin produced significantly more anticholinergic side effects, sedation, and confusion.

(Continued)

TABLE 1 Randomized Controlled Trial of Pharmacotherapy of Acute Late Life Depression (*Continued*)

Studies	Drugs	*n*	Mean dose or dose range (mg/day)	Age range or mean age	Duration (weeks)	Outcome scales	Results
Eklund K (24)	Mianserin Imipramine	25 25	45 105	60–88	4	HAM-D CGI VASD	There was no significant difference of antidepressant efficacy between the drugs. Significantly more anticholinergic side effects were observed in imipramine group.
Evans M (25)	Fluoxetine Placebo	38 38	20	75–85 Mean 80.4	8	HAM-D	No difference was found between the response rates of two groups. There was a trend for the results in the fluoxetine group to continue to improve with time. Patients with serious illness who completed 5 weeks of treatment had lower HAM-D scores than those receiving placebo.
Fairweather DB (26)	Fluoxetine Amitriptyline	Total: 66	20 75	Mean 69.9	7	MADRS	Both drugs reduced the depression significantly and there was no difference between two groups in terms of antidepressant efficacy.
Falk WE (27)	Fluoxetine Trazodone	14 13	48 350	Mean 68.3	7	HAM-D CGI	Both drugs were equally effective in treating depression. There was a trend to report more insomnia in the fluoxetine group.
Feighner JP (29)	Fluoxetine Doxepin	78 79	55 135	61–90	6	HAM-D RDS CAS CGI	Both drugs were equally effective in improving the mean end point score compared with baseline for all efficacy measures.
Feighner JP (28)	Desipramine Adinazolam	15 15	94 38	60–85 Mean 68.17	8	HAM-D MADRS CGI	HAM-D score were significantly decreased at the end of the study for both groups. The decrease in adinazolam group was significantly higher than fluoxetine group. There was no difference in the number of responders.

Finkel SI (98)	Sertraline Fluoxetine	42 33	80.4 30	70–93 Mean 74.5	12	HAM-D CGI HAM-A	End point scores of efficacy measure revealed no difference among the groups but the number of responders was greater in sertraline group than fluoxetine. There was no difference in remission rates. The only adverse effect observed to be more frequent in sertraline group was "shaking." There was no other difference in side effect profiles.
Finkel SI (30)	Sertraline Nortriptyline	39 37	102 68	70–89 Mean 74.5	12	HAM-D CGI POMS Q-LES-Q	Both drugs significantly decreased depression scores. Reduction of depression scores and rate of responders greater and side effects less frequent with sertraline.
Forlenza OV (32)	Sertraline Imipramine	28 27	50 150	Mean 68.5	6	MADRS	Both groups had a significant decrease in MADRS scores compared to baseline. There was no difference of antidepressant efficacy between groups. The overall tolerability of both drugs was similar.
Forlenza OV (31)	Sertraline Imipramine	27 28	50 150	Mean 68.5	8	MADRS	The response and remission rates for both groups were similar. Side effects were more frequent among patients treated with imipramine.
Georgotas A (33)	Nortriptyline Phenelzine Placebo	25 22 28	79 53.9	Mean 64.6	7	HAM-D ZSS CGI	HAM-D reductions were significantly greater with both nortriptyline and phenelzine when compared to placebo. There was no significant difference in treatment effect between two drugs. The most frequently reported side effects were anticholinergic and were present significantly more often in nortriptyline group.

(*Continued*)

TABLE 1 Randomized Controlled Trial of Pharmacotherapy of Acute Late Life Depression (*Continued*)

Studies	Drugs	*n*	Mean dose or dose range (mg/day)	Age range or mean age	Duration (weeks)	Outcome scales	Results
Geretsegger C (34)	Paroxetine Amitriptyline	44 47	22.7 109.5	Mean 75.15	6	HAM-D MADRS CGI	Both groups showed similar good antidepressant efficacy. There was no significant difference of side effect frequency between groups.
Gerner R (35)	Trazodone Imipramine Placebo	18 23 19	305 145	60–90	4	HAM-D BDS	HAM-D scores significantly lower at the end of the study when compared to the baseline scores for both drug groups. Both drugs were significantly better than placebo in treating the depression. Anticholinergic side effects were significantly frequent in imipramine group, compared to placebo and trazodone.
Goldstein SE (36)	Amitriptyline Nomifensine	18 15	75–150 75–150	64–89 Mean 71.7	4	HAM-D PGRS CGI	There was a significant decrease of HAM-D scores for each of the drug groups. There was no significant difference between groups.
Guelfi JD (60)	Fluoxetine Tianeptine	122 115	20 25–37.5	Mean 77.5	12	NDS MADRS GDS CGI	Both drugs effective and tolerable in treating depression. Reduction in depression score and rate of responders were greater in fluoxetine.
Guilibert E (37)	Paroxetine Clomipramine	40 39	30 75	>60	6	HAM-D	No significant difference was found for any of the efficacy measures between the groups. Nervous system side effects reported in the paroxetine group were significantly higher while the anticholinergic side effect incidence was higher in clomipramine group.

Gwirtsman HE (38)	Maprotiline Doxepin	24 25	144 129	Mean 63.78	6	HAM-D ZSS	Marked improvement was observed with both antidepressants, and maprotiline group showed significantly greater improvement than doxepin group. No significant difference was observed between groups with respect to side effects.
Halikas J (39)	Mirtazapine Trazodone Placebo	49 48 49	28.7 219.5	55–81 Mean 62	6	HAM-D MADRS	The reduction in HAM-D score was significantly greater in mirtazapine than in the placebo group. The difference between trazodone and placebo did not reach the significance. The frequency of dry mouth and somnolence was significantly higher in both drug groups compared to placebo.
Hoyberg OJ (40)	Mirtazapine Amitriptyline	56 59	37.3 73.8	60–85 Mean 70.5	6	HAM-D MADRS CGI	There was no difference in HAM-D reduction between drug groups. They were both effective in treating depression. There was no significant difference in the frequency of reported side effects between the groups.
Hutchinson DR (41)	Paroxetine Amitriptyline	58 32	30 100	Mean 71.75	6	HAM-D CGI	There was a significant decrease of HAM-D score from baseline to the end of the study for both groups, with no difference between treatments. Significantly lower patients taking paroxetine reported side effects. The anticholinergic side effects were significantly lower in paroxetine group.
Jansen W (42)	Nomifensine Placebo	46 43	100	Mean 75	4	HAM-D	Nomifensine treated patients showed significant improvement over the placebo group. Nomifensine was well tolerated.

(*Continued*)

TABLE 1 Randomized Controlled Trial of Pharmacotherapy of Acute Late Life Depression (*Continued*)

Studies	Drugs	*n*	Mean dose or dose range (mg/day)	Age range or mean age	Duration (weeks)	Outcome scales	Results
Jarvik LF (43)	Doxepin Imipramine Placebo	10 12 10	NR NR	55–81	26	HAM-D	The average improvement in both drug groups was significantly greater than placebo. Differences between these two groups were not significant.
Kane JM (44)	Imipramine Bupropion High Bupropion Low Placebo	13 13 11 7	146 323 150	55–77 Mean 63.8	4	HAM-D ZSS CGI	Imipramine was superior to placebo as well as to both low- and high-dose bupropion, but only on Zung scale. No difference between groups was found on other measures.
Kasper S (61)	Escitalopram Fluoxetine Placebo	173 164 180	10 20	65–93 Mean 75	8	MADRS CGI	Response rates did not differ meaningfully between escitalopram, fluoxetine, and placebo. Rate of withdrawal due to side effects was higher for both drugs compared to placebo.
Katona C (46)	Imipramine Reboxetine	171 176	80.8 4.5	Mean 74.15	8	HAM-D CGI-S	The reduction in HAM-D scores was comparable between the groups. There were fewer serious side effects in reboxetine group.
Katz IR (48)	Nortriptyline Placebo	18 12	62.5	NR	7	HAM-D CGI GDS	Significant drug–placebo differences were apparent in CGI-I, HAM-D, but not in GDS.
Kivela SL (49)	Sulpiride Placebo	35 31	200	65–86 Mean 74.65	20	HAM-D	The effect of sulpiride on depressive symptoms did not differ from the effect of placebo.
Kok RB (91)	Venlafaxine XR Nortriptyline	40 41	156 94.5	Mean 72.2	12	MADRS HAM-D GDS CGI	Both drugs equally effective in terms of remission rates and other secondary measures and equally tolerable.

Kretschmar JH (50)	Amitriptyline Mianserin	17 20	125 50	59–86 Mean 71.5	3	HAM-D CGI	CGI-I showed a significant better response in favor of mianserin but there was no difference on HAM-D scores between the groups at the end of the study.
Kyle, CJ (51)	Citalopram Amitriptyline	179 186	24.3 51.6	Mean 73.75	8	HAM-D MADRS CGI	Both drugs produced equivalent time-related declines in severity of depression. Amitriptyline produced greater overall incidence of side effects.
La Pia S (52)	Fluoxetine Mianserin	20 20	20 40	60–80 Mean 71.8	6	HAM-D GDS	Both drugs significantly decreased the HAM-D scores. Patients in the fluoxetine group showed significant improvement in HAM-D symptom clusters of nuclear symptoms, sleep disorders, slowing-down, agitation, and somatization; while the improvement in mianserin group was only significant for nuclear symptoms.
Lakshmanan M (53)	Doxepin Placebo	Total: 29	13.6	70–88	3	HAM-D GDS HVID	Doxepin group had significantly greater reduction in depressive symptoms when compared to placebo. There was no difference between placebo and doxepin groups in regard to side-effect profile.
Mahapatra SN (57)	Venlafaxine XR Dothiepin	44 48	100 100	64–87 Mean 74	7	HAM-D MADRS CGI	Depression scores decreased significantly from baseline in both groups although there was no difference between groups. There was no difference between the frequencies of adverse events between the groups.
Merideth CH (58)	Imipramine Nomifensine Placebo	22 20 19	150 150	Mean 68.79	5	CGI HAM-D BPRS HSC	Both drugs were superior to placebo in treating the depression, although they did not differ significantly from each other. Nomifensine was associated with less anticholinergic and sedative side effects than imipramine.

(*Continued*)

TABLE 1 Randomized Controlled Trial of Pharmacotherapy of Acute Late Life Depression (*Continued*)

Studies	Drugs	*n*	Mean dose or dose range (mg/day)	Age range or mean age	Duration (weeks)	Outcome scales	Results
Moller HJ (62)	Imipramine Brofaromine	62 127	87 85	Mean 68	8	HAM-D VZSS	Brofaromine showed comparable efficacy to imipramine in treating depression. Anticholinergic side effects were more abundant in imipramine while restlessness, sleep disturbance, and headache were more frequent with brofaromine. In the global evaluation of tolerability there was an advantage for brofaromine.
Mulsant BH (63)	Nortriptyline Paroxetine	54 62	51.4 23	Mean 72.15	12	HAM-D	There were no significant differences between groups in term of efficacy and tolerability.
Nair NP (64)	Moclobemide Nortriptyline Placebo	36 38 35	400 75	60–90	7	HAM-D CGI	There was no significant difference between moclobemide and placebo in terms of efficacy, while nortriptyline was found to be superior to placebo. Anticholinergic side effects occurred more often with nortriptyline than either moclobemide or placebo.
Navarro V (65)	Citalopram Nortriptyline	29 29	33.4 61.1	Mean 70.69	12	HAM-D	A significantly higher remission rate to nortriptyline than to citalopram was demonstrated, particularly if severe patients were assessed. The autonomic side effects were significantly higher for nortriptyline than for citalopram.
Nelson JC (92)	Duloxetine Placebo	EA:90 TA: 209	60	55–82 EA:Mean 63.4 TA: Mean 62.8	9	HAM-D CGI PGI	Reanalysis of subjects older than 55 years from three studies. Decrease in depression measure and remission rates significantly better than placebo. Dropouts due to adverse events significantly greater with duloxetine.

Newhouse PA (66)	Sertraline Fluoxetine	117 119	71.5 29.1	Mean 67.5	12	HAM-D CGI MADRS	Both drug were equally effective in decreasing the HAM-D scores. Sertraline treated patients showed greater improvement on cognitive measures. Both drugs were equally well tolerated.
Nugent D (67)	Amitriptyline Viloxazine	25 25	150 300	60–78 Mean 67.65	4	HAM-D WSAS	Citalopram treated patients improved more then placebo patients. Both cognitive and emotional functioning improved significantly more in citalopram group. The side-effect ratings of citalopram and placebo were not different at the end of the study.
Nyth AI (68)	Citalopram Placebo	98 51	30	65–91	6	HAM-D MADRS CGI	Citalopram treated patients improved more than placebo treated patients. There was no difference of side effect rating between the groups at the end of the study.
Pancheri P (69)	Imipramine Moclobemide	15 15	96.6 533.3	60–85 Mean 77.9	8.5	HAM-D HAM-A RDI	Both drugs induced an improvement in depressive and anxious symptoms with moclobemide showing a faster onset.
Pelicier Y (70)	Paroxetine Clomipramine	41 42	20 60	Mean 70.65	5	MADRS ZSS	Both drugs equally effective and tolerable
Phanjoo AL (72)	Fluvoxamine Mianserin	25 25	170 60	65–87 Mean 76.5	6	MADRS CGI	Both drugs were equally effective. The only difference between groups was in CGI score at week 2 in favor of fluvoxamine. At the end of the study, the difference was not statistically significant. Both drugs were equally tolerated.
Rahman MK (73)	Fluvoxamine Dothiepin	26 26	157 159	61–86 Mean 74	6	MADRS	There were no significant differences in efficacy between drugs at any assessment measures. Both drugs were equally well tolerated, without any significant difference at their side-effect profiles.

(Continued)

TABLE 1 Randomized Controlled Trial of Pharmacotherapy of Acute Late Life Depression (*Continued*)

Studies	Drugs	*n*	Mean dose or dose range (mg/day)	Age range or mean age	Duration (weeks)	Outcome scales	Results
Raskin J (93)	Duloxetine Placebo	207 104	60	65–90 Mean 72	8	GDS HAM-D CGI	Reduction in depression scores, rate of response, and remission greater with duloxetine. It is as tolerable as placebo.
Reynolds CF III (74)	Nortriptyline Placebo	43 39	66	Mean 64.4	8	HAM-D	Nortriptyline was superior to placebo in achieving remission of bereavement-related major depressive episode.
Rossini D (94)	Sertraline Fluvoxamine	48 40	150 200	Mean 68	7	HAM-D	The decrease in depression score was faster with fluvoxamine, but responder rate was similar to sertraline. Both were equally tolerable.
Salloway S (77)	Sertraline Placebo	30 29	50–100	Mean 69.59	8	HAM-D CGI	Elderly with high and low hyperintensities on the MRI scan were treated with placebo and sertraline. Efficacy of sertraline was not different form placebo and severity of hyperintensity was not a factor determining response rate.
Schatzberg AF (78)	Paroxetine Mirtazapine	120 126	26.5 25.7	Mean 71.85	8	HAM-D CGI	Both drugs decreased the HAM-D scores significantly. Mirtazapine group had a faster decrease in HAM-D scores. The median time to achieving the response was shorter, and the mean change from base line was greater in mirtazapine group. Significantly more patients in paroxetine group discontinued the therapy because of side effects.

Schatzberg A (95)	Venlafaxine IR Fluoxetine Placebo	104 100 96	37.5–225 20–60	Mean 71	8	MADRS HAM-D CGI	There were a significant decrease in depression scores with both drugs and placebo. There were no statistical difference between three groups in terms of reduction of depression scores and remission rates. The incidence of adverse events was greater in venlafaxine than fluoxetine and placebo.
Schone W (79)	Paroxetine Fluoxetine	54 52	20–40 20–60	65–85 Mean 74	6	HAM-D MADRS SCAGS	There was no difference between drugs in HAM-D change from baseline at the end of the study. However there was a significant difference at week 3 in favor of paroxetine. There was no significant difference in terms of side effects.
Schneider LS (99)	Sertraline Placebo	350 366	50–100	59–97 Mean 68.8	8	HAM-D CGI PGI	Sertraline was effective and well tolerated. Drug–placebo difference was not large.
Schweiser E (100)	Imipramine Buspirone Placebo	60 57 60	89 38	65–89 Mean 72	8	HAM-D CGI	Antidepressant effect of imipramine was earlier and more robust than comparators. Imipramine was better than placebo but improvement with buspirone was not different than placebo.
Seigfried K (80)	Maprotiline Mainserin Nomifensine	25 25 25	100 40 100	67–83 Mean 74	4	HAM-D CFFT	All treatment groups showed a significant reduction in depression scores. At the end of the study, both nomifensine and mianserin were superior to maprotiline. The frequency of side effects was higher in maprotiline than both mianserin and nomifensine.
Smeraldi E (96)	Venlafaxine IR Clomipramine Trazodone	55 58 57	75–150 50–100 50–300	Mean 71.3	6	MADRS HAM-D CGI	Decreases in depression scores greater with venlafaxine IR and clomipramine than with trazodone. Fewer side effects with venlafaxine than with comparators.

(*Continued*)

TABLE 1 Randomized Controlled Trial of Pharmacotherapy of Acute Late Life Depression (*Continued*)

Studies	Drugs	*n*	Mean dose or dose range (mg/day)	Age range or mean age	Duration (weeks)	Outcome scales	Results
Tignol J (82)	Milnacipran Imipramine	219	100 100	65–93 Mean 74.1	8	HAM-D MADRS CGI	Both drugs equally effective in terms of response, remission, and decrease in depression measures. Significantly greater number of side effects, especially anticholinergic side effects observed with amitriptyline.
Tiller J (83)	Moclobemide Mianserin	11 11	412 85	60–83 Mean 69.6	8	HAM-D CDRS HAM-A	A sequential analysis of paired subjects. Both drugs equally effective in decreasing depression ratings. Dropouts due to side-effect rates were similar for both drugs.
Tollefson GD (84)	Fluoxetine Placebo	335 336	20	60 Mean 67.75	6	HAM-D GDS CGI	Fluoxetine was significantly more efficacious than placebo in overall response and remission. There was no significant difference in dropout rates due to side effects between two groups.
Waite J (85)	Amitriptyline Dothiepin Mianserin	17 15 13	NR NR NR	Mean 76.23	6	HAM-D VAS	No treatment showed a significant superiority over the others, nor was there any difference in tolerance.
Wakelin JS (86)	Fluvoxamine Imipramine Placebo	33 29 14	161 160	60–71 Mean 64	4	HAM-D CGI	Both drugs were superior then placebo in treating depression. Imipramine was associated with significant postural fall in diastolic blood pressure compared to placebo. There was no such difference between fluvoxamine and placebo.
Weihs KL (87)	Paroxetine Bupropion	52 48	22 197	60–88 Mean 70.1	6	HAM-D CGI	No significant HAM-D scores were found between groups at any week. There was no difference between treatment-response rates between the groups.

Depression Comorbid wityh Dementia						
Karlsson I (45)	Citalopram Mianserin	157 163	28 40	65–95	MADRS	The treatments were equivalent with respect to MADRS scores. Patients with dementia showed a smaller decrease of depression scores compared to non-demented patients.
Katona CL (47)	Paroxetine Imipramine	99 99	24.9 60.3	60–98 Mean 76.6	MADRS CGI	Both paroxetine and imipramine were equally effective in treating depression. Anticholinergic and nonfatal serious side effects were reported by more patients treated with Imipramine.
Lyketsos CG (55)	Sertraline Placebo	12 10	50–150	Mean 77	HAM-D CSD	Sertraline is superior to placebo in reducing depression in patients with Alzheimer disease. There was no difference in side effects between groups.
Magai C (56)	Sertraline Placebo	17 14	100	Mean 89.25	CSD GS	Sertraline had no significant benefit over placebo
Petracca GM (71)	Fluoxetine Placebo	17 24	40	Mean 70.75	HAM-D CGI	Both fluoxetine and placebo showed a significant decline in HAM-D scores of depressed Alzheimer patients. Fluoxetine was well tolerated and most of the side effects were mild.
Roth M (76)	Moclobemide Placebo	Total: 694	400	60–90	HAM-D	Moclobemide produced significant decrease in depression scores of both demented and depressed patients when compared to placebo. There was no significant difference in side effects between groups.
Taragano FE (81)	Fluoxetine Amitriptyline	18 19	10 25	Mean 72.05	HAM-D	The efficacy was similar for both drugs. There were more dropouts in amitriptyline group than in fluoxetine group.

(*Continued*)

TABLE 1 Randomized Controlled Trial of Pharmacotherapy of Acute Late Life Depression (*Continued*)

Studies	Drugs	*n*	Mean dose or dose range (mg/day)	Age range or mean age	Duration (weeks)	Outcome scales	Results
Poststroke Depression							
Lipsey JR (54)	Nortriptyline Placebo	14 20	100	Mean 61	HAM-D ZSS		There was a significant improvement of depression in poststroke patients treated with nortriptyline when compared to placebo.
Robinson RG (75)	Fluoxetine Nortriptyline Placebo	23 16 17	40 100	Mean 67.33	HAM-D		Nortriptyline produced a significantly higher response rate than fluoxetine and placebo in treating depression and in treating the anxiety symptoms and in poststroke patients. Fluoxetine in increasing dose of 10–40 mg/day led to weight loss that was not seen with placebo or nortriptyline.
Wiart L (88)	Fluoxetine Placebo	16 15	20	Mean 67.6	MADRS		End point MADRS scores of fluoxetine group was significantly lower than those of placebo. Response rate of fluoxetine group was significantly higher compared to placebo.

Abbreviations: BDS, Beck depression scale; BPRS, brief psychiatric rating scale; CAS, Covi anxiety scale; CDRS, Carroll depression rating scale; CGI, Clinical global impression; CSD, Cornell scale for depression; ECP, Evaluation clinique de la personalite; GDS, Geriatric depression scale; GS, Gestalt scale; HSC, Hopkins symptom checklist; HVID, Highland view index of dependency; MADRS, Montgomery Asberg Rating Scale; PGRS, plutchik geriatric rating scale; POMS, profile of mood states; RDI, Rome depression inventory; NR, not reported; RDS, raskin depression scale; SCAGS, Sandoz clinical assessment geriatric scale; SRT, Symptoms rating test; STAI, State-trait anxiety inventory; WSAS, Wakefield self-assessment scale; VAS, Visual analogue scale; VAS-D, Visual analogue scale–depression; VZSS, Von Zerssen self-rating score; PGI, Patient global impression; Q-LES-Q, Quality of life enjoyment and satisfaction–questionnaire; NDS, Newcastle depression scale; AJRS, Aubin Jouvent rating scale; ZSS, Zung self-rating scale; EA, Efficacy analysis; TA, Tolerability analysis.

moclobemide, mianserin, reboxetine, tianeptine, adinazolam, sulpiride, viloxazine, brofaromine, or nomifensine.

The evidence base is limited for studies regarding the treatment of depression in demented elders. Only seven of the studies noted here relate to that important population. Similarly, we located only three studies carried out in a cohort of post-stroke subjects with depression. There is clearly a need for more investigation in both these areas, given the high frequency of depression in demented individuals and following a cerebrovascular accident (CVA).

Another area of weakness in our evidence base relates to the settings of these studies. Only four were carried out exclusively among residents of long-term care settings. Among the others, 32 drew upon outpatient populations, 15 obtained subjects solely from an inpatient population, 20 studied a mix of inpatients and outpatients, and no setting was described for the remaining 21 studies.

The term "geriatric" lumps together very distinct subclasses of older adults, ranging from retirement-age individuals to those who have lived for more than a century. Since depression and its treatment may differ between younger and older populations of the elderly, it is notable that our evidence base is skewed toward the "young old" and is relatively sparse regarding the "old old" aged 70 years and beyond. None of these studies that we include reported a mean age less than 60 years. Minimum age among the studies we reviewed was 50, while the maximum reported age extended to 98 years.

Depression is more prevalent among women than men, and life expectancy is greater among women. These facts may account for our observation that more than 80% of the trial cohorts we reviewed contained more women than men. The mean proportion of women among samples was 65%. Given the high rate of late-life suicide and its predominance among men, these figures emphasize the need not only for studies of the high prevalence female population but also for more data on the high suicide-risk male population. The exclusion of acutely suicidal or severely medically ill individuals from the most antidepressant studies further limits our understanding of the treatment of high-risk elderly subpopulations.

Given findings that response to an antidepressant is slower among older cohorts, the need for longer study durations is apparent in this age group. The durations of these trials varied from 3 to 52 weeks, with a mean of only 8.5 weeks. Only half of the studies (50%) exceeded six weeks in duration.

The number of subjects receiving a specific agent varied greatly among studies, from 7 to 366, with a mean of 69. A variety of rating scales was used to assess response, most frequently the Hamilton Depression Rating Scale and/or the Montgomery Asberg Depression Rating Scale.

Heterocyclic Antidepressants (HCAs)

HCA studies in the elderly have been most frequently reported in medically healthy, relatively young populations. Our literature search identified 49 placebo-controlled trials or comparison trials in which a heterocyclic was administered to acutely depressed elderly subjects. Amitriptyline and imipramine were the most frequently studied agents, with 15 trials apiece. There were 11 nortriptyline trials, 5 doxepin trials, 3 trials each for dothiepin and clomipramine, 2 trials for maprotiline, and 1 for desipramine. No randomized-controlled trials were identified for protriptyline or trimipramine.

The heterocyclics inhibit the presynaptic reuptake of the monoamine neurotransmitters serotonin and norepinephrine. This class includes the tricyclic antidepressants and a solitary tetracyclic agent, maprotiline that is similar in its properties.

Among the tricyclic antidepressants, available agents are characterized as tertiary or secondary amines. The tertiary amines—amitriptyline, imipramine, trimipramine, doxepin, clomipramine, and amoxapine—are in general more highly sedating, anticholinergic, and associated with postural hypotension. In elderly patients, these effects are of great importance if they increase the likelihood of severe constipation with impaction, urinary retention in men with preexisting prostatic hypertrophy, or a hip-fracturing fall. Their many extraneous pharmacodynamic effects have earned for amitriptyline, at least, the designation of "polypharmacy in a pill" and the recommendation by some authorities that amitriptyline should be avoided in elderly patients (106). Clomipramine, a tertiary amine recognized as effective in treating depression and also obsessive compulsive disorder, was compared to paroxetine in one controlled geriatric study and found to be similarly efficacious but associated with more severe adverse effects (37). In general, the tertiary amine heterocyclics, although historically important, are not commonly used now for treatment of depression in the elderly.

In contrast to the tertiary amines, the secondary amines—nortriptyline, desipramine, and protriptyline—are regarded as relatively effective and safe agents for treating elderly depressed patients. Nortriptyline in particular has substantial evidence to support its use, although in general the use of tricyclics has waned with growing popularity of the newer antidepressants.

Nortriptyline, which is associated with less severe anticholinergic and orthostatic effects than the tertiary amine tricyclics, is the tricyclic most often considered for use in elderly patients. Meaningful standards have been established to guide its dosing (as well as the dosing of imipramine and desipramine), and plasma levels are of practical value in older patients because of the reduced margin of safety between therapeutic and toxic drug levels. When its use is optimized by monitoring serum levels, nortriptyline is as well tolerated as serotonin reuptake inhibitors and as effective. Roose and Suthers (107) caution that nortriptyline treatment is associated with significant anticholinergic effects, an increase in heart rate, and less improvement of quality of life than was associated with sertraline in one comparison study. On the other hand, nortriptyline has demonstrated significant efficacy in a nursing home cohort (48), a population in which it is particularly difficult to show antidepressant effects that surpass those of a placebo; furthermore, two studies show nortriptyline to be well tolerated and efficacious in the less-often studied "old-old" population, adults greater than 70 years of age (30,108). Beyond nortriptyline and desipramine, the latter studied in one randomized-controlled geriatric depression trial, the use of heterocyclic antidepressants in the elderly is increasingly limited as treatment alternatives increase.

Maprotiline, a tetracyclic relative of the tricyclics, is considered similarly effective and also shares a similar spectrum of side effects. Maprotiline's major disadvantages, which are of particular concern in older adults, are its long half-life (which would imply slower development of a steady-state serum level and lengthier toxicity following overdose) and its increased association with seizures, especially when dosage is increased with excessive rapidity. In addition, maprotiline has been linked with a relatively higher frequency of a reversible skin rash that clears after discontinuation of the drug.

Many clinicians consider the side-effect profile of heterocyclics problematic for older patients. Use of heterocyclic antidepressants can be accompanied by side effects including sedation, confusion, urinary retention, exacerbation of glaucoma, blurred vision, dry mouth, constipation, fatigue, dizziness, falls, gait disturbance, toxicity in overdose, and cardiovascular effects.

The cardiovascular side effects of heterocyclics have attracted particular attention and are of special concern in older patients (104). Heterocyclic antidepressants possess a quinidine-like property of slowing cardiac conduction that renders them undesirable for treatment of patients with bundle branch disease. Orthostatic hypotension, which may endanger elderly individuals with unstable gait or marginal perfusion of heart or brain, is characteristic of the heterocyclics but appears to be less pronounced with nortriptyline than other members of the class (109). These properties do not contraindicate the use of heterocyclics in older patients, but they do emphasize the necessity for attentive monitoring of adverse effects and appropriate use of serum levels to guide achievement of therapeutic blood levels while minimizing administration of excessively large, potentially toxic doses. Monitoring of nortriptyline levels, by reducing excessive dosing, also helps to reduce accumulation of cardiotoxic hydroxy-metabolites that may endanger older patients, particularly those with renal impairment (8).

Surprisingly, cardiovascular adverse effects were reported by very few patients in both groups in a meta-analysis of side effects of SSRIs and HCAs in elderly patients (110). An earlier expert consensus guideline group, however, suggested reserving first-line use of heterocyclics only for "severe depression," in which nortriptyline is designated a highly ranking alternate to the SSRIs. Studies in which nortriptyline's use was accompanied by monitoring of plasma levels have shown particularly good outcomes, and the consensus guideline recommends starting at 10 to 30 mg/day and aiming for target plasma levels between 50 and 150 ng/mL, usually achieved at doses between 40 and 100 mg/day. Dosing recommendations for other heterocyclics are listed in Table 2.

Four meta-analyses of antidepressant treatment in late-life depression have supported the prevailing clinical opinion that newer agents are as effective in older patients as the heterocyclics, though data generally supporting the view that newer agents are more tolerable have not consistently reached statistical significance. One recent meta-analysis of side effects from seven studies comparing an SSRI to a TCA, however, reported that TCAs were associated with significantly greater side effect–related discontinuation rates, and the gastrointestinal side effects, dizziness, and drowsiness common with TCAs were emphasized in this context. SSRIs, however, were not free of side effects. Seventeen percent of SSRI recipients, for example, were reported to experience nausea and vomiting (110).

Monoamine Oxidase Inhibitors (MAOIs)

MAOIs are prescribed less frequently these days because of their potential for toxic drug–drug or drug–food interactions; nonetheless, their effectiveness remains on a par with other agents for treatment of unipolar major depressive disorder. In cases of atypical depression, often with concomitant panic attacks, the MAOIs may be of particular value. This class of antidepressants works by competitively binding the monoamine oxidase (MAO) enzyme, a protein responsible for destroying catecholamines and indoleamines in presynaptic neurons and in the synapses. MAO located in the intestines also destroys ingested neurotransmitter-like chemicals,

TABLE 2 Antidepressants for Use in Late-Life Depression

Generic name	Brand name	Available dosage forms	Starting dose range (mg/day)	Usual geriatric dose range (mg/day)	Notes
Heterocyclic Antidepressants (HCA)					
Nortriptyline	Pamelor Aventyl and others	10-, 25-,50-,75-mg tablets	10–25	25–100	TCA with least postural hypotension Follow plasma levels: Therapeutic window 50–150 ng/mL (Response is likely to decrease beyond therapeutic range maximum)
Desipramine	Norpramin Pertofrane and others	10-, 25-, 50-, 75-, 100-, 150-mg tablets	10–25	25–150	TCA with least anticholinergic effect Therapeutic blood range 75–150 ng/mL (Response is less likely to improve above therapeutic range maximum)
Doxepin	Sinequan and others	10-, 25-, 50-, 75-, 100-, 150-mg tablets and oral solution	NR	NR	Strong anticholinergic and sedative effect Plasma level: efficacy relation is not established Strong antihistaminic (H_2) effect
Protriptyline	Vivactyl and others	5-,10-mg tablets	NR	NR	One of the least sedating of heterocyclics Orthostatic hypotension, cardiovascular toxicity, and anticholinergic side effects Very long elimination half-life (140 hr)
Imipramine	Tofranil and others	10-, 25-, 50-mg tablets and injectable solution	NR	NR	Sedative and anticholinergic effects less severe then amitriptyline Frequently causes postural hypotension Therapeutic blood range 75–150 ng/mL (Response is unlikely to improve above therapeutic range maximum)
Amitriptyline	Elavil and others	10-, 25-, 50-, 75-, 100-, 150-mg tablets and injectable solution	NR	NR	Strong sedative effect Frequent anticholinergic effects Low doses and monitoring of plasma levels can reduce anticholinergic side effects
Clomipramine	Anafranil and others		NR	NR	Strong sedative, anticholinergic, hypotensive, and cardiac side effects

Trimipramine	Surmontil	25-, 50-, 100-mg tablets	NR	NR	Strong anticholinergic and sedative effect Strong H_2 blocker
Monoamine Oxidase Inhibitors (MAOI)					
Phenelzine	Nardil	15-mg tablet	15	15–45	Requires restrictions of diet and coadministered medications
Tranylcypromine	Parnate	10-mg tablet	10	10–40	
Isocarboxazid	Marplan	10-mg tablet	10	10–40	
Selegiline	Emsam transdermal	6-, 9-, 12-mg patch	6	Undetermined	MAOI diet restriction may not be required at lowest dose. Coadministration with various medications remains contraindicated
Moclobemide	Not available in U.S.A.		150	150–300	MAOI diet restriction may not be required at usual doses. Coadministration with various medications remains contraindicated
Selective Serotonin Reuptake Inhibitors (SSRI)					
Fluoxetine	Prozac and others	10-, 20-, 40-mg capsule 20 mg/5ml oral solution	10	10–40	Oral solution available
	Prozac Weekly	90-mg enterically coated cap	90 once weekly		Initiate after establishment of daily regimen of 20 mg/day, waiting 1 week after last daily dose
Sertraline	Zoloft and others	25-, 50-, 100-mg tablet 20 mg/mL oral solution	25	50–200	Oral solution available
Fluvoxamine	Luvox and others	25-, 50-, 100-mg tablet	25	50–200	
Paroxetine	Paxil and others	10-, 20-, 40-mg tablet 10 mg/5 mL oral solution	10	10–40	Possesses mild anticholinergic effects
Paroxetine CR	Paxil CR	12.5-, 25-mg CR tablet	12.5	12.5–25	
Citalopram	Celexa and others	20-, 40-mg tablet 10 mg/5 mL solution	10	10–40	
Escitalopram	Lexapro		5–10	10–20	
Serotonin Norepinephrine Reuptake Inhibitor (SNRI)					
Venlafaxine	Effexor and others	25-, 37.5-, 50-, 75-, 100-mg tablet	25	50–225	Blood pressure elevation associated with higher dose range

(*Continued*)

TABLE 2 Antidepressants for Use in Late-Life Depression (*Continued*)

Generic name	Brand name	Available dosage forms	Starting dose range (mg/day)	Usual geriatric dose range (mg/day)	Notes
	Effexor XR	37.5-, 75-, 150-mg capsule	37.5	50–300	
Duloxetine	Cymbalta	20-, 30-, 60-mg capsule	40	40–120	
Desvenlafaxine	Pristiq	50-mg tablet	50	Undetermined	
Milnacipran	Not available in U.S.A.		50	50–100	Dose should be adjusted in case of renal impairment
Noradrenergic and Specific Serotonergic Antidepressant (NaSSA)					
Mirtazapine and others	Remeron	15-, 30-, 45-mg tablet 15-, 30-mg orally disintegrating tablet	7.5–15	15–45	
Serotonin Antagonist and Reuptake Inhibitor (SARI)					
Nefazodone and others	Serzone	50-, 100-, 150-, 200-, 250-mg tablet	50 bid	100–500	Sedating for many patients and associated with rare hepatic fatalities
Trazodone	Desyrel	50-, 100-, 150-mg tablet	25–50*	25–200*	*Dose range applies to trazodone's common use, as a hypnotic agent often combined with another antidepressant
Norepinephrine Dopamine Reuptake Inhibitor (NDRI)					
Bupropion	Wellbutrin and others	75-, 100-mg tablet	75	100–300	Contraindicated with eating disorders, caution with seizure disorders
	Wellbutrin SR and others	100-, 150-mg SR tablet	100	100–450	
	Wellbutrin XL	150 and 300 mg tablets			
Norepinephrine Reuptake Inhibitor (NRI)					
Reboxetine	Not available in U.S.A.		4	4–8	Caution with adrenergic side effects

Serotonine Reuptake Enhancer					
Tianeptine	Not available in U.S.A.		25	25	Inadequate information about the efficacy and tolerability
Stimulants					
Methylphenidate	Ritalin	5-, 10-, 20-mg v	2.5	10 bid	
	Ritalin SR	20-mg SR capsule 20-mg SR tablet	NR	20 (may be substituted once the dose of methylphenidate is established)	Several new preparations of extended release methylphenidate are also available
Dexedrine	Dextrostat	15-mg capsule 5 mg/5 mL oral solution	2.5	10 bid	

*Available Generically.
Source: The antidepressant classification system is adapted from reference 176. The content of this table is adapted from references 8 and 177.

protecting the central nervous system against their potential effects. When MAO is inhibited, the body loses its defenses against such "false neurotransmitters," rendering it vulnerable to the "hypertensive crisis" reaction, which is the most serious MAOI adverse effect. Researchers have now delineated with some clarity the foods or medications which must be avoided by a patient taking an MAOI, making this adverse effect more preventable (Table 3). It is worth emphasizing that these interacting foods and medications should be avoided several days before starting an MAOI and 7 to 10 days after stopping an MAOI. Switching between MAOIs and other antidepressants, even other MAOIs, requires appropriate timing. Fluoxetine, the most slowly eliminated antidepressant, should be stopped a full five weeks prior to an MAOI trial. The washout of an MAOI prior to starting another antidepressant should be given for two weeks.

Important MAOI side effects include increased appetite and weight gain, induction of mania or hypomania, orthostatic hypotension, sexual dysfunction including inhibition of orgasm, swelling of the ankles or feet, increased sweating, skin rash, constipation, drowsiness, dry mouth, insomnia, nightmares, or fatigue. Because MAOIs can produce transaminase elevations, periodic measurements of liver enzymes are appropriate.

Among the eight randomized-controlled geriatric depression trials we identified for monoamine oxidase inhibitors, the treatment in six was moclobemide, a reversible inhibitor of MAO A not available in United States. One trial investigated another MAOI unavailable in the United States, brofaromine, and only one trial addressed the use of phenelzine. No studies of tranylcypromine, isocarboxazid, or transdermal selegiline in the elderly were identified. Thus, the use of the four MAOIs available in the United States (Table 2) appropriately maintains a secondary role in the treatment of late-life depression. The availability of a transdermal MAOI offers a possible advantage to the rare patient who is depressed, but unable to take or tolerate an orally administered medication.

Selective Serotonin Reuptake Inhibitors (SSRIs)

SSRI studies in depressed elderly subjects, similarly to those of HCAs, have most frequently been carried out in medically healthy, relatively young elderly cohorts. Our literature search identified 45 placebo-controlled or comparison trials in which an SSRI was administered to acutely depressed elderly subjects.

SSRIs have become the most frequently prescribed antidepressants in the United States, primarily as a result of their ease of use and generally well-tolerated side-effect profile. Fluoxetine (Prozac, Prozac Weekly, and others), sertraline (Zoloft and others), paroxetine (Paxil, Paxil CR, Pexeva, and others), fluvoxamine (Luvox and others), citalopram (Celexa and others), and escitalopram (Lexapro) comprise the SSRIs. These antidepressants possess distinctly different properties from the heterocyclics or MAOIs, although their efficacy in treating depression is considered comparable. Their receptor selectivity confers a more specific neurotransmitter effect, so in general they lack some pharmacodynamic effects that may produce adverse clinical responses. In particular, the SSRIs lack significant antiadrenergic effects responsible for postural hypotension, antihistaminic effects associated with sedation and increased appetite, and with the exception of paroxetine the SSRIs lack anticholinergic effects associated with dry mouth, constipation, urinary hesitancy or retention, and erectile dysfunction. At therapeutic dosing levels, cardiac

TABLE 3 Foods and Medications Interacting with Monoamine Oxidase Inhibitors

Foods containing tyramine	
Avocados	Particularly if overripe
Bananas	Reactions can occur if eaten in large amounts; tyramine levels high in peel
Bean curd	Fermented bean curd, fermented soy bean, soy bean pastes, soy sauces, and miso soup, prepared from fermented bean curd, all contain tyramine in large amounts; miso soup has caused reactions.
Beer and ale	Major domestic brands do not contain appreciable amounts; some imported brands have had high levels; nonalcoholic beer may contain tyramine and should be avoided
Caviar	Safe if vacuum packed and eaten fresh or refrigerated only briefly
Cheese	Reactions possible with most, except unfermented varieties such as cottage cheese; in others, tyramine concentration is higher near rind and close to fermentation holes
Figs	Particularly if overripe
Fish	Safe if fresh, dried products should not be eaten; caution required in restaurants; vacuum-packed products are safe if eaten promptly or refrigerated only briefly
Liver	Safe if very fresh, but rapidly accumulates tyramine; caution required in restaurants
Milk products	Milk and yogurt appear to be safe
Protein extracts	See also Soups; avoid liquid and powdered protein dietary supplements
Meat	Safe if known to be fresh; caution required in restaurants
Sausage	Fermented varieties such as bologna, pepperoni, and salami have a high tyramine content
Shrimp paste	Contains large amounts of tyramine
Soups	May contain protein extracts and should be avoided
Soy sauce	Contains large amounts of tyramine; reactions have occurred with teriyaki
Wines	Generally do not contain tyramine, but many reactions have been reported with chianti, champagne, and other wines
Yeast extracts	Dietary supplements, e.g., Marmite, contain large amounts; yeast in baked goods, however, is safe
Food not containing tyramine	
Caffeine	A weak pressor agent; large amounts may cause reactions
Chocolate	Contains phenylethylamine, a pressor agent that can cause reactions in large amounts
Fava beans (broad beans, "Italian" green beans)	Contain dopamine, a pressor amine, particularly when overripe
Ginseng	Some preparations have caused headache, tremulousness, and manic-like symptoms
Liqueurs	Reactions reported with some, e.g., Chartreuse and Drambuie; cause unknown
New Zealand prickly spinach	Single case report; patient ate large amounts
Whiskey	Reactions have occurred; cause unknown
Medications to avoid	
Decongestants or cough suppressant	Sympathomimetics contained in OTC medications for respiratory symptoms or for dietary aids (e.g., phenylpropanolamine, pseudoephedrine), or the cough suppressant dextromethorphan
Pain relievers[a]	Meperidine is VERY dangerous
CNS depressants	Local and general anesthetics[a]

(*Continued*)

TABLE 3 Foods and Medications Interacting with Monoamine Oxidase Inhibitors (*Continued*)

Stimulants[a]	Amphetamine, cocaine, methylphenidate,
Monoamines or related compounds	L-dopa[a], L-tryptophan, L-tyrosine, phenylalanine
Antihypertensives[a] (including β-blockers and thiazide diuretics)	Exaggerated hypotensive effect may occur
Other antidepressants[a]	Especially SRIs
Some herbal preparations	Containing ginseng or ma huang

[a] May be usable with precautions and careful monitoring
Source: Adapted from Refs. 8 and 179.

toxicity is inconsequential, and overdoses with SSRIs are less dangerous than with heterocyclics or monoamine oxidase inhibitors.

Though considered more tolerable than previous antidepressants by many clinicians, SSRIs are not completely without adverse effects. Furthermore, the frequency of their adverse effects among elderly subjects is similar to that seen with heterocyclic antidepressants (101,111). Their most frequent adverse effects are nausea, anxiety, anorexia, diarrhea, dizziness, nervousness, headache, or insomnia. Not infrequently, they reduce libido and/or impair sexual performance. They appear capable of inducing mania in bipolar individuals. Hyponatremia, a rare SRI adverse effect in general, is more frequently seen among elderly patients. Extrapyramidal side effects such as akathisia are occasionally observed. Weight loss, an early concern with fluoxetine, is thought to be associated with pretreatment high body mass index (112). Paroxetine's anticholinergic properties, nonlinear kinetics, and association with discontinuation symptoms have been considered relative disadvantages in comparison to the other SSRIs.

From the SSRI studies, several generalizations can be made. First, nearly all comparisons of SSRIs to placebo show the SSRI to be more efficacious than placebo. Second, the comparisons of SSRIs to heterocyclics or other antidepressants show similar efficacy among agents. Finally, a number of the comparisons of SSRIs with heterocyclics demonstrate or opine that the SSRIs are better tolerated. Within the SSRIs, however, a qualitative overview of studies does not readily suggest one to be superior to the others in elderly subjects. Only six randomized-controlled trials, in fact, compare one SSRI to another (16,30,61,66,79,94).

A consensus guideline drawing upon the expertise of a panel of acknowledged experts in geriatric psychopharmacology (105) endorsed the first-line use of SSRIs in geriatric depression on the basis of their proven efficacy and possibly greater tolerability, and rated citalopram and sertraline most highly as treatments of choice while paroxetine and fluoxetine received lower ratings. Citalopram and sertraline have both been shown effective in geriatric populations. Both are generically available agents that interact minimally with the cytochrome P450 enzyme system and possess an elimination half-life sufficiently long to justify once-daily dosing. In the absence of cost considerations, escitalopram might also be recommended as a first-line choice, since it shares many properties with citalopram. Further studies will be needed, however, to examine escitalopram's efficacy in older adults, since the two currently available RCTs show good tolerability but no statistical superiority of escitalopram over placebo in elderly depressed adults (61,90). In the RCT that compares escitalopram to fluoxetine, the high placebo response in the fluoxetine comparison cohort (47%) and the substantial disproportionate early consent withdrawal rate for fluoxetine may have impacted on the findings of that study. The "last observation carried forward" analysis of results brought high depression scores of early fluoxetine discontinuers into the final efficacy determination, resulting in statistical superiority of escitalopram over fluoxetine but of neither antidepressant over placebo (61).

In agreement with the consensus guideline, our recommendation for an initial citalopram dose is 10 to 20 mg/day and for an initial sertraline dose we recommend 25 to 50 mg/day. Care must then be taken to increase the dose adequately, aiming for resolution of depressive symptoms without inducing intolerable side effects. This result is most likely to be achieved, in our experience, at final dosing levels of 20 to 40 mg/day for citalopram and 50 to 150 mg/day for sertraline, levels higher than the expert consensus guideline's average dosing recommendations but consistent with FDA indications.

Serotonin Norepinephrine Reuptake Inhibitors (SNRIs)

Venlafaxine, milnacipran, duloxetine, and desvenlafaxine (a separately marketed active metabolite of venlafaxine) differ from the SSRIs in that they block the presynaptic reuptake of both norepinephrine and serotonin. Although this dual action effect calls to mind the tricyclic antidepressants' effects, the SNRIs as a class lack α_1 adrenergic antagonism, and they do not significantly antagonize histaminic or cholinergic neurotransmission. Venlafaxine acts like an SSRI at lower dosages but exerts a dual reuptake inhibition beyond the lower dose range. Duloxetine, milnacipran, and desvenlafaxine, on the other hand, exert similar antagonistic effects on serotonin and norepinephrine reuptake even at low doses. Venlafaxine's and milnacipran's tendencies at higher dose levels to increase blood pressure is regarded by some clinicians as a relative drawback when treating the elderly, many of whom already have elevated blood pressure. Venlafaxine, duloxetine, and desvenlafaxine are the SNRIs currently available in the United States, and the former two have been studied in elderly cohorts.

Although some data suggest the association of greater antidepressant efficacy with dual action agents in comparison to SSRIs, their superiority over SSRIs remains to be demonstrated in the elderly. SNRIs have been assessed in elderly cohorts in eight published studies (57,82,89,91–93,95,96). Desvenlafaxine, the most recently released antidepressant in the United States, has not yet been specifically studied as a treatment for late-life depression. Milnacipran, not currently available in the United States, was compared in one published randomized-controlled trial with imipramine in an elderly depressed cohort and showed comparable efficacy with more tolerable side effects (82). More data are available regarding venlafaxine and duloxetine.

The benefits and side effects of venlafaxine XR in older adults have been found similar to those observed in younger populations; however, Schatzberg and colleagues were not able to find any significant differences among venlafaxine IR, fluoxetine, and placebo in efficacy but did note a relatively high rate of discontinuations due to side effects in the venlafaxine IR cohort (95). The authors of this study questioned the sensitivity of their scale for measurement of response and remission, noted that placebo should be viewed as an "active" drug in comparator studies about the treatment of depression, and reiterated the finding that drug comparison studies often report higher remission rates than "placebo-controlled" trials. In light of these considerations, they concluded that venlafaxine IR should not be considered inactive despite its similar efficacy in this study to placebo treatment (95). Although one (57) of the above mentioned studies reported the emergence of hypertension in only 2% of subjects treated with venlafaxine, blood pressure increases have been reported in other venlafaxine studies and suggest the prudence of appropriate blood pressure monitoring in elderly patients. Our clinical experience and a consensus guideline suggest venlafaxine XR as a rational choice for patients who fail to respond an initial SSRI regimen.

Randomized-controlled trials evaluating the efficacy and tolerability of duloxetine 60 mg/day in treating late-life depression found duloxetine to be more effective than placebo. The rates of dropouts due to side effects and changes in vital signs were similar to those observed in placebo groups (92,93). An interesting finding was that duloxetine not only reduced depressive symptoms, but also significantly decreased some pain-related measures in comparison to placebo. Duloxetine, if supported by further evidence, may be a useful agent for treating depression in the elderly that is accompanied by certain forms of chronic pain, although at present the FDA indication for analgesic use specifies only the pain syndromes of diabetic polyneuropathy and fibromyalgia.

Noradrenergic and Specific Serotonergic Antidepressant (NaSSA)

Mirtazapine is the only available NaSSA in the United States. It combines antagonism of presynaptic noradrenergic α_2 autoreceptors and heteroreceptors with antagonism of H_1, 5-HT_2, and 5-HT_3 receptors. The resulting clinical effect is a depression-reducing increase in synaptic norepinephrine levels accompanied by sedation, appetite-enhancement, and minimal nausea. This combination of effects might be anticipated to be most specifically helpful in treating anxious, insomniac, anorexic elderly depressives.

Mirtazapine has been assessed in three trials in elderly depressed subjects. In these trials, mirtazapine was as effective and well tolerated as either amitriptyline, trazodone, or paroxetine (39,40,78). Schatzberg has reported an earlier antidepressant effect onset for mirtazapine as compared to paroxetine (78). Clinicians are advised to resist the temptation to begin mirtazapine therapy at doses less than 15 mg/day, since excessively low dosing can be associated with a predominantly sedating, antihistaminic effect that may deter the patient from proceeding further with the course of treatment. Patients may question the counterintuitive notion, though it appears to be supported by clinical observations, that higher doses of this antidepressant are less sedating than lower doses.

Serotonin Antagonist/Reuptake Inhibitors (SARIs)

Nefazodone and trazodone share the same effect of weak serotonin reuptake inhibition combined with a potent postsynaptic $5HT_{2A}$ receptor-blocking activity, a characteristic thought to mitigate some SSRI side effects, such as anxiety or sexual dysfunction. Nefazodone has in addition a weak norepinephrine reuptake inhibition and weak α_1 receptor-blocking effect while trazodone has α_1 and histamine receptor-blocking activities.

Although trazodone is primarily used in the elderly as a hypnotic agent or as a non-antipsychotic pharmacotherapy for agitation in demented patients (97), its antidepressant efficacy and tolerability are shown in seven RCTs (9,11,12,27,35,

39,96). In general, trazodone's efficacy was similar to that of other antidepressants, though greater effects were noted with venlafaxine or clomipramine in comparison trials. Trazodone's side effects are no less severe than those of venlafaxine or clomipramine, although its specific side-effect profile may be relatively well tolerated by older patients. Trazodone use as an antidepressant is limited by its side effects, primarily sedative and orthostatic effects, and because of the rare but serious complication of priapism (113).

Nefazodone, by contrast, has not been studied in the treatment of late-life depression. It may be useful in some anxious elderly patients who fail the initial SSRI trial but because of its CYP3A4 inhibition and in light of recent reports (114,115) and an FDA warning (116), linking its use with several cases of liver failure, it should be used with caution and not considered among the first-line choices for elderly patients.

Norepinephrine and Dopamine Reuptake Inhibitor (NDRI)

Bupropion is the only currently available NDRI in the United States. It is unique among available antidepressants in its nonserotonergic and weak dopamine and norepinephrine reuptake blocking mechanism. Although unavailable for some years after its initial marketing because of concern about increased seizure risk, its seizure-inducing rate among patients with no history of seizures, coadministered seizure-facilitating drugs, or other risk factors, is considered acceptably low. The slow and extended release preparations (bupropion SR and presumably bupropion XL) are associated with a lower risk of seizures than the IR form. Though an infrequent complication, the seriousness of seizures requires that this risk be discussed among the potential adverse effects reviewed with a patient considering a bupropion trial.

Bupropion has been investigated to some extent in elderly depressed subjects. Its minimal effects on weight gain or sexual function make it especially suitable for some patients, and it is usually nonsedating. Bupropion's mechanism of action does not suggest an antianxiety effect, yet a comparison of bupropion SR to paroxetine in elderly depressed subjects showed no increased rate of treatment-emergent anxiety with bupropion (87).

Bupropion is not regarded as a first-line choice when treating psychotic depression, which is more common in older than in younger adults. Preliminary findings in a small sample of younger adults suggested less risk of a switch to mania with bupropion when treating bipolar depression in younger adults (117) but the robustness of this finding or its importance in the elderly are not clear. As noted in Table 2, bupropion IR can be initiated at 75 mg/day and bupropion SR at 100 mg/day. In order to decrease the seizure risk the IR form of bupropion should be administered on a three-times daily regimen or the SR form on a twice daily regimen, with no greater than 450 mg/day total IR dose or 400 mg/day total SR dose per day and with no single dose exceeding 200 mg, except with XL forms, which may be given up to 300 mg at a single dose and up to 450 mg/day. Dose increases spaced at least a week apart will allow equilibration of blood levels to each new steady state. The elderly are predisposed to accumulate bupropion and its metabolites (118) and these may contribute to bupropion's side effects, the most frequent of which are headache, somnolence, insomnia, agitation, dizziness, diarrhea, dry mouth, or nausea. An unusual side effect reported in several elderly patients on bupropion was the tendency to fall backwards (119).

Norepinephrine Reuptake Inhibitor (NRI)

Reboxetine, marketed and used in Europe but not in the United States, is the only clinically available potent and selective norepinephrine reuptake inhibitor. It does not have any significant effect on other neurotransmitter systems or receptors and thus is largely free of side effects frequently encountered with HCAs. It was assessed in only one study of late-life depression (46), and found as effective as imipramine. Patients treated with reboxetine reported less cardiac side effects and side effects related to hypotension but more insomnia compared to imipramine group. Adrenergic side effects such as dry mouth, constipation, insomnia, increased sweating, tachycardia, and urinary hesitancy/retention are experienced but usually well tolerated.

Serotonin Reuptake Enhancer (SRE)

Tianeptine, not available in the United States, is the only compound currently in this category of antidepressants. It has no direct significant action on noradrenergic pre- or postsynaptic receptors. It enhances serotonin reuptake in the cortex and hippocampus. It may also alter the norepinephrine system indirectly via its action on the serotonin system. Its mechanism of action in the treatment of depression is beyond the scope of this chapter, but it is reported that it decreases the expression of serotonin mRNA and reduces the number of serotonin transporter binding sites (120,121). Tianeptine's most common side effects are nausea, constipation, abdominal pain, headache, dizziness, and altered dreaming. Limited data from two randomized-controlled comparison trials(59,60) in the elderly make it preliminary to recommend this medication or suggest a specific starting dosage (although 25 mg/day has been recommended) for the treatment of depression in later life.

Stimulants

Some compounds not regarded as appropriate for antidepressant monotherapy, such as the stimulants, are nonetheless considered by some clinicians to be capable of augmenting an antidepressant. Amphetamines or methylphenidate, despite the frequency of their use, are supported as antidepressant agents in the elderly only by very limited controlled data (122). Methylphenidate's use as a monotherapy for late-life depression is advocated on the basis of one very brief controlled trial among medically ill depressed geriatric subjects (123) and other uncontrolled clinical series that suggest significant response rates and limited adverse reactions. Stimulants are not recommended for first-line treatment by the expert consensus panel, but factors that may justify a stimulant trial for the treatment of depression typically include apathy or psychomotor retardation, concurrent medical illness, intolerance of standard antidepressants, and the need for a rapid response. In addition, a recent retrospective chart review from Japan raised the possibility that methylphenidate might have a beneficial role in the treatment of vascular depression (124).

ACUTE PHASE OF LATE-LIFE DEPRESSION TREATMENT

Data from antidepressant trials of longer duration support the claim that, compared with younger adults, older subjects require longer intervals of treatment in order to achieve full antidepressant effectiveness. Georgotas and colleagues (125), for example, reported results from a comparison of phenelzine and nortriptyline among middle-aged and older adults that demonstrated significant improvement of most symptoms during and after the fourth week of treatment. In a late-life depression study using nortriptyline (126), Dew and colleagues found that a significant subgroup of drug-responsive elderly subjects did not meet criteria for recovery until the 10th week. Acute antidepressant treatment response in older depressed patients should be anticipated to take 3 to 10 weeks, perhaps, and this extended duration of a drug trial is consistent with the recommendation of the expert consensus guideline (105), which endorses waiting a minimum of two to three weeks but as long as 7.5 weeks before considering an antidepressant trial adequate. In line with this suggestion, a reanalysis of data from two clinical studies found that week 4 of an antidepressant trial was the critical time at which to predict antidepressant response in elderly. Only 35% and 16.5% of patients who had not achieved at least 30% reduction in baseline HAM-D score by week 4 achieved remission as defined by either HAM-D $\leq$ 10 or HAM-D $\leq$ 6 at the end of 12 weeks (127). Based on this finding, authors suggest that improvement in the first four to six weeks identifies patients who are highly likely to benefit from continuing the treatment and that a change in regimen should be considered for others.

CONTINUATION AND MAINTENANCE PHASES OF LATE-LIFE DEPRESSION TREATMENT

Following acute response and/or remission of depression to antidepressant treatment, a continuation phase begins. As with younger patients, lowering of the effective antidepressant dose is discouraged and monitoring of side effects and treatment adherence remains important. In contrast to the recommended 4- to 6-month continuation phase recommended in the treatment of younger adults, expert opinion suggests a period of 6 to 12 months to be appropriate for older patients. The goal of this treatment phase is to consolidate gains and prevent relapse, which is defined as reemergence of depressive symptoms associated with the treated episode.

Following continuation treatment, some patients should be advised to enter a maintenance phase of treatment. There is as yet no clear consensus about the optimal criteria for patient selection or for duration of maintenance pharmacotherapy in the elderly, but consensus supports a lower threshold for inclusion and the use of lengthier maintenance treatments than in younger depressives. Repeatedly, undertreatment has been shown to be a factor in poor outcome and early relapse. Maintenance treatment, on the other hand, has been shown to be effective in older patients and should be pursued actively. Factors such as the number and severity of depressive episodes, response to treatment, concomitant anxiety symptoms (105), and delayed response to treatment during the first episode (128) may be important ones to consider in planning the duration of maintenance treatment. The expert consensus guideline recommends that treatment extends for one year or longer after a severe first episode, and for three or more years following a third or subsequent episode (105). Additional research is needed to guide and assess the effectiveness of maintenance antidepressant treatment in the medically ill, very old, or cognitively impaired elderly. The value of maintenance treatment and the studies supporting its effectiveness are addressed in detail in chapter 19 of this book.

SIDE EFFECTS OF PARTICULAR IMPORTANCE IN ELDERLY

Antidepressants are well known to have cardiovascular, gastrointestinal, and neuropsychiatric side effects that may negatively influence the success of antidepressant treatment. Side effects that may merely inconvenience younger adults can be of much more dire importance in the elderly. The most significant of these are reviewed here.

Falls

Although rarely seen or of minor clinical importance in younger populations, falls may be particularly disturbing and even life-threatening in elderly populations. The incidence of falls increases with age (129). Although falls are attributed to a confluence of risk factors, the risk ratio for recurrent falls in elderly psychotropic drug users compared to nonusers has been reported to be 1.97, after controlling for depression, dementia, and other risk factors (130). For amitriptyline or its equivalent in doses of greater than or equal to 50 mg/day, the risk ratio for falling was elevated to 2.4, yet fluoxetine 20 mg/day or more (or its equivalent) was associated with a similar risk ratio of 1.9 (131). A review of 28 observational studies and one RCT strengthened the validity of the association between psychotropics and increased risk of falls in the elderly patients and emphasized that SSRIs may be as potent or even greater risk factors than the HCAs (132). Evidence about the negative impact of depression on bone mineral density (BMD) should heighten our attention to optimizing bone density and reducing fall risk factors in older patients. Diem and colleagues reported a decrease in mean total hip BMD of 0.69% per year in women with a geriatric depression scale (GDS) score of less than 6 on the 15-item version, compared with 0.96% per year in women with a GDS score of 6 or greater. Depression severity was independently associated with a higher rate of BMD loss in elderly women even after the exclusion of those treated with antidepressants (133).

Hyponatremia

Hyponatremia, a relatively rare but potentially hazardous SSRI/SNRI side effect, is more frequent among older adults than in a younger population. Hyponatremia can lead to lethargy, confusion, convulsion, coma, delirium, and even death in severe cases. The clinical presentation of hyponatremia depends on its severity and abruptness of its onset. Chronic hyponatremia may go clinically undetected but abrupt falls in sodium levels are usually symptomatic. Studies of young depressed patients report that serotonergic agents are more frequently associated with hyponatremia than other antidepressants (134). After controlling for sex, age, depression status, consumption of other drugs that may cause hyponatremia, and medical illness severity, patients using SSRIs or venlafaxine showed an odds ratio of 3.5 for hyponatremia compared to patients not taking these drugs (135). A review of studies on hyponatremia associated with SSRIs reports the incidence varying from 0.5% to 32% (136). Older patients, females, patients using concomitant diuretics, low body weight, and lower baseline sodium level were found to be the risk factors increasing the likelihood of hyponatremia with SSRIs. Hyponatremia was found to develop in the first few weeks of treatment and to resolve within two weeks of SSRI discontinuation.

There are only a few reports of rechallenge with same or other compounds from the same class. Hyponatremia recurred in some but not all (136). Our suggestion is to measure baseline sodium level for patients at greater risk of developing hyponatremia and repeat the measurement after the first month of the therapy. Those on diuretics, and particularly those who are also restricting sodium intake, may be at particular risk and should have their sodium levels monitored more closely.

Weight Alterations

Weight alterations can be associated with serious health consequences in the elderly. Depression is the most common cause of weight loss in ambulatory elderly (137), and further weight loss due to gastrointestinal or appetite-suppressing adverse effects of antidepressants may have serious detrimental effects on already fragile individuals. Significant weight gain, on the other hand, can also be associated with health-related risk such as increased risk for hypertension, interference with glycemic control, and adverse effects on lipid metabolism.

Clinical experience in younger adults, and findings of worsened glycemic control in association with HCA treatment (138) suggest that this class of drugs might increase weight in the elderly, but a study assessing the impact of antidepressants on weight alterations in nursing home residents found that HCAs were not associated with clinically significant weight gain and, after adjustment, for other confounding factors (139). Use of an SSRI, in this same study, was also not associated with significant weight gain. Mirtazapine, due to its histamine$_2$ receptor-blocking activity, is known to increase weight in younger adults, but evidence to show that this is a risk in the elderly, is lacking. One study comparing the effect of mirtazapine with other non-HCA drugs in nursing home residents concluded that its impact on weight was not different from comparators after controlling for other factors (140). In our clinical experience, however, mirtazapine may increase weight significantly. Although these findings do not emphasize an association between SSRIs, HCAs, mirtazapine, and weight alterations, the interactions of antidepressant use with other important factors like baseline weight, severity of depression, and metabolic risk factors are largely unknown. Thus, we suggest monitoring the weight of elderly treated with antidepressants regardless of the compound.

Discontinuation Symptoms

Abrupt reduction or cessation of SSRIs or SNRIs may result in a discontinuation syndrome characterized by symptoms such as dizziness, lethargy, nausea, depressed mood, anxiety, agitation, irritability, insomnia, vivid dreams, and headache. This description is based on the data from younger populations, and the effect of SSRI or SNRI discontinuation on an older patient is assumed but not proven to be similar. Discontinuation symptoms may emerge even after skipping one daily dose when the antidepressant's elimination half-life is short, as with paroxetine or venlafaxine. The symptoms may be mistaken for anxiety or for worsening of depression, leading to unhelpful treatment interventions. Clinicians may be able to limit the occurrence of discontinuation symptoms by discussing and monitoring treatment adherence, and by educating the patient and family about the circumstances that will lead to their appearance. For patients who have finished a course of treatment and are due to discontinue their antidepressant, discontinuation symptoms may present an obstacle to final cessation of an antidepressant. In some cases, replacement of a shorter-acting antidepressant with one possessed of a lengthy elimination half-life will allow easier tapering and discontinuation.

Bleeding

Serotonin plays an essential role in platelet aggregation and in the modulation of vascular tone. Serotonergic antidepressants, which can decrease the serotonin content of platelets, have been observed to increase the risk of bleeding (141). An important mixed-age cohort study showed that upper gastrointestinal bleeding risk was increased 2.6-fold by SSRIs compared to other antidepressants, weakly supported by the findings of a subsequent large observational cohort study (142,143). Walraven and colleagues, in a large scale retrospective cohort study, reported that the SSRIs were most likely to increase risk for upper gastrointestinal bleeding in the oldest patients studied (octogenarians) and those with previous gastrointestinal bleeding (144). Concurrent use of nonsteroidal antiinflamatory drugs (NSAIDs) with SSRIs is also reported to increase bleeding risk when compared to non-SSRI NSAID users. Based on these data we suggest being attentive to risk factors or reports of hemorrhage when prescribing SSRIs to elderly patients, especially those with a prior history of gastrointestinal bleeding and/or NSAID use. Reasoning by anxious analogy, one might wonder whether serotonergic antidepressants increase the risk of intracranial bleeding, but a population-based case-control study in a mixed-age cohort reported no association of SSRI use with hemorrhagic or ischemic strokes (145) and an additional study, comparing the effects of SSRIs with those of HCAs, showed no increase in the risk for cerebrovascular events (146).

SHORTCOMINGS OF THE CURRENT EVIDENCE BASE FOR TREATMENT OF LATE-LIFE DEPRESSION

In our attempt to determine an optimal treatment approach for late-life depression, we have explored ways of pooling or meta-analyzing data from the available evidence base. The obstacles we have encountered are the same ones earlier faced by the authors of the meta-analyses already published on the pharmacotherapy of geriatric depression (101–104). To circumvent the obstacles created by comparing or pooling data from trials that vary so greatly, several of the meta-analytic reports rely upon drastically pared-down subsamples of published studies in reaching their conclusions. This approach, though it sacrifices much useful information, has been considered necessary because the published treatment studies differ so greatly in statistical methods, thoroughness of reporting, treatment parameters, and sample definition. Some of the key methodological issues will be described here for the purpose of illustrating ways in which future studies can be made more comparable.

To begin with, the studies that have served to demonstrate antidepressants' superiority to placebo are not equally well suited to determine whether one antidepressant is superior to another antidepressant of similar efficacy. A comparison between two effective antidepressants, as Thase (147) has pointed out, may require detection of a mean endpoint difference of as little as two HAM-D points. Such a small difference is unreliably detected by studies enrolling fewer than 120 subjects per treatment group, accounting in part for the large number of negative trials in small treatment groups. The differences between active agents are presumably even smaller and more difficult to demonstrate (147).

Even when treatment differences among groups might be more conspicuous, an appropriate outcome measure must be chosen to detect them. No current diagnostic instrument is ideally matched to this task. The HAM-D, which is most frequently chosen, was not designed for elderly patients and may be excessively influenced by the presence of nonspecific somatic symptoms. Though typically used as an outcome measure for early antidepressant trials in demented, depressed subjects, the HAM-D is now often supplemented or replaced by newer scales such as the Cornell Scale for Depression in Dementia (CSDD), which relies on behavioral observations and collateral reports, because demented patients may lack the ability to provide a detailed self-report. Another improvement in more recent studies is the inclusion of an instrument that measures quality of life, since conclusions based solely on a changed rating of depressive symptoms may paint an incomplete picture of a patient's degree of meaningful improvement.

The design and quality of individual RCTs exploring antidepressant treatment of late-life depression vary greatly from study to study. We noted particularly a great deal of variation in thoroughness of reporting, dosing levels, and trial durations. In addition to employing small samples, some studies fail to report information necessary to a meta-analysis, such as standard error of the mean changes in depression measurements over the course of the treatment trial. Antidepressant dosage magnitude, too, varies across a wide range. Mittman, in her meta-analysis (103), converted antidepressant doses to a standardized Defined Daily Dose (DDD) that represented the average dose of the drug per day for adults, when it is prescribed for its main indication. Assigning a value of 1.0 to an "appropriate daily dose," she reported study doses ranging from 0.33 to 3.0 for tricyclic antidepressants, and 0.33 to 4 for SSRIs.

Duration of trials, too, has varied dramatically. Mittman calculated average trial durations for trials with tricyclics (5.3 ± 1.2 weeks), SSRIs (5.7 ± 1.0 weeks), and placebo (5.3 ± 1.3 weeks). Our own analysis (which included additional studies) found an average overall trial duration of 8.5 ± 6.7 weeks. Valuable additional information can be obtained from longer trials, given older patients' more prolonged recoveries.

As a final observation regarding the hazards of antidepressant treatment in the elderly, we reiterate the well-known observation that pharmacotherapy studies among older subjects have not adequately addressed the inherent diversity of the elderly population. Elderly cohorts include individuals whose ages span a range of more than 3 decades. There may be important differences between the drug-response pattern and optimal dosing strategy, the pharmacokinetics and the drug interactions for a 65-year old as compared to a 95-year old. Beyond the changes associated with normal aging, many elderly depressed individuals are also affected by one or more chronic illnesses that may influence antidepressant choice or drug response. Elders affected by such neurologic processes as Alzheimer Disease, other dementias, stroke, or cerebrovascular disease may respond differently than healthy elders to a specific antidepressant. The syndromes of vascular depression, for example, may represent variant depressive syndromes that are associated with a different pathophysiology, symptoms, and responses to therapeutic interventions. The presence of comorbid medical diseases such as cardiovascular disease or diabetes may further alter the pharmacokinetics and pharmacodynamics of a prescribed antidepressant, affecting the patterns of responsiveness and of adverse outcomes (see Chapter 11). The oldest patients, those with more severe medical illnesses, the demented, and those sequestered in long-term care facilities may be the most challenging to treat and are certainly the least-extensively studied. We will include here, therefore, some recommendations tailored to treatment of specific geriatric depressive subgroups: those with psychotic depression, depression with dementia, depression in long-term care settings, depression comorbid with medical illness, and treatment-resistant depression. Further discussion of depression with cognitive impairment can be found in Chapters 9 and 10.

SPECIAL ISSUES IN THE TREATMENT OF LATE-LIFE DEPRESSION

Depression with psychotic features, termed psychotic depression or delusional depression after its most typical presenting symptom, is more prevalent among older individuals than among younger individuals with major depression (148). The standard of treatment for delusional depression has been to combine an antidepressant with an antipsychotic agent, although elderly patients often experience difficulty with the side effects produced by a sufficiently high level of antipsychotic medication. ECT, a nonpharmacologic approach covered in Chapter 16, is often considered the optimal treatment for delusional depression in older patients because of its proven efficacy and tolerability, which may exceed that of combination pharmacotherapy. Although Mulsant reports that the effect of adding perphenazine to nortriptyline was not significantly superior to that of nortriptyline and placebo in the treatment of psychotic depression of late life (149), controlled studies of olanzapine or another atypical antipsychotic may in time justify their preferred use in treating late-life delusional depression. Olanzapine has already been shown effective in younger delusionally depressed subjects (150,151) and the effect of the combination of olanzapine and sertraline on a mixed-age cohort of psychotic depressed patients is soon to be reported by the investigators of the STOP-PD project. Although a strong evidence base does not exist to guide maintenance treatment for psychotic depression in the elderly, a reasonable approach based on current thinking is to continue both the antidepressant and antipsychotic medication (152). Whether the mortality and morbidity issues identified with antipsychotic agents among demented psychotic patients and highlighted in a boxed warning on prescribing information apply equally to nondemented depressed elders is not known, but prudence would suggest prescribing these medications at the lowest effective dose and for the briefest appropriate duration. Antipsychotic agents for use in geriatric mood disorders are summarized in Table 4.

The *interface between dementia and depression* is addressed in detail in Chapters 9 and 10. Pharmacotherapy issues relevant to this discussion will be touched upon here. Among demented patients, perhaps half will develop significant depression, but this depression comorbid with dementia is often overlooked by clinicians. Apathy, passivity, decreased initiative, and poor concentration are associated with both depression and dementia and, therefore, diagnostically nonspecific. Several, but not all, placebo-controlled trials (153) have shown antidepressant treatment beneficial in groups of depressed demented subjects. Streim and colleagues (154) noted a preferential response to low-dose nortriptyline rather than standard dose treatment in a cognitively impaired subgroup of depressed, frail nursing home subjects. The expert consensus guideline on depressive disorders in older adults emphasizes the importance of concurrent psychosocial intervention and recommends as preferred antidepressants citalopram, sertraline, or venlafaxine XR (105). Although venlafaxine is recommended by experts, one RCT found no significant advantage of this antidepressant over placebo in the treatment of depression comorbid with dementia. The study cohort, however, was relatively small ($n = 31$) and the primary outcome measure was the MADRS, which may be an inaccurate tool for measuring depression in demented subjects (155). Another RCT using the Cornell Scale for Depression in Dementia reported sertraline to be significantly more effective than placebo in treating depression in a group of demented elders (156), but this finding is in contrast to the report by Magai and colleagues, whose depressed late-stage Alzheimer disease patients responded no better to sertraline than to placebo (56). Nyth and colleagues, reporting the findings of a 6-week multicenter double-blind trial in 149 depressed elderly patients with somatic disorders and/or dementia, concluded that citalopram treatment produced significant improvement in both cognitive and emotional functioning (68). For practical reasons regarding the difficulty of defining depression in demented patients and carrying out a study in such a

TABLE 4 Selected Antipsychotic Agents for Use in Late-Life Mood Disorders

Generic name	Trade name	Starting dose range (mg/day)	Treatment dose range (mg/day)	Notes
Typical antipsychotic agents (high potency)				
Haloperidol	Haldol and others	0.5	2–10	Available as oral solution, IM injection, IV injection
	Haldol decanoate and others	12.5 IM q 14–28 days	50–200 IM q 28 days	Depot injectable preparation
Perphenazine	Trilafon and others	2	4–32	Available as oral solution or IM injection
Fluphenazine	Prolixin and others	0.5	2–10	Available as oral solution or IM injection
	Prolixin decanoate and others	12.5 IM q 7–14 days	12.5–50 IM q 14–21 days	Available as depot injectable preparation
	Prolixin enanthate			
Atypical antipsychotic agents				
Risperidone	Risperdal and others	0.25	0.5–6	Available as oral solution
Olanzapine	Zyprexa	2.5	2.5–15	Available also as orally disintegrating tablet
Quetiapine	Seroquel	25	50–500	Sedative
Clozapine	Clozaril	6.25	25–200	Anticholinergic, Low in EPS
Ziprasidone	Geodon	20	20 bid–60 bid	Monitoring of QTc suggested Available for IM injection
Aripiprazole	Abilify	5–10	Undetermined	

population, the evidence base in this area remains weak. Our treatment suggestion, which is to assess patients with the Cornell Scale and treat with sertraline or perhaps citalopram, is in line with the consensus guideline.

The treatment of comorbid dementia and depression often takes place in *long term care facilities* (LTCF), home to 5% of the U.S.'s elderly population. Many LTCF residents suffer from clinically significant depressive symptoms or a full-blown major depressive disorder. A recent study, however, reported that only 55% of the depressed LTCF residents assessed were receiving antidepressants and 32% of these were treated with subtherapeutic dosing (157). In a study assessing the rate of depression in an LTCF where a comprehensive evaluation was performed at admission and during the course of stay, the incidence of depression was 19.9% at admission. The majority of those depressed at admission (15%) remained depressed at a 6-month reassessment, while fewer than half (7.5%) remained depressed at 12 months. These data indicate the importance of psychiatric evaluation and appropriate treatment of depression in LTCFs (158), yet many questions remain. We have identified only four RCTs for pharmacotherapy of major depression in which subjects were recruited solely from LTCFs. Of these, one compared nortriptyline to placebo (48), one compared sertraline to placebo (56), one compared amitriptyline to nomifensine (36), and one compared two doses of nortriptyline (154). Study durations were 7-, 8-, 4- and 10 weeks, respectively. Nortriptyline was found to be superior to placebo, but authors noted that only two in three subjects could complete the trial and emphasized the need for close monitoring of side effects (48). Streim and colleagues, who reported a relationship between plasma levels of nortriptyline and clinical improvement, hypothesized the existence of a therapeutic window that is lower for cognitively impaired than cognitively intact elders (154). Placebo, however, performed as effectively as sertraline in one LTCF study of depressed patients with late-stage Alzheimer disease (56). In the remaining study (36), nomifensine was judged as superior in treating reactive depression and amitriptyline for endogenous depression. The most significant conclusion to draw from these studies is that more investigations are needed in long-term care settings.

Late-life depression comorbid with physical illness can present a variety of difficult choices to a clinician. Often, an already complex presentation of late-life depression is further complicated by the presence of comorbid medical illness' symptoms. Pharmacodynamic and pharmacokinetic changes of late life, vulnerability to drug interactions, and antidepressant side effects that may worsen the comorbid medical condition also require consideration. A comprehensive approach to the treatment of late-life depression comorbid with medical illness is beyond the scope of this chapter and the reader is referred to Chapter 11 in this book for a fuller discussion; however, we suggest consideration of an antidepressant's side effect profile, pharmacokinetics and pharmacodynamics, interactions with other drugs, and accessibility or cost when choosing the appropriate antidepressant for any older patient, including those with significant comorbid medical illness. Clinicians also should keep in mind that the treatment of depression comorbid with particular medical illness necessitates an individualized approach that takes into account individual patient factors, the comorbid illness's status and severity, the issues related to collaboration with a medical treatment team, and support of the patient's family system. For further detail, readers may wish to consult several comprehensive discussions of geriatric psychopharmacology (5–8) or of physical illness and depression in older adults (159) as well as chapter 9 of this book.

Too often, the first and second antidepressants tried are unsuccessful or poorly tolerated and a patient acquires the diagnosis of *treatment resistant depression*. Even in well-designed research trials that should achieve optimal outcomes, response rates for late-life depression are typically in the 50% to 65% range (versus 25 to 30% for placebo) and remission rates are in the 30% to 40% range (versus 15% for placebo) (160) Clinicians, therefore, must become familiar with treatment options available after initial treatment failure(s). The initial step, in general, should be to reassess the patient's diagnosis and treatment, perhaps guided by the following mnemonic of **A-B-C-D**: "A" refers to the need to assess prior treatment Adequacy, especially whether an appropriate medication was chosen and whether it was prescribed at a proper dose for an adequate duration. "B" reminds us to consider Behavioral factors that can impede treatment response, such as concurrent pain or illness, financial stress, recent losses or bereavement, an unsatisfactory living environment, or victimization by a spouse or other caregiver. "C," which refers to Compliance (though "adherence" is a more current term because it conveys a less submissive patient role) and reminds us to verify that the patient actually took the medication as prescribed. "D," finally, prompts a Diagnostic review to consider whether psychosis, severe and/or independent anxiety, substance abuse, personality disorder, or a range of medical illnesses might be interfering with treatment response. The patient who has failed two antidepressant trials and is "A-B-C-D Negative" is most likely a treatment-resistant depressive and should be considered for one of the limited range of choices available: optimization, switching, augmenting, coprescribing, or addition of a nonpharmacologic intervention.

Optimization refers not only to achieving the appropriate dose of an antidepressant but also includes management of side effects and simplification of a prescribing regimen in order to support treatment adherence. Adverse effects of sedation, insomnia, gastrointestinal responses such as diarrhea or constipation, sexual dysfunction, and altered weight should be explored and can be addressed in most cases by altering a medication's dose or timing or by adding an additional medication. Regimen simplification can be achieved by consolidating doses, limiting the total number of pills by using the most efficient dosing combination, and associating the pill-taking with a regularly scheduled event such as breakfast or bedtime so that the patient is reminded each day to take the medication. As explored in Chapter 6, it's also important to understand the medication's cost to the patient, and this may require direct inquiry.

Switching is the intervention of choice for elders with treatment-resistant depression who have not tolerated a specific drug or who have shown no response despite an adequate trial. Switching is particularly appropriate when improvement is a less urgent matter, for example, in outpatients with good support systems and relative stability, because in exchange for a longer transition to a new treatment it results in a simpler, less costly regimen that is less likely to be associated with drug interactions than augmenting. The STAR∗D study results have suggested that it is not necessary to switch to a different class of antidepressant as was often previously recommended. Nonetheless, after two failed SSRI trials it would not be unreasonable to switch to an SNRI, bupropion, or mirtazapine, basing the choice on a variety of factors including medical risk factors, degree of sedation or activation, formulary availability, and the matching of a side-effect profile to a specific patient's preferences. None of the antidepressants have been determined to be more efficacious than others in this switch process. Following failure of this strategy, use of nortriptyline or an MAO inhibitor may be appropriate, recognizing that some additional responses will occur but at the risk of a less tolerable side-effect profile.

In partial responders, an augmentation strategy is often pursued, though no study demonstrates its superiority over switching to a different antidepressant. Augmentation strategies aim for a rapid response, suitable for the hurried pace of inpatient treatment, but introduce a more complex and expensive regimen with greater potential for drug interactions. The use of any augmenting or coprescribed agent in a treatment-resistant depressed elder should be regarded as an "off label" use since no medication is specifically indicated for this purpose, although (see below) aripiprazole has received an FDA indication for adjunctive treatment of depression in adults. Off label use is permitted when clinically justified, but the need for patient understanding, awareness, and informed acceptance of such a treatment is heightened when a clinician departs from the well-traveled path of "indicated" treatments that should be used first.

Lithium carbonate (Li_2CO_3) augmentation, the most credibly documented augmentation strategy in younger adults, can successfully augment an antidepressant at blood levels between 0.4 and 0.8 mmol/L (6). In an open label study, 33.3% of an elderly cohort diagnosed with treatment resistant depression achieved remission with Li_2CO_3 augmentation (161). Lithium's use for augmentation can be effective, and lithium may have beneficial neuroprotective effects, but patients can be deterred by its side effects, which can include cognitive dysfunction, gastrointestinal symptoms, or annoyance with the cost and inconvenience of the required intermittent blood tests. Another augmentation strategy in younger adults is the addition of triiodothyronine (162). In younger adults, doses from 5 to 50 mcg/day are used to drive TSH into the lower quartile of the normal laboratory reference range, but older adults' treatment can be accompanied even at low-T3 doses by unpleasantly stimulating symptoms that may include increased anxiety, insomnia, tremor, and even anginal pain.

In practice, many clinicians reserve lithium and T3, though a more substantial evidence base describes their use in young adults, until trials of several other medications have been explored. Broadly, these medications can be divided into *activators* and *sedaters*. Activators are preferred for fatigued, anergic partial responders, and sedaters for anxious or agitated partial responders. For all of these, evidence for use in late-life depression is sparse compared to support for use in younger adults (though here, too, the evidence base is limited). The beneficial effect of the addition of methylphenidate (5–20 mg/day) to a preexisting antidepressant regimen in elderly patients diagnosed with vascular depression was reported in a small retrospective chart review recently (124), adding support to the earlier finding of Lavretsky and colleagues of accelerated response to citalopram by addition of methylphenidate demonstrated in a placebo-controlled double-blind trial (163). No controlled studies describe the use of other stimulants as augmenters in the treatment of late-life depression, but the addition of modafinil (200 mg/day) to an SSRI in partial responders with persistent fatigue and sleepiness was investigated in a nongeriatric, multicenter, placebo-controlled trial that concluded this to be a helpful combination. In geriatric populations, modafinil has not been subjected to sufficient study as an augmenter, but one case report describes its benefits in the treatment of one depressed geriatric "failure-to-thrive" inpatient (164). The other prominent activating augmentor is bupropion, which has safely been used to enhance the effects of serotonergic antidepressants in medically frail elderly subjects (165). In a naturalistic study that explored the use of several augmentors (166) in treatment-resistant late-life depressives, bupropion performed on a par with nortriptyline or lithium, each of which might be regarded as more sedating (or perhaps anxiolytic) augmenters. An even more sedating augmentor than nortriptyline is mirtazapine, anecdotally helpful and widely used in conjunction with other antidepressants in doses from 7.5 to 45 mg at bedtime. Mirtazapine has been studied as one augmenting strategy in the STAR*D, but geriatric studies are also needed. Despite the warnings from the FDA with respect to atypical antipsychotic medications' mortality-increasing effects on psychotic demented patients, the use of augmenting antipsychotics has become common in late-life treatment resistant depressives. Only limited data are available to support this use, but many clinicians believe these medications to be sufficiently safe and tolerable in this role to justify their use with appropriate patient education about this off-label intervention. The only controlled trial to date in an older cohort examined the use of risperidone augmentation to prevent relapse in treatment resistant depressed subjects (167). The subjects were depressed adults aged 55 years and older who failed to respond to an adequate trial of citalopram at 20 to 40 mg/d. After four to six weeks of additional treatment with open label risperidone (0.25 to 1 mg/d), remitted subjects entered a 24 week double blind maintenance phase that compared risperidone augmentation of citalopram with placebo augmentation of citalopram. The authors concluded that significantly more risperidone-augmented patients remitted during the open-label phase, but risperidone augmentation was associated with only a nonsignificant statistical trend toward delayed time to relapse during the double blind maintenance phase. An earlier open-label study of aripiprazole augmentation (maximum dose 15 mg/day) in nonremitting late-life depressives reported a high rate of symptom reduction and remission but with a 25% dropout rate and significant side effects, primarily dry mouth, agitation, and drowsiness (168). Though an open study, credibility is increased by the availability of two 6-week, double-blind, randomized placebo-controlled trials in younger adults sufficiently positive to justify an FDA indication for use as an adjunctive, or add-on treatment of major depressive disorder (169,170).

In addition to these activating and sedating augmenters, three hormonal treatments should be mentioned in this discussion. In postmenopausal depressed elderly women, Schneider and colleagues (171) demonstrated an augmenting effect when estrogen replacement therapy (ERT) was added to fluoxetine 20 mg/day, but this use of estrogen is rare in the wake of studies raising concerns about estrogen's safety in elderly women. In one intriguing, unreplicated report, a brief pulse of dexamethasone enhanced treatment outcome of two elderly patients with resistant depression (172). Finally, testosterone augmentation appears a promising augmenting strategy in hypogonadal elderly treatment-resistant depressed men (173), though perhaps not in eugonadal men (174). Use of testosterone should be avoided in men with medical contraindications including prostate cancer or liver disease.

In some patients with treatment-resistant depression, no response occurs despite optimization, switching, or augmentation. The decision, then, may be to add psychotherapy (particularly one of the validated approaches described in chapter 17) or suggest ECT (described fully in Chapter 16). These interventions, of course, could be added at an earlier stage of treatment resistance, since there is at present no clear evidence-based guideline that clarifies optimal sequencing of these treatments. In chapter 16, some additional treatments (vagal nerve stimulation, repetitive transcranial magnetic stimulation, and deep brain stimulation) are described. Although neither thoroughly studied nor widely available at present, these approaches may in the future provide additional treatment choices.

CONCLUSION

As this chapter makes clear, the ideal antidepressant for treating late-life depression remains to be identified. Experience with available agents, however, has identified some desirable characteristics for superior results with older patients. These are indicated in Table 5, adapting DeVane's approach (175). Although no currently available agents matches this list of ideal characteristics, the growth of our elderly population and the likelihood that late-life depression will become more prevalent makes it important to determine and promote optimal pharmacotherapy practices for specialists and primary care clinicians treating late- life depression. Identifying superior agents and establishing meaningful comparison data among them will require more standardized and more powerful approaches than those used in many of the studies we reviewed. Currently available studies only partially answer our questions, largely because they lack statistical power, comparable design, or sufficiently thorough reporting. Underpowered studies make it difficult to assume that "not significantly different from" is synonymous with "equal to" (147).

TABLE 5 Characteristics of an Ideal Antidepressant for Late-Life Depression

Efficacy characteristics
Alleviates symptoms, producing response or remission
Produces therapeutic benefits rapidly
Achieves effectiveness with all or most patients
Maintains effectiveness in continuation and maintenance phases of treatment
Safety and tolerability characteristics
Remains affordable even when not covered by insurance
Produces only infrequent or mild adverse effects
Induces minimal toxicity in overdose
Improves or does not impair cognition
Enhances quality of life and functionality
Pharmacokinetic characteristics
Possesses minimal anticholinergic, antidopaminergic, antiadrenergic, antihistaminic, or cardiotoxic effects
Yields predictable dose–effect relationship
Follows consistent and predictable pattern of disposition
Has a wide therapeutic index
Is inactivated/eliminated by multiple pathways
Has an elimination half-life suitable for once-daily dosing
Participates rarely in pharmacokinetic (including CYP450) drug-drug interactions

Source: Adapted from Ref. 175.

Furthermore, our identification of very few published studies in which an investigated drug showed no efficacy (61,65,71,75,77,90,95) suggests a systematic bias against the availability of negative studies, the so-called "file drawer effect" by which positive studies find their way more easily into circulation. In the future, we would hope to see more studies designed with sufficient statistical power to detect reliably the possible differences among compared drugs, standardized measures for efficacy and side effects that would promote greater comparability among studies, special attention to groups about whom less is known such as the "old old," demented, poststroke, treatment resistant, and those with the vascular depression syndromes; a standard format for reporting methods and results that would include f and t statistics, standard deviations, and standard errors; and reporting of negative as well as positive trials. In this way, our effectiveness in treating late-life depression can be improved, resulting in better acute- and longer-term outcomes, increased survival, and enhanced quality of life for our patients.

REFERENCES

1. Rowe JW, Andres R, Tobin JD, et al. The effect of age on creatinine clearance in men: A cross-sectional and longitudinal study. J Gerontol 1976; 31(2):155–163.
2. Turnheim K. Drug dosage in the elderly. Is it rational? Drugs Aging 1998; 13(5):357–379.
3. Raskind MA, Peskind ER, Holmes C, et al. Patterns of cerebrospinal fluid catechols support increased central noradrenergic responsiveness in aging and Alzheimer's disease. Biol Psychiatry 1999; 46(6):756–765.
4. Nobler MS, Mann JJ, Sackeim HA. Serotonin, cerebral blood flow, and cerebral metabolic rate in geriatric major depression and normal aging. Brain Res Brain Res Rev 1999; 30(3):250–263.

5. Jacobson S, Pies R, Greenblat D. Handbook of Geriatric Psychopharmacology. Washington, D.C.: American Psychiatric Press Inc., 2002.
6. Katona C. Depression in Old Age. Chichester, UK: John Wiley & Sons, 1994.
7. Nelson J. Geriatric Psychopharmacology. New York, NY: Marcel Dekker, 1998.
8. Salzman C. Clinical Geriatric Psychopharmacology. 4th Edition. Baltimore, MD: Williams & Wilkins, 2004.
9. Altamura AC, Mauri MC, Rudas N, et al. Clinical activity and tolerability of trazodone, mianserin, and amitriptyline in elderly subjects with major depression: A controlled multicenter trial. Clin Neuropharmacol 1989; 12(suppl 1):S25–S33; S34–S37
10. Altamura AC, Percudani M, Guercetti G, et al. Efficacy and tolerability of fluoxetine in the elderly: A double-blind study versus amitryptiline. Int Clin Psychopharmacol 1989; 4(suppl 1):103–106.
11. Ather SA, Ankier SI, Middleton RS. A double-blind evaluation of trazodone in the treatment of depression in the elderly. Br J Clin Pract 1985; 39(5):192–199.
12. Bayer AJ, Pathy MS, Cameron A, et al. A comparative study of conventional and controlled-release formulations of trazodone in elderly depressed patients. Clin Neuropharmacol 1989; 12(suppl 1):S50–S55; discussion S56–S57.
13. Bocksberger JP, Gachoud JP, Richard J, et al. Comparison of the efficacy of moclobemide and fluvoxamine in elderly patients with a severe depressive episode. Eur Psychiatry 1993; 8:319.
14. Bondareff W, Alpert M, Friedhoff AJ, et al. Comparison of sertraline and nortriptyline in the treatment of major depressive disorder in late life. Am J Psychiatry 2000; 157(5):729–736.
15. Branconnier RJ, Cole JO, Ghazvinian S, et al. Clinical pharmacology of bupropion and imipramine in elderly depressives. J Clin Psychiatry 1983; 44(5Pt 2):130–133.
16. Cassano GB, Puca F, Scapicchio PL, et al. Paroxetine and fluoxetine effects on mood and cognitive functions in depressed nondemented elderly patients. J Clin Psychiatry 2002; 63(5):396–402.
17. Cohn CK, Shrivastava R, Mendels J, et al. Double-blind, multicenter comparison of sertraline and amitriptyline in elderly depressed patients. J Clin Psychiatry 1990; 51(suppl B):28–33.
18. Cohn JB, Varga L, Lyford A. A two-center double-blind study of nomifensine, imipramine, and placebo in depressed geriatric outpatients. J Clin Psychiatry 1984; 45(4Pt 2):68–72.
19. Dalery J, Aubin V. Comparative study of paroxetine and mianserin in depression in elderly patients: Efficacy, tolerance, serotonin dependence. Encephale 2001; 27(1):71–81.
20. De Ronchi D, Rucci P, Lodi M, et al. Fluoxetine and amitriptyline in elderly depresed patients, a 10-week, double-blind study on course of neurocognitive adverse events and depressive symptoms. Arch Gerontol Geriatr 1998;6(suppl):125–140.
21. De Vanna M, Kummer J, Agnoli A, et al. Moclobemide compared with second-generation antidepressants in elderly people. Acta Psychiatr Scand Suppl 1990; 360:64–66.
22. Dorman T. Sleep and paroxetine: A comparison with mianserin in elderly depressed patients. Int Clin Psychopharmacol 1992; 6(suppl 4):53–58.
23. Dunner DL, Cohn JB, Walshe T, III, et al. Two combined, multicenter double-blind studies of paroxetine and doxepin in geriatric patients with major depression. J Clin Psychiatry 1992; 53(suppl):57–60.
24. Eklund K, Dunbar GC, Pinder RM, et al. Mianserin and imipramine in the treatment of elderly depressed patients. Acta Psychiatr Scand Suppl 1985; 320:55–59.
25. Evans M, Hammond M, Wilson K, et al. Placebo-controlled treatment trial of depression in elderly physically ill patients. Int J Geriatr Psychiatry 1997; 12(8):817–824.
26. Fairweather D, Kerr J, Harrison D. A double-blind comparison of the effects of fluoxetine and amitriptyline on cognitive functioning in elderly depressed patients. Hum Psychopharm 1993; 8:41–47.
27. Falk WE, Rosenbaum JF, Otto MW, et al. Fluoxetine versus trazodone in depressed geriatric patients. J Geriatr Psychiatry Neurol 1989; 2(4):208–214.

28. Feighner JP, Boyer WF, Hendrickson GG, et al. A controlled trial of adinazolam versus desipramine in geriatric depression. Int Clin Psychopharmacol 1990; 5(3):227–232.
29. Feighner JP, Cohn JB. Double-blind comparative trials of fluoxetine and doxepin in geriatric patients with major depressive disorder. J Clin Psychiatry 1985; 46(3Pt 2):20–25.
30. Finkel SI, Richter EM, Clary CM. Comparative efficacy and safety of sertraline versus nortriptyline in major depression in patients 70 and older. Int Psychogeriatr 1999; 11(1):85–99.
31. Forlenza OV, Almeida OP, Stoppe A, Jr, et al. Antidepressant efficacy and safety of low-dose sertraline and standard-dose imipramine for the treatment of depression in older adults: Results from a double-blind, randomized, controlled clinical trial. Int Psychogeriatr 2001; 13(1):75–84.
32. Forlenza OV, Stoppe Junior A, Hirata ES, et al. Antidepressant efficacy of sertraline and imipramine for the treatment of major depression in elderly outpatients. Sao Paulo Med J 2000; 118(4):99–104.
33. Georgotas A, McCue RE, Hapworth W, et al. Comparative efficacy and safety of MAOIs versus TCAs in treating depression in the elderly. Biol Psychiatry 1986; 21(12):1155–1166.
34. Geretsegger C, Stuppaeck CH, Mair M, et al. Multicenter double blind study of paroxetine and amitriptyline in elderly depressed inpatients. Psychopharmacology (Berl) 1995; 119(3):277–281.
35. Gerner R, Estabrook W, Steuer J, et al. Treatment of geriatric depression with trazodone, imipramine, and placebo: A double-blind study. J Clin Psychiatry 1980; 41(6):216–220.
36. Goldstein SE, Birnbom F, Laliberte R. Nomifensine in the treatment of depressed geriatric patients. J Clin Psychiatry 1982; 43(7):287–289.
37. Guilibert E, Pelicier Y, Archambault J. A double-blind, multicentre study of paroxetine versus clomipramine in depressed elderly patients. Acta Psychiatr Scand 1989; 80(suppl 350):132–134.
38. Gwirtsman HE, Ahles S, Halaris A, et al. Therapeutic superiority of maprotiline versus doxepin in geriatric depression. J Clin Psychiatry 1983; 44(12):449–453.
39. Halikas J. Org 3770 (mirtazapine) versus trazodone: A placebo controlled trial in depressed elderly patients. Hum Psychopharm 1995; 10:S125–S133.
40. Hoyberg OJ, Maragakis B, Mullin J, et al. A double-blind multicentre comparison of mirtazapine and amitriptyline in elderly depressed patients. Acta Psychiatr Scand 1996; 93(3):184–190.
41. Hutchinson D, Tong S, Moon C. Paroxetine in the treatment of elderly depressed patients in general practice: A double-blind comparison with amitriptyline. Br J Clin Res 1991; 2:43–57.
42. Jansen W, Siegfried K. Nomifensine in geriatric inpatients: A placebo-controlled study. J Clin Psychiatry 1984; 45(4Pt 2):63–67.
43. Jarvik LF, Mintz J, Steuer J, et al. Treating geriatric depression: A 26-week interim analysis. J Am Geriatr Soc 1982; 30(11):713–717.
44. Kane JM, Cole K, Sarantakos S, et al. Safety and efficacy of bupropion in elderly patients: Preliminary observations. J Clin Psychiatry 1983; 44(5Pt 2):134–136.
45. Karlsson I, Godderis J. Augusto De Mendonca Lima C, et al. A randomised, double-blind comparison of the efficacy and safety of citalopram compared to mianserin in elderly, depressed patients with or without mild to moderate dementia. Int J Geriatr Psychiatry 2000; 15(4):295–305.
46. Katona C, Bercoff E, Chiu E, et al. Reboxetine versus imipramine in the treatment of elderly patients with depressive disorders: A double-blind randomised trial. J Affect Disord 1999; 55(2–3):203–213.
47. Katona CL, Hunter BN, Bray J. A double-blind comparison of the efficacy and safety of paroxetine and imipramine in the treatment of depression with dementia. Int J Geriatr Psychiatry 1998; 13(2):100–108.
48. Katz IR, Simpson GM, Curlik SM, et al. Pharmacologic treatment of major depression for elderly patients in residential care settings. J Clin Psychiatry 1990; 51(suppl):41–47; discussion 48.
49. Kivela S, Lehtomaki E. Sulpride and placebo in depressed elderly outpatients: A double-blind study. Int J Geriatr Psychiatry 1987; 2:255–260.

50. Kretschmar J. Mianserin and amitriptyline in elderly hospitalized patients with depressive illness: A double-blind trial. Curr Med Ther Opin 1980; 6(suppl 7):144–151.
51. Kyle CJ, Petersen HE, Overo KF. Comparison of the tolerability and efficacy of citalopram and amitriptyline in elderly depressed patients treated in general practice. Depress Anxiety 1998; 8(4):147–153.
52. La Pia S, Giorgio D, Ciriello R. Evaluation of the efficacy, tolerability, and theraputic profile of fluoxetine versus mianserin in the treatment of depressive disorders in the elderly. Curr Ther Res 1992; 52(6):847–858.
53. Lakshmanan M, Mion LC, Frengley JD. Effective low dose tricyclic antidepressant treatment for depressed geriatric rehabilitation patients. A double-blind study. J Am Geriatr Soc 1986; 34(6):421–426.
54. Lipsey JR, Robinson RG, Pearlson GD, et al. Nortriptyline treatment of post-stroke depression: A double-blind study. Lancet 1984; 1(8372):297–300.
55. Lyketsos CG, Sheppard JM, Steele CD, et al. Randomized, placebo-controlled, double-blind clinical trial of sertraline in the treatment of depression complicating Alzheimer's disease: Initial results from the Depression in Alzheimer's Disease study. Am J Psychiatry 2000; 157(10):1686–1689.
56. Magai C, Kennedy G, Cohen CI, et al. A controlled clinical trial of sertraline in the treatment of depression in nursing home patients with late-stage Alzheimer's disease. Am J Geriatr Psychiatry 2000; 8(1):66–74.
57. Mahapatra SN, Hackett D. A randomised, double-blind, parallel-group comparison of venlafaxine and dothiepin in geriatric patients with major depression. Int J Clin Pract 1997; 51(4):209–213.
58. Merideth CH, Feighner JP, Hendrickson G. A double-blind comparative evaluation of the efficacy and safety of nomifensine, imipramine, and placebo in depressed geriatric outpatients. J Clin Psychiatry 1984; 45(4Pt 2):73–77.
59. Brion S, Audrain S, de Bodinat C. Major depressive episodes in patients over 70 years of age. Evaluation of the efficiency and acceptability of tianeptine and mianserin. Presse Med 1996; 25(9):461–468.
60. Guelfi JD, Bouhassira M, Bonett-Perrin E, et al. The study of the efficacy of fluoxetine versus tianeptine in the treatment of elderly depressed patients followed in general practice. Encephale 1999; 25(3):265–270.
61. Kasper S, de Swart H, Friis Andersen H. Escitalopram in the treatment of depressed elderly patients. Am J Geriatr Psychiatry 2005; 13(10):884–891.
62. Moller HJ, Volz HP. Brofaromine in elderly major depressed patients—A comparative trial versus imipramine. Eur Neuropsychopharmacol 1993; 3(4):501–510.
63. Mulsant BH, Pollock BG, Nebes R, et al. A twelve-week, double-blind, randomized comparison of nortriptyline and paroxetine in older depressed inpatients and outpatients. Am J Geriatr Psychiatry 2001; 9(4):406–414.
64. Nair NP, Amin M, Holm P, et al. Moclobemide and nortriptyline in elderly depressed patients. A randomized, multicentre trial against placebo. J Affect Disord 1995; 33(1):1–9.
65. Navarro V, Gasto C, Torres X, et al. Citalopram versus nortriptyline in late-life depression: A 12-week randomized single-blind study. Acta Psychiatr Scand 2001; 103(6):435–440.
66. Newhouse PA, Krishnan KR, Doraiswamy PM, et al. A double-blind comparison of sertraline and fluoxetine in depressed elderly outpatients. J Clin Psychiatry 2000; 61(8):559–568.
67. Nugent D. A double-blind study of viloxazine and amitriptyline in depressed geriatric patients. Clin Trials J 1979; 16:13–16.
68. Nyth AL, Gottfries CG, Lyby K, et al. A controlled multicenter clinical study of citalopram and placebo in elderly depressed patients with and without concomitant dementia. Acta Psychiatr Scand 1992; 86(2):138–145.
69. Pancheri P, Delle Chiaie R, Donnini M, et al. Effects of moclobemide on depressive symptoms and cognitive performance in a geriatric population: A controlled comparative study versus imipramine. Clin Neuropharmacol 1994; 17(suppl 1):S58–S73.

70. Pelicier Y, Schaeffer P. Multicenter double-blind study comparing the efficacy and tolerance of paroxetine and clomipramine in reactive depression in the elderly patient. Encephale 1993; 19(3):257–261.
71. Petracca GM, Chemerinski E, Starkstein SE. A double-blind, placebo-controlled study of fluoxetine in depressed patients with Alzheimer's disease. Int Psychogeriatr 2001; 13(2):233–240.
72. Phanjoo AL, Wonnacott S, Hodgson A. Double-blind comparative multicentre study of fluvoxamine and mianserin in the treatment of major depressive episode in elderly people. Acta Psychiatr Scand 1991; 83(6):476–479.
73. Rahman MK, Akhtar MJ, Savla NC, et al. A double-blind, randomised comparison of fluvoxamine with dothiepin in the treatment of depression in elderly patients. Br J Clin Pract 1991; 45(4):255–258.
74. Reynolds CF, III, Miller MD, Pasternak RE, et al. Treatment of bereavement-related major depressive episodes in later life: A controlled study of acute and continuation treatment with nortriptyline and interpersonal psychotherapy. Am J Psychiatry 1999; 156(2):202–208.
75. Robinson RG, Schultz SK, Castillo C, et al. Nortriptyline versus fluoxetine in the treatment of depression and in short-term recovery after stroke: A placebo-controlled, double-blind study. Am J Psychiatry 2000; 157(3):351–359.
76. Roth M, Mountjoy CQ, Amrein R. Moclobemide in elderly patients with cognitive decline and depression: An international double-blind, placebo-controlled trial. Br J Psychiatry 1996; 168(2):149–157.
77. Salloway S, Boyle PA, Correia S, et al. The relationship of MRI subcortical hyperintensities to treatment response in a trial of sertraline in geriatric depressed outpatients. Am J Geriatr Psychiatry 2002; 10(1):107–111.
78. Schatzberg AF, Kremer C, Rodrigues HE, et al. Double-blind, randomized comparison of mirtazapine and paroxetine in elderly depressed patients. Am J Geriatr Psychiatry 2002; 10(5):541–550.
79. Schone W, Ludwig M. A double-blind study of paroxetine compared with fluoxetine in geriatric patients with major depression. J Clin Psychopharmacol 1993; 13(6 suppl 2):34S–39S.
80. Siegfried K, O'Connolly M. Cognitive and psychomotor effects of different antidepressants in the treatment of old age depression. Int Clin Psychopharmacol 1986; 1(3):231–243.
81. Taragano FE, Lyketsos CG, Mangone CA, et al. A double-blind, randomized, fixed-dose trial of fluoxetine vs. amitriptyline in the treatment of major depression complicating Alzheimer's disease. Psychosomatics 1997; 38(3):246–252.
82. Tignol J, Pujol-Domenech J, Chartres JP, et al. Double-blind study of the efficacy and safety of milnacipran and imipramine in elderly patients with major depressive episode. Acta Psychiatr Scand 1998; 97(2):157–165.
83. Tiller J, Maguire K, Davies B. A sequential double-blind controlled study of moclobemide and mianserin in elderly patients. Int J Geriatr Psychiatry 1990; 5:199–204.
84. Tollefson GD, Bosomworth JC, Heiligenstein JH, et al. A double-blind, placebo-controlled clinical trial of fluoxetine in geriatric patients with major depression. The Fluoxetine Collaborative Study Group. Int Psychogeriatr 1995; 7(1):89–104.
85. Waite J, Grundy E, Arie T. A controlled trial of antidepressant medication in elderly in-patients. Int Clin Psychopharmacol 1986; 1(2):113–126.
86. Wakelin JS. Fluvoxamine in the treatment of the older depressed patient; double-blind, placebo-controlled data. Int Clin Psychopharmacol 1986; 1(3):221–230.
87. Weihs KL, Settle EC, Jr, Batey SR, et al. Bupropion sustained release versus paroxetine for the treatment of depression in the elderly. J Clin Psychiatry 2000; 61(3):196–202.
88. Wiart L, Petit H, Joseph PA, et al. Fluoxetine in early poststroke depression: A double-blind placebo-controlled study. Stroke 2000; 31(8):1829–1832.
89. Allard P, Gram L, Timdahl K, et al. Efficacy and tolerability of venlafaxine in geriatric outpatients with major depression: A double-blind, randomised 6-month comparative trial with citalopram. Int J Geriatr Psychiatry 2004; 19(12):1123–1130.

90. Bose A, Li D, Gandhi C. Escitalopram in the acute treatment of depressed patients aged 60 years or older. Am J Geriatr Psychiatry 2008; 16(1):14–20.
91. Kok RM, Nolen WA, Heeren TJ. Venlafaxine versus nortriptyline in the treatment of elderly depressed inpatients: A randomised, double blind, controlled trial. Int J Geriatr Psychiatry 2007:DOI: 10.1002/gps.182.
92. Nelson JC, Wohlreich MM, Mallinckrodt CH, et al. Duloxetine for the treatment of major depressive disorder in older patients. Am J Geriatr Psychiatry 2005; 13(3):227–235.
93. Raskin J, Wiltse CG, Siegal A, et al. Efficacy of duloxetine on cognition, depression, and pain in elderly patients with major depressive disorder: An 8-week, double-blind, placebo-controlled trial. Am J Psychiatry 2007; 164(6):900–909.
94. Rossini D, Serretti A, Franchini L, et al. Sertraline versus fluvoxamine in the treatment of elderly patients with major depression: A double-blind, randomized trial. J Clin Psychopharmacol 2005; 25(5):471–475.
95. Schatzberg A, Roose S. A double-blind, placebo-controlled study of venlafaxine and fluoxetine in geriatric outpatients with major depression. Am J Geriatr Psychiatry 2006; 14(4):361–370.
96. Smeraldi E, Rizzo F. Double-blind, randomized study of venlafaxine, clomipramine and trazodone in geriatric patients with major depression. Prim Care Psychiatry 1998; 4:189–195.
97. Sultzer DL, Gray KF, Gunay I, et al. A double-blind comparison of trazodone and haloperidol for treatment of agitation in patients with dementia. Am J Geriatr Psychiatry 1997; 5(1):60–69.
98. Finkel SI, Richter EM, Clary CM, et al. Comparative efficacy of sertraline vs. fluoxetine in patients age 70 or over with major depression. Am J Geriatr Psychiatry 1999; 7(3):221–227.
99. Schneider LS, Nelson JC, Clary CM, et al. An 8-week multicenter, parallel-group, double-blind, placebo-controlled study of sertraline in elderly outpatients with major depression. Am J Psychiatry 2003; 160(7):1277–1285.
100. Schweizer E, Rickels K, Hassman H, et al. Buspirone and imipramine for the treatment of major depression in the elderly. J Clin Psychiatry 1998; 59(4):175–183.
101. Gerson S, Belin TR, Kaufman A, et al. Pharmacological and psychological treatments for depressed older patients: A meta-analysis and overview of recent findings. Harv Rev Psychiatry 1999; 7(1):1–28.
102. Klawansky S. Meta-analysis on the treatment of depression in late life. In: Schneider L, et al., ed. Diagnosis and Treatment of Depression in Late Life, Results of the NIH Consensus Development Conference. Washington, D.C.: American Psychiatric Press Inc., 1994:333–352.
103. Mittmann N, Herrmann N, Einarson TR, et al. The efficacy, safety and tolerability of antidepressants in late life depression: A meta-analysis. J Affect Disord 1997; 46(3):191–217.
104. Mottram P, Wilson K, Strobl J. Antidepressants for depressed elderly. Cochrane Database Syst Rev 2006; (1):CD003491.
105. Alexopoulos G, Katz I, Reynolds CI, et al. The expert consensus guideline series pharmacotherapy of depressive disorders in older patients. Postgrad Med Spec Rep 2001; (Oct.):1–88.
106. Beers MH. Explicit criteria for determining potentially inappropriate medication use by the elderly. An update. Arch Intern Med 1997; 157(14):1531–1536.
107. Roose SP, Suthers KM. Antidepressant response in late-life depression. J Clin Psychiatry 1998; 59(suppl 10):4–8.
108. Oslin DW, Streim JE, Katz IR, et al. Heuristic comparison of sertraline with nortriptyline for the treatment of depression in frail elderly patients. Am J Geriatr Psychiatry 2000; 8(2):141–149.
109. Roose SP, Glassman AH, Siris SG, et al. Comparison of imipramine- and nortriptyline-induced orthostatic hypotension: A meaningful difference. J Clin Psychopharmacol 1981; 1(5):316–319.

110. Wilson K, Mottram P. A comparison of side effects of selective serotonin reuptake inhibitors and tricyclic antidepressants in older depressed patients: A meta-analysis. Int J Geriatr Psychiatry 2004; 19:754.
111. Wilson K, Mottram P, Sivanranthan A, et al. Antidepressant versus placebo for depressed elderly. Cochrane Database Syst Rev 2001; (2):CD000561.
112. Goldstein DJ, Hamilton SH, Masica DN, et al. Fluoxetine in medically stable, depressed geriatric patients: Effects on weight. J Clin Psychopharmacol 1997; 17(5):365–369.
113. Rothschild AJ. The diagnosis and treatment of late-life depression. J Clin Psychiatry 1996; 57(suppl 5):5–11.
114. Aranda-Michel J, Koehler A, Bejarano PA, et al. Nefazodone-induced liver failure: Report of three cases. Ann Intern Med 1999; 130(4Pt 1):285–288.
115. Schirren CA, Baretton G. Nefazodone-induced acute liver failure. Am J Gastroenterol 2000; 95(6):1596–1597.
116. Schwetz BA. From the Food and Drug Administration. JAMA 2002; 287(9):1103.
117. Sachs GS, Lafer B, Stoll AL, et al. A double-blind trial of bupropion versus desipramine for bipolar depression. J Clin Psychiatry 1994; 55(9):391–393.
118. Sweet RA, Pollock BG, Kirshner M, et al. Pharmacokinetics of single- and multiple-dose bupropion in elderly patients with depression. J Clin Pharmacol 1995; 35(9):876–884.
119. Szuba MP, Leuchter AF. Falling backward in two elderly patients taking bupropion. J Clin Psychiatry 1992; 53(5):157–159.
120. Kuroda Y, Watanabe Y, McEwen BS. Tianeptine decreases both serotonin transporter mRNA and binding sites in rat brain. Eur J Pharmacol 1994; 268(1):R3–R5.
121. Watanabe Y, Sakai RR, McEwen BS, et al. Stress and antidepressant effects on hippocampal and cortical 5-HT1A and 5-HT2 receptors and transport sites for serotonin. Brain Res 1993; 615(1):87–94.
122. Satel SL Nelson JC. Stimulants in the treatment of depression: A critical overview. J Clin Psychiatry 1989; 50(7):241–249.
123. Wallace AE, Kofoed LL, West AN. Double-blind, placebo-controlled trial of methylphenidate in older, depressed, medically ill patients. Am J Psychiatry 1995; 152(6):929–931.
124. Mantani A, Fujikawa T, Ohmori N, et al. Methylphenidate in the treatment of geriatric patients with vascular depression: A retrospective chart review. Am J Geriatr Psychiatry 2008; 16(4):336–337.
125. Georgotas A, McCue RE, Friedman E, et al. Response of depressive symptoms to nortriptyline, phenelzine and placebo. Br J Psychiatry 1987; 151:102–106.
126. Dew MA, Reynolds CF, III, Houck PR, et al. Temporal profiles of the course of depression during treatment. Predictors of pathways toward recovery in the elderly. Arch Gen Psychiatry 1997; 54(11):1016–1024.
127. Sackeim HA, Roose SP, Burt T. Optimal length of antidepressant trials in late-life depression. J Clin Psychopharmacol 2005; 25(4 suppl 1):S34–S37.
128. Flint AJ, Rifat SL. The effect of treatment on the two-year course of late-life depression. Br J Psychiatry 1997; 170:268–272.
129. van Weel C, Vermeulen H, Van Den Bosch W. Falls, a community care perspective. Lancet 1995; 345(8964):1549–1551.
130. Thapa PB, Gideon P, Fought RL, et al. Psychotropic drugs and risk of recurrent falls in ambulatory nursing home residents. Am J Epidemiol 1995; 142(2):202–211.
131. Thapa PB, Gideon P, Cost TW, et al. Antidepressants and the risk of falls among nursing home residents. N Engl J Med 1998; 339(13):875–882.
132. Hartikainen S, Lonnroos E, Louhivuori K. Medication as a risk factor for falls: Critical systematic review. J Gerontol A Biol Sci Med Sci 2007; 62(10):1172–1181.
133. Diem SJ, Blackwell TL, Stone KL, et al. Depressive symptoms and rates of bone loss at the hip in older women. J Am Geriatr Soc 2007; 55(6):824–831.
134. Movig KL, Leufkens HG, Lenderink AW, et al. Association between antidepressant drug use and hyponatraemia: A case-control study. Br J Clin Pharmacol 2002; 53(4):363–369.
135. Kirby D, Harrigan S, Ames D. Hyponatraemia in elderly psychiatric patients treated with selective serotonin reuptake inhibitors and venlafaxine: A retrospective controlled study in an inpatient unit. Int J Geriatr Psychiatry 2002; 17(3):231–237.

136. Jacob S, Spinler SA. Hyponatremia associated with selective serotonin-reuptake inhibitors in older adults. Ann Pharmacother 2006; 40(9):1618–1622.
137. Thompson MP, Morris LK. Unexplained weight loss in the ambulatory elderly. J Am Geriatr Soc 1991; 39(5):497–500.
138. Lustman PJ, Griffith LS, Clouse RE, et al. Effects of nortriptyline on depression and glycemic control in diabetes: Results of a double-blind, placebo-controlled trial. Psychosom Med 1997; 59(3):241–250.
139. Rigler SK, Webb MJ, Redford L, et al. Weight outcomes among antidepressant users in nursing facilities. J Am Geriatr Soc 2001; 49(1):49–55.
140. Mihara IQ, McCombs JS, Williams BR. The impact of mirtazapine compared with non-TCA antidepressants on weight change in nursing facility residents. Consult Pharm 2005; 20(3):217–223.
141. Skop BP, Brown TM. Potential vascular and bleeding complications of treatment with selective serotonin reuptake inhibitors. Psychosomatics 1996; 37(1):12–16.
142. de Abajo FJ, Rodriguez LA, Montero D. Association between selective serotonin reuptake inhibitors and upper gastrointestinal bleeding: Population based case-control study. BMJ 1999; 319(7217):1106–1109.
143. Layton D, Clark DW, Pearce GL, et al. Is there an association between selective serotonin reuptake inhibitors and risk of abnormal bleeding? Results from a cohort study based on prescription event monitoring in England. Eur J Clin Pharmacol 2001; 57(2):167–176.
144. van Walraven C, Mamdani MM, Wells PS, et al. Inhibition of serotonin reuptake by antidepressants and upper gastrointestinal bleeding in elderly patients: Retrospective cohort study. BMJ 2001; 323(7314):655–658.
145. Bak S, Tsiropoulos I, Kjaersgaard JO, et al. Selective serotonin reuptake inhibitors and the risk of stroke: A population-based case-control study. Stroke 2002; 33(6):1465–1473.
146. Barbui C, Percudani M, Fortino I, et al. Past use of selective serotonin reuptake inhibitors and the risk of cerebrovascular events in the elderly. Int Clin Psychopharmacol 2005; 20(3):169–171.
147. Thase ME. The next step forward: A move toward evidence, and away from fear of the industry. Psychopharmacol Bull 2002; 36(4):4–5.
148. Meyers BS, Greenberg R. Late-life delusional depression. J Affect Disord 1986; 11(2):133–137.
149. Mulsant BH, Sweet RA, Rosen J, et al. A double-blind randomized comparison of nortriptyline plus perphenazine versus nortriptyline plus placebo in the treatment of psychotic depression in late life. J Clin Psychiatry 2001; 62(8):597–604.
150. Konig F, von Hippel C, Petersdorff T, et al. First experiences in combination therapy using olanzapine with SSRIs (citalopram, paroxetine) in delusional depression. Neuropsychobiology 2001; 43(3):170–174.
151. Rothschild AJ, Bates KS, Boehringer KL, et al. Olanzapine response in psychotic depression. J Clin Psychiatry 1999; 60(2):116–118.
152. Flint AJ, Rifat SL. Two-year outcome of psychotic depression in late life. Am J Psychiatry 1998; 155(2):178–183.
153. Olin JT, Katz IR, Meyers BS, et al. Provisional diagnostic criteria for depression of Alzheimer disease: Rationale and background. Am J Geriatr Psychiatry 2002; 10(2):129–141.
154. Streim JE, Oslin DW, Katz IR, et al. Drug treatment of depression in frail elderly nursing home residents. Am J Geriatr Psychiatry 2000; 8(2):150–159.
155. de Vasconcelos Cunha UG, Lopes Rocha F, Avila de Melo R, et al. A placebo-controlled double-blind randomized study of venlafaxine in the treatment of depression in dementia. Dement Geriatr Cogn Disord 2007; 24(1):36–41.
156. Lyketsos CG, DelCampo L, Steinberg M, et al. Treating depression in Alzheimer disease: Efficacy and safety of sertraline therapy, and the benefits of depression reduction: The DIADS. Arch Gen Psychiatry 2003; 60(7):737–746.
157. Brown MN, Lapane KL, Luisi AF. The management of depression in older nursing home residents. J Am Geriatr Soc 2002; 50(1):69–76.

158. Payne JL, Sheppard JM, Steinberg M, et al. Incidence, prevalence, and outcomes of depression in residents of a long-term care facility with dementia. Int J Geriatr Psychiatry 2002; 17(3):247–253.
159. Schulberg HC, Schultz R, Miller MD, et al. Depression and physical illness in older primary care patients: Diagnostic and treatment issues. In:Williamson GM, Shaffer DR, Parmelee PA, eds. Physical Illness and Depression in Older adults: A Handbook of Theory, Research, and Practice. New York, NY: Kluwer Academic Publishers, 2002:239–256.
160. Shanmugham B, Karp J, Drayer R, et al. Evidence-based pharmacologic interventions for geriatric depression. Psychiatr Clin North Am 2005; 28(4):821–835, viii.
161. Kok RM, Vink D, Heeren TJ, et al. Lithium augmentation compared with phenelzine in treatment-resistant depression in the elderly: An open, randomized, controlled trial. J Clin Psychiatry 2007; 68(8):1177–1185.
162. Nierenberg AA, Fava M, Trivedi MH, et al. A comparison of lithium and T(3) augmentation following two failed medication treatments for depression: A STAR*D report. Am J Psychiatry 2006; 163(9):1519–1530; quiz 1665.
163. Lavretsky H, Park S, Siddarth P, et al. Methylphenidate-enhanced antidepressant response to citalopram in the elderly: A double-blind, placebo-controlled pilot trial. Am J Geriatr Psychiatry 2006; 14(2):181–185.
164. Schillerstrom JE, Seaman JS. Modafinil augmentation of mirtazapine in a failure-to-thrive geriatric inpatient. Int J Psychiatry Med 2002; 32(4):405–410.
165. Spier SA. Use of bupropion with SRIs and venlafaxine. Depress Anxiety 1998; 7(2):73–75.
166. Whyte EM, Basinski J, Farhi P, et al. Geriatric depression treatment in nonresponders to selective serotonin reuptake inhibitors. J Clin Psychiatry 2004; 65(12):1634–1641.
167. Alexopoulos GS, Canuso CM, Gharabawi GM, et al. Placebo-controlled study of relapse prevention with risperidone augmentation in older patients with resistant depression. Am J Geriatr Psychiatry 2008; 16(1):21–30.
168. Rutherford B, Sneed J, Miyazaki M, et al. An open trial of aripiprazole augmentation for SSRI non-remitters with late-life depression. Int J Geriatr Psychiatry 2007; 22(10):986–991.
169. Berman RM, Marcus RN, Swanink R, et al. The efficacy and safety of aripiprazole as adjunctive therapy in major depressive disorder: A multicenter, randomized, double-blind, placebo-controlled study. J Clin Psychiatry 2007; 68(6):843–853.
170. Marcus RN, McQuade RD, Carson WH, et al. The efficacy and safety of aripiprazole as adjunctive therapy in major depressive disorder: A second multicenter, randomized, double-blind, placebo-controlled study. J Clin Psychopharmacol 2008; 28(2):156–165.
171. Schneider LS, Small GW, Hamilton SH, et al. Estrogen replacement and response to fluoxetine in a multicenter geriatric depression trial. Fluoxetine Collaborative Study Group. Am J Geriatr Psychiatry 1997; 5(2):97–106.
172. Bodani M, Sheehan B, Philpot M. The use of dexamethasone in elderly patients with antidepressant-resistant depressive illness. J Psychopharmacol 1999; 13(2):196–197.
173. Seidman SN, Rabkin JG. Testosterone replacement therapy for hypogonadal men with SSRI-refractory depression. J Affect Disord 1998; 48(2–3):157–161.
174. Seidman SN, Miyazaki M, Roose SP. Intramuscular testosterone supplementation to selective serotonin reuptake inhibitor in treatment-resistant depressed men: Randomized placebo-controlled clinical trial. J Clin Psychopharmacol 2005; 25(6):584–588.
175. DeVane CL. Pharmacologic characteristics of ideal antidepressants in the 21st century. J Clin Psychiatry 2000; 61(suppl 11):4–8.
176. Stahl SM. Essential Psychopharmacology, 2nd ed. New York, NY: Cambridge University Press, 2001.
177. Ellison JM, Gottlieb G: Recognition and management of late life mood disorders. In: Sirven JI, Malamut BL (eds): Clinical Neurology of the Older Adult. Philadelphia, Lippincott Williams & Wilkins, 2002; pp. 447–462.
178. Food interacting with MAO inhibitors. Med Lett Drugs Ther 1989; 31(785):11–12.
179. Ellison JM. Medications for mental disorders: A brief history and an overview of current uses. In: Ellison JM, ed. The Psychotherapist's Guide to Pharmacotherapy. Chicago, IL: Year Book Medical Publishers, 1989:119–143.

16 Electroconvulsive Therapy and Neurotherapeutic Treatments for Late-Life Mood Disorders

Stephen Seiner
ECT Clinic, McLean Hospital, Belmont, Massachusetts, U.S.A.

Anna Burke
Geriatric Psychiatry Program, McLean Hospital, Belmont, Massachusetts, U.S.A.

INTRODUCTION

Electroconvulsive therapy (ECT) is well established as one of the most powerful and evidence-based treatments for severe mood disorders, and yet it remains underutilized. Limitations of early ECT technique, adverse media portrayal, and a lack of education about the procedure have stigmatized ECT for decades, and significant advances in the procedure have not completely eliminated that stigma. Patients and family members are often surprised to learn that the procedure still is used, and may even be offended to have it recommended. This reaction may be particularly common among geriatric patients who remember the early stigma of ECT.

Severe depression, however, is a debilitating and often life-threatening disorder. Some patients with late-life depression respond poorly to standard psychotherapeutic and pharmacotherapeutic treatments. The geriatric patient is also more sensitive to the side effects of medications, due to changes in drug metabolism, protein binding, and receptor sensitivity associated with aging. Even when treatment might otherwise succeed, elderly patients' nonadherence can present an obstacle to a successful outcome. As a result, geriatric patients often require encouragement from their family members to get and keep them in treatment. Unfortunately, their support may not be mobilized until the patient has irretrievably lost many social supports and the family feels desperate. It is often out of this desperation that these patients and their family members are finally referred for an ECT consultation. They are usually frightened of the procedure but reassured when provided with the facts about ECT's good safety record, impressive efficacy, and relatively mild side effects in most patients.

While ECT is often a very effective and appropriate choice for treating late-life depression, it must be administered with great care. The risks associated with ECT are higher in elderly patients with significant underlying medical disease; however, with thoughtful evaluation and planning, most patients; even those with significant medical disease can undergo ECT with considerable safety.

INDICATIONS FOR ECT

Major Depression

Depression in the geriatric population requires special attention in several respects. The severity of geriatric depression can lead to increased medical morbidity and even mortality (1–3). The individuals often have lesser physical reserves to weather the poor nutrition and weight loss associated with depression, fewer social supports, and a decreased ability to rebuild their social network after isolating themselves during an episode of depression. They also have a higher suicide rate, as discussed elsewhere in this book (4,5). These factors combine to increase the urgency of successfully treating the depression. This urgency, compounded with the frequent medication intolerance observed in depressed elders (6,7), suggests that ECT should be routinely considered as a treatment for severely depressed older adults.

Efficacy data in geriatric patients strongly support the use of ECT. Several studies have reported that the elderly may have higher response rates to ECT than the general population (8). In a large, prospective, multisite study of 268 patients, Tew and colleagues reported a response rate of 54% for patients younger than 60 years, 73% for patients from 60 to 74 years, and 67% for those older than 75 years (8). Other studies also support the use of ECT in the "old old" population (older than 75 years of age), finding ECT to be a relatively safe, well-tolerated, and effective treatment in this age group, with response rates reaching as high as 85% (9,10). In a large, multisite, longitudinal study that reported remission rates for patients in different age groups receiving bilateral ECT for major depression, those aged 65 and older had a 90% remission rate while those aged 45 and younger showed a 70% remission rate (11).

The efficacy of ECT for depression in patients with concurrent dementia remains inadequately explored. Rao and Lyketsos, however, did study the effects of ECT on hospitalized patients who suffered from both dementia and depression (12) and found that ECT improved mood significantly by the time of discharge from the hospital. Although close to half of these patients developed delirium, there was a mean improvement in initial mini-mental status exam (MMSE) scores of 1.62 points by the time of discharge, suggesting that ECT did not worsen, and indeed might relieve, some of the cognitive impairment in these patients.

In small case studies and a recent preliminary retrospective study, ECT has also been reported to be effective in treating agitation and aggression in demented patients (13,14), This deserves further investigation and would be an important contribution to the field, as currently there are no FDA-indicated treatments for agitation in dementia. While behavioral interventions and/or medications can help many, there are patients for whom current treatments are inadequate and whose quality of life is unacceptable. These preliminary studies suggest that closely supervised ECT may be a reasonable option in those patients.

Psychotic Depression

ECT has consistently been shown to be an effective treatment for psychotic depression in the general population (15,16), and has been proposed by some as the first-line treatment for this condition when symptoms are severe or when oral medications are not an option (17). A study by Petrides and colleagues demonstrated that mixed-age psychotic depressed patients responded more quickly and robustly to ECT (bilateral) than did nonpsychotic depressed patients (18), with response rates as high as 95%. Literature reviews and meta-analyses support ECT as being at least as effective in treating psychotic depression as "combination medication" treatment—a combination of antidepressant and antipsychotic medications. They further support ECT as being significantly more effective than either antidepressant or antipsychotic monotherapy (19). In a study of late-life psychotic depression, ECT was shown to be significantly more effective than combination medication treatment (20). The paucity of data on newer pharmacologic options for treating psychotic depression highlights the need for systematic studies, including prospective comparisons to ECT.

OTHER SYNDROMES ASSOCIATED WITH LATE-LIFE DEPRESSION

Several syndromes, some of which are more prevalent in the geriatric population and related to depression in later life, are responsive to ECT. Parkinson disease has an extremely high rate of comorbid depression, reaching as high as 40% in some studies (21). ECT, by virtue of its ability to increase CNS dopamine turnover, may be uniquely effective in treating both the mood and the movement components of this condition (22–24). Maintenance ECT has also been reported to be helpful in case reports of patients with intractable or difficult-to-treat Parkinson disease (25,26).

Catatonia secondary to comorbid psychiatric conditions has also been shown to respond well to ECT, although ECT's effectiveness in treating catatonia due to medical or neurologic conditions has been less thoroughly studied (27). Possible neurologic and medical disorders underlying catatonia should be investigated thoroughly and treated as aggressively as possible prior to the use of ECT (27). A severe form of catatonia, known as malignant catatonia, has high associated rates of morbidity and mortality. ECT, which has been shown effective in treating malignant catatonia (28), should be considered an early treatment option. Neuroleptic malignant syndrome (NMS) may be related to malignant catatonia (29) and has been shown to be responsive to ECT in a review of the limited cases reported in the literature (30).

BIPOLAR DISORDER/BIPOLAR DEPRESSION

ECT has been shown to be effective for treatment of mania (31), mixed affective states (32), and bipolar depression (33) in mixed-age populations. The severity of bipolar episodes and the frequency with which affected individuals cycle between manic and depressive episodes tend to increase as bipolar patients age (34), making treatment more challenging and sometimes more urgent. Unfortunately, studies of ECT in geriatric bipolar patients are limited.

Mukherjee and colleagues reviewed 50 years of treatment of acute manic episodes with ECT, and concluded that ECT is associated with remission or marked improvement in approximately 80% of mixed-age manic patients, and can be helpful for manic patients who have not responded to pharmacologic treatments (31). The optimal placement of electrodes remains controversial, with some research supporting the preferential use of bilateral ECT for mania (35), while other studies have found right unilateral treatment to be effective as well (36).

Mixed bipolar mood states can be difficult to diagnose and particularly challenging to treat pharmacologically. Few studies have assessed ECT in mixed states, but the existing evidence appears to support its use in these patients. Devanand and colleagues found that 80% of patients with mixed affective states responded well to ECT, but they required longer hospital stays and a greater number of ECT treatments than bipolar depressed patients (32). Ciapparelli, however, in a larger study, found that medication nonresponsive patients with mixed symptoms responded well to ECT and demonstrated a more rapid and robust response than bipolar depressed patients (33). The differences in the results of these two studies may reflect differences in electrode placement. All patients received bilateral ECT in the latter study, whereas in the former some received unilateral while others received bilateral ECT or a combination.

In general adult populations, ECT has also been shown to be effective in bipolar depression (31,36). There is some evidence that bipolar depression may show a more rapid response and require fewer treatments than unipolar depression (37). Patients who appear to be responding early should be monitored closely for symptoms of emerging mania because all antidepressant treatments can occasionally precipitate mania (38).

SPECIAL ECT CONSIDERATIONS IN THE ELDERLY

The older patient presents some unique medical risks and psychologic concerns that the treatment team must assess prior to initiating ECT. Complex medical conditions including cardiac risk factors combined with pulmonary and orthopedic difficulties are often the rule rather than the exception. Dementia can certainly complicate the picture further, and often imposes an increased burden on the family, which may be required to assist with treatment decisions. Special attention needs to be paid to the family dynamics when an elderly parent is being treated with ECT.

Medical Concerns

In the general population, ECT is a very safe procedure. Its reported mortality rate is approximately 4 deaths per 100,000 treatments (39). There are no absolute contraindications to ECT, but several conditions increase the risks associated with treatment. These risks, however, must be weighed against the risks of untreated depression, which include increased cardiac risk (40), increased suicide risk (11,41), and increased overall medical morbidity and mortality (1–3). Without treatment, patients with unresponsive catatonia or severe psychotic depression often present a significant mortality and morbidity risk. In contrast, Philibert and colleagues reported that geriatric patients who received ECT had lower mortality rates at follow-up than those who had not received ECT (42).

Cardiac Illness

Perhaps the most common medical consideration in the elderly patients evaluated for ECT is cardiac disease. The rare deaths that occur during ECT are most often cardiac in nature (39). With careful planning, informed consent, and appropriate medical backup, patients with severe cardiac disease can be treated with relative safety. Zielinski and colleagues studied a series of depressed patients with serious cardiac disease who underwent ECT (43) and found a significantly increased rate of cardiac complications. Of 40 patients, they found 8 "major" complications including "persistent ECG changes lasting hours to days, accompanied by chest pain, asystole or persistent arrhythmias." Importantly though, they had no deaths, and 38 of the 40 patients were able to complete the study. In a retrospective study, Rice and colleagues examined 80 patients with cardiac risk factors who received ECT. They found that the high cardiac risk group had more minor complications, but no major complications (44).

Successful treatment of the depressed elderly patient with cardiac disease begins with a thorough history of cardiovascular symptoms, disease, and treatments. ECT affects the heart through the autonomic nervous system via the vagus nerve, sympathetic tract, and circulating catecholamines sequentially (45). This results in predictable fluctuations in cardiac rhythm, pulse, and blood pressure, during an average treatment.

Patients with major cardiac risk factors such as unstable or severe angina, recent myocardial infarction, significant arrhythmias, severe valvular disease, or decompensated congestive heart failure (46), present the greatest treatment-associated safety concerns. These patients should have medical stabilization, cardiology consultation, evaluation of ischemia and left ventricular function, and correction of the underlying pathology if possible, before ECT is performed (47). The nonevasive evaluation can include an exercise tolerance test or a pharmacologic stress test if the patient is unable to exercise, and, if needed, an echocardiogram. A thallium study as part of the stress test can be particularly helpful in determining the amount of myocardial tissue at risk. In patients with an intermediate risk profile (46), such as mild angina, prior (not recent) myocardial infarction, compensated congestive heart failure, or diabetes mellitus, a determination of functional status should take place. If the patient has good functional status, ECT can take place along with appropriate medical treatment (47). If functional status is poor, then a reassessment of the risk to benefit analysis is warranted. Cardiology consultation on these patients can help determine whether medical intervention to improve functional status should take place before ECT is attempted.

Immediately post-MI, vulnerable myocardial tissue and increased irritability and risk of arrhythmia need to be considered. ECT can transiently increase cardiac output and demand, stressing vulnerable tissue; therefore, it is preferable to avoid ECT in the immediate post-MI period. What constitutes the immediate post-MI period is unclear. The American College of Cardiology National Database Library defines a recent MI as one that occurred more than seven days, but less than one month ago (46). In general, the longer one can allow for the myocardial tissue to heal before ECT is initiated, the better. Given the high rate of post-MI depression and increased mortality associated with it (48,49), however, ECT may have to be considered in extreme cases during the post-MI period. Consultation with a cardiologist and careful planning with anesthesiology can make ECT an option in a controlled general hospital setting.

Hypertension is a frequent risk factor among geriatric ECT patients. Ideally, the patient's blood pressure should be optimized with daily medication before beginning ECT. For patients with a history of hypertension already controlled with blood pressure medication, it is usually best to continue the medication as scheduled throughout the ECT treatment period. Premedication with a β-blocker may help attenuate the hyperdynamic response of ECT (50,51), and can be considered in patients with excessively high blood pressures or tachycardia during ECT, especially in patients with known cardiovascular disease (52). Such measures, however, should be employed with caution as overly aggressive treatment of hypertension or tachycardia can contribute to asystole, bradycardia, or hypotension during phases of the treatment when parasympathetic tone is prominent.

Another potential complicating cardiac factor is the presence of an internal pacemaker or automatic implantable cardiac defibrillator. In general, ECT does not significantly affect pacemakers, but a magnet must be immediately accessible to override any abnormal signals, if necessary (52). Prior to a course of ECT, an automatic implantable cardiac defibrillator function should be turned off during treatments, although the pacemaker function should generally be left on (53).

Atrial fibrillation can be a concern as ECT may convert atrial fibrillation to normal sinus rhythm, at least transiently (54). For this reason, anticoagulation is a reasonable prophylactic measure to prevent a mural thrombus from embolizing.

Anticoagulation of some patients, for example, those at high risk for falls or gastrointestinal bleeding, may present an unacceptable risk. In these cases, and when the anticoagulation may not have been consistently at the proper level, transesophogeal echocardiogram can be helpful in identifying whether there is a mural thrombus that could increase the risk of embolic events. Whereas some have raised concerns regarding the risk of intracerebral hemorrhage with patients taking warfarin and receiving ECT (55), available data suggest low intracerebral hemorrhage risk for ECT in patients whose international normalized ratio is at a therapeutic level (54,56).

In summary, the presence of significant cardiac disease should alert the clinician to the need for a careful assessment to fully assess and minimize the risks of treatment with ECT. Consultation with a cardiologist and careful planning with the anesthesiologist usually lower the risk sufficiently to allow these patients to be treated successfully.

Pulmonary Illness

The use of a muscle relaxant during ECT necessitates that the patient be ventilated during the procedure, usually with simple masked ventilation. Preexisting lung pathology, however, can complicate this otherwise routine task. Any pulmonary complaint by elderly patients prior to or during a course of treatment with ECT must be evaluated.

Chronic obstructive pulmonary disease (COPD), asthma, pneumonia, bronchitis, and other lung diseases can increase the difficulty of maintaining adequate oxygen saturation, elevate the risk of bronchospasm, and increase demands on the heart. Pretreatment with bronchodilators can be helpful in treating patients with COPD and asthma (57). However, theophylline increases the risk of prolonged seizures and status epilepticus (58–60) and should be discontinued unless absolutely necessary. The treatment team should make every effort to optimize pulmonary function. This could include the use of inhalers or nebulizers to improve air exchange for COPD or asthma, preoxygenation for low oxygen saturation, and proper antibiotic treatment for infectious lung disease.

Gastrointestinal Disease

Peptic ulcer disease, gastritis, gastric reflux disease, or swallowing difficulties secondary to stroke or other neurologic disease can increase the risk of aspiration and/or laryngospasm in the elderly. Every effort should be made to limit aspiration risk as much as possible prior to the initiation of ECT. Examples include pretreatment with sodium citrate (antacid) to neutralize gastric contents, metoclopramide to increase gastric emptying, and H2 blockers or proton pump inhibitors to decrease acid production (53). Cricoid pressure is sometimes applied during the treatment to reduce the risk of aspiration in selective cases, but the effectiveness of this is uncertain (61). Pretreatment intubation can help to protect the airway during treatment of patients with more severe aspiration risk or with severe underlying lung disease, although this must be weighed against the risks of multiple intubations during a treatment course.

Musculoskeletal Disease

Since the adoption of muscle relaxants and anesthesia as routine elements of ECT, the risks of long bone fractures and other complications have dropped significantly.

Because of the relative fragility of bones, joints, and especially vertebrae in the elderly, careful attention must be paid to the timing and degree of muscle relaxation. Prior to treatment, it is important to evaluate and compensate for active vertebral disc disease, recent fractures, or significant spinal stenosis. Consultation with a neurologist or orthopedist may be appropriate. In many patients with musculoskeletal problems of these types, adequate dosing of the muscle relaxant can decrease complications and limit the risk of ECT (53).

Posttreatment falls are a potential side effect of ECT, possibly due to confusion, sedation, orthostasis due to pretreatment β-blockade, or memory loss. DeCarle and colleagues found the number of ECT treatments and a diagnosis of Parkinson disease to be two independent risk factors for falls in the elderly receiving ECT (62). Patients should be monitored closely prior to and during a course of ECT treatments to balance difficulties, confusion, orthostasis, sedation, and other signs that they may be at increased risk for falling.

Neurologic Disease

ECT alters regional blood flow to the brain (63) and brain metabolism (64), and it is unclear how these changes affect patients who have suffered a recent cerebrovascular accident (CVA).How soon ECT can safely be performed after a CVA, is unknown. Canine studies have suggested that it may take nine weeks for the margins of the infarction to fully heal; (65) in clinical practice, however, patients have been successfully treated with ECT within one month of having a CVA (66,67). One case report of ECT as early as 7 to 14 days poststroke has been reported (68). A retrospective study of 19 geriatric poststroke patients who received ECT showed acute improvement in 95% (69). Although five patients developed ECT-related medical complications, none experienced exacerbation of preexisting neurologic deficits. In another study, ECT produced marked improvement in 12 of 14 patients with depression and a history of stroke, and none showed worsening of their neurologic status (67). There are case reports of neurologic deficits arising during post-ECT recovery. These deficits, however, are rare and often transient (70).

Intracranial vascular lesions such as aneurysms or vascular malformations, space occupying lesions, or other causes of increased intracranial pressure should be considered to be associated with "substantially increased" risk according to the APA task force on ECT (53). The risks of herniation, intracranial bleed, or other neurologic complications, need to be weighed carefully against potential benefits of treatment. In some cases, provision of ECT may still be the most appropriate treatment option. A review by Salaris and colleagues, for example, found no adverse outcome during the ECT treatment of eight reported cases of patients with intracranial vascular masses (71). Instances of successful ECT have also been reported in patients with brain tumors and elevated intracranial pressure (72). Under such unusual and potentially hazardous circumstances, ECT typically requires an experienced anesthesiologist and consultation with a neurologist and/or neurosurgeon in order to assess and control the risk as much as possible. Further study is needed to fully understand the risks that brain tumors pose for patients undergoing ECT. With these patients, the psychiatrist, patient, and family need to consider carefully the risks and benefits associated with ECT, an alternative treatment, or no treatment.

In general, Parkinson disease responds positively to ECT treatment, as already described. Several studies have demonstrated that ECT can be helpful in treating not only the depression that is seen very commonly with Parkinson disease, but also that it can transiently relieve many of the neurologic symptoms as well. The effects of ECT on progressive supranuclear palsy are not as clear. Other neurologic illnesses such as multiple sclerosis, polio, and paralysis can present anesthesia risks, and input from the anesthesiologist is crucial to defining the degree of risk. While challenging, patients with these neurologic illnesses can often be treated effectively with ECT. There are case reports of ECT-precipitating episodes of neurologic deterioration in multiple sclerosis (73), but many multiple sclerosis patients have been successfully treated without short-term neurologic complication (74). The long-term effect of ECT on the course of multiple sclerosis is unknown. This should be part of the risk to benefit ratio calculation when assessing a depressed multiple sclerosis patient for ECT.

Malignancies

Depression is common in cancer patients, occurring in as many as a quarter of them (75), and ECT has been used to treat depression successfully in patients with various forms of cancer (76,77). One major concern that arises in using ECT in patients with systemic cancer is the risk of treating when cerebral metastases may affect safety. When there is evidence of current or even a history of cancers with a high likelihood of metastasis to the brain, especially lung cancer, breast cancer, and melanoma (78), it is particularly prudent to consider neuroimaging of the brain. While special attention needs to be paid to tumors that have high rates of central nervous system metastasis, other systemic tumors may also raise clinicians' concern. As the treatment of systemic tumors continues to improve and patients survive longer, the incidence of central nervous system involvement can be expected to rise for most types of tumors (78), and neuroimaging, therefore, may be considered in patients with other types of systemic tumors as well. Focal neurologic findings on physical examination of any patient with a history of systemic cancer should raise serious concern about central nervous system metastases, warranting further neurologic assessment, likely to include neuroimaging. As depression can be a secondary neurologic symptom of a brain tumor, it is reasonable to image the brain of any patient with a history of systemic cancer and new onset of depression.

Because ECT has been performed in patients with brain lesions, the discovery of a brain metastasis does not absolutely prohibit ECT treatment. Of course, if a brain lesion is discovered in the pre-ECT workup, the potential prognosis and specific treatment of the lesion must be addressed, as well as the possibility that the lesion may be contributing to the mood symptoms that initially prompted the ECT consultation. The oncology team may feel that treatment of the tumor is a priority in increasing the overall chances of survival. Should the decision be made to proceed with ECT, knowledge of the existence of a brain metastasis can help the treatment team to prepare appropriately for ECT.

Memory Loss

Memory loss is perhaps the most frequent concern expressed by patients and family members who are contemplating ECT, regardless of age. Typically, the memory loss is mild and usually resolves after the ECT has ended. In some studies that have examined patients several months after ECT, no sustained cognitive disturbances were found (79–81). A review of 39 papers addressing the long-term memory effects of ECT found that the majority of studies suggested that ECT does not typically cause long-term memory deficits, although a small number of studies did find some deficits months after ECT, particularly in personal autobiographic material (82). A more recent prospective naturalistic study examined ECT practiced in the community, and found that sustained autobiographic memory loss was found more often with bilateral ECT than with unilateral brief pulse ECT (83). When seen with bilateral ECT, the amount of memory loss did correlate with number of treatments. While geriatric patients are thought to be at higher risk for memory loss during ECT due to a presumed decrease in cognitive reserve, studies have shown elderly patients often tolerate the cognitive effects of ECT very well (84,85). Perhaps because cognition can be adversely affected by severe depression, some studies have shown improved cognition after ECT (86,87).

The risk of memory loss becomes an even bigger concern when patients already have some memory loss or dementia at baseline. ECT can be performed when patients have dementia, but particular care has to be taken to monitor memory throughout the course of treatment and respond to the emergence of short-term confusion or frank delirium that may develop. While there is no clear consensus on the best way to reduce ECT-associated memory loss in the elderly with baseline cognitive impairment, the following basic guidelines should be considered:

1. *Prescreen cognitive functioning:* Documenting baseline cognitive impairment, if present, allows for reasonable expectations regarding post-ECT memory function and prevents preexisting memory deficits from being attributed to ECT. The form of cognitive testing depends on the patient and can range from simple memory testing to formal neuropsychological testing.
2. *Monitor memory throughout treatment:* This can include formal testing, but observations of caregivers can be even more important. More frequent episodes of getting lost, forgetting things, or becoming confused are important to note. Helpful questions to ask the patient routinely include questions about recent events, daily activities, and orientation. These can easily be incorporated into the standard discussion about mood and overall improvement with the patient prior to each treatment.
3. *Consider decreasing the frequency of treatments:* When significant and disruptive memory loss is noted, or if considerable memory loss was present prior to treatments, it is very reasonable to decrease the frequency of the treatments in the acute course from three times weekly to twice or even once a week. There is evidence that twice-a-week treatment can be as effective with less memory loss than three-times-a-week treatment, although the response to treatment may be less rapid (88,89). With increasing pressure to decrease the length of hospitalization stays, treatment teams are sometimes reluctant to slow down treatment, but it should be remembered that marked confusion can interrupt ECT and result in longer hospitalizations when it is necessary to wait for a patient to re-stabilize cognitively. Some patients can also be treated as outpatients if adequate supports can be arranged.
4. *Favor unilateral over bilateral treatment when reasonable:* Unilateral treatments are associated with less memory loss and little confusion (90,91), and should be used preferentially, if possible. Mixed or manic episodes, a history of nonresponse to unilateral treatments, or very high seizure thresholds, however, may lead to preferential treatment with bilateral placement. In such patients, strong consideration should be given to a decreased frequency of treatment in dementia patients undergoing bilateral ECT. More recently, ultrabrief pulse unilateral

ECT has been gaining popularity in order to limit the cognitive effects of ECT (92). Despite limited controlled data, many centers are using this technique of reducing the width of the pulse delivered to 0.3 ms, while compensating with adjustments in the frequency and duration of the stimulus train. This technique attempts to deliver a more efficient seizure and better control the effects on cognition. While some centers are reporting significant success (93,94), the question of whether this technique is as effective as typical brief pulse, unilateral has not been clearly answered. Moreover, elderly patients, especially those with some degree of cortical atrophy, as in dementia, are expected to have higher seizure thresholds, and it is unknown whether ultrabrief pulse would be as effective under these circumstances. Minimal data for the geriatric population, especially those with dementia, are available to guide treaters. Controlled trials are desperately needed in order to validate the use of this technique in the cognitively impaired elderly.

5. *Set expectations with patient and family:* This is advisable in all cases, and of special importance for patients with dementia. Worsening memory loss and/or confusion is very upsetting to most patients and families, and education about this possibility ahead of time as well as reassurance during the course of treatment can be extremely helpful and is a good clinical practice.

PSYCHOLOGICAL ISSUES

The following sections address psychological issues, including making the decision about ECT and family involvement in the ECT process.

Making the Decision

Suggesting ECT to a geriatric patient can present formidable challenges for a number of reasons. Geriatric patients spent much of their adult lives during a time when the idea of "shock treatments" was even more stigmatized than it is now. In addition, geriatric depression may be hidden behind somatic symptoms, making it more difficult to diagnose. Perhaps the most difficult obstacle occurs when patients have somatic ruminations or delusions, and refuse ECT because they feel their difficulties are all medical rather than psychiatric. Providing education, establishing an alliance between the patient and treatment team, and involving the family can be helpful with delusional patients.

Patients, family, and physicians are often indecisive about somatic treatment of depressive symptoms when the patient's circumstances, which may for example, include multiple recent losses, bring into question the appropriateness of a diagnosis of major depressive disorder. While it is important to acknowledge losses, a patient who shows symptoms of a complicated bereavement including depressed mood, severe vegetative symptoms, suicidal ideation, and/or psychosis warrants a diagnosis of major depressive disorder and aggressive intervention. When ECT is performed in such patients, particular attention has to be paid to limit memory loss as much as possible, as patients worry about losing recent memories about their loved ones. If the loss is a very recent one, it may be worthwhile to delay ECT, if possible, to decrease the risk of jeopardizing these memories. Occasionally, patients will forget about the loss of their loved one immediately after an ECT treatment, and then feel retraumatized as the memory soon returns. These issues need to be discussed carefully with the patient and family before proceeding with ECT.

Some patients may have had complications during ECT they received years ago, before the introduction of anesthesia and muscle relaxants. Others may have seen movies from decades ago that portrayed ECT without anesthesia or used as a punitive procedure. They will need education about the advances in ECT and anesthesia, as well as its clinical indications, in order to make an informed decision.

Family Involvement

Depressed patients frequently worry about being a "burden" to their families, and do not want their families to be concerned or involved. While it is important to respect patient's decisions about this, in general it is very important to have the family involved in the decision about ECT. Sometimes family members disagree about ECT—a situation better addressed early rather than ignored. A family meeting that educates about ECT and addresses family concerns can be very helpful. Otherwise, family members may not realize and may disagree until partway through the ECT course, when this disagreement may escalate and cause an interruption or cessation of the ECT. A patient's refusal of ECT in order to pacify family members who disagree about the need for this procedure can sometimes be avoided with simple family education.

Whenever there are conflicts between the wishes of the patient and those of the family, the patient's preference takes precedence as long as the patient has demonstrated the capacity to provide a valid informed consent. When the patient is not competent to make such decisions, an authorized health care representative such as a health care proxy, guardian, or judge should become involved in making this decision. Legal consultation around this issue usually defines the pertinent statutes and issues to be addressed prior to proceeding with treatment. In general, every effort should be made to bring the patient, treatment team, and family together with a unified plan.

MAINTENANCE TREATMENT

One of the biggest challenges for the ECT practitioner is to determine how to keep the patient better, once improved with the acute ECT course. Some patients may have a course of ECT and need no further pharmacologic or ECT treatment, but they are the minority. Most patients referred for ECT have had multiple medication trials and often have long histories of recurrent depression. Therefore, relapse rates following ECT can be very high (95). For patients with relapsing or recurrent mood disorders, some form of maintenance treatment is usually warranted, and this may include antidepressant pharmacologic treatment, intensive psychotherapy or psychosocial intervention, maintenance ECT, or some combination of these.

Pharmacologic Maintenance

Medications are the most typical form of maintenance treatment following ECT. Given that many ECT patients have already failed multiple medication trials, however, it can be difficult to choose an effective medication regimen. Relapse rates of patients receiving medication maintenance following ECT appears to be related to medication resistance prior to ECT (96,97). If the pre-ECT regimen has been ineffective, it is usually advisable to switch or augment the regimen following ECT. Combination medication strategies, such as nortriptyline and lithium salts, have been shown to have some success in reducing post-ECT relapse rates in medication resistant or psychotic depressed patients (95), decreasing relapse rates from

84% to 39% at 24 weeks post-ECT. Such combinations, however, can sometimes be difficult for elderly patients to tolerate. Because many patients have not had trials with monoamine oxidase inhibitors (MAOIs) that can be effective in cases of treatment-resistant depression (TRD) (98,99), this class of drugs may be appropriate to consider for post-ECT maintenance pharmacologic treatment. In addition, ECT can be used to treat the depression during the washout period needed to switch from another antidepressant to an MAOI. MAOIs can be difficult to tolerate due to the orthostatic effects, and great care needs to be taken in monitoring elderly patients initiated on this type of medication. This is especially true given that the potential short term memory loss from ECT may interfere with adherence to the dietary modifications required with MAO inhibitor treatment. Therefore, it is often advisable to have a family member helping to monitor the medication and diet at home, and who can alert the physician if there are problems managing these issues. Many geriatric patients, however, tolerate MAOIs without difficulty.

In general, psychotic depression has a higher relapse rate than nonpsychotic depression (100,101), and this appears to hold true in the geriatric population as well (93). Therefore, aggressive treatment following ECT is appropriate. Some evidence suggests that early withdrawal of the antipsychotic medication post-ECT may result in higher relapse rates in these patients (102). Therefore, in patients with psychotic depression, antipsychotic treatment following ECT for some extended maintenance period of several months, or even years in some cases, is usually helpful, and when withdrawn, should be tapered slowly with very close monitoring.

Maintenance or Continuation ECT

Some patients who have demonstrated medication resistance or intolerance of medication side effects choose to continue with ECT on a continuation or maintenance ECT basis. The aim of continuation ECT is very much like tapering a medication after successful treatment. The rate of the taper should be tailored to each individual patients needs, but often consists of weekly treatments following the acute course for two to four weeks, and then tapering that as tolerated. The goal of this may vary. For many patients, the aim is to prolong the ECT effect until an adequate maintenance medication regimen can be found. If the patient begins to show signs of relapse when the time between treatments is extended, it may represent the need for medication adjustment. The advantage of the continuation ECT in this example is that the ECT can be used to prevent relapse and rehospitalization while the medication adjustment is made. Once a patient appears stable on medication without relapse with monthly or greater intervals between ECT, the ECT is discontinued. Other patients are tired of multiple medication trials and side effects and are content to receive monthly maintenance treatments indefinitely. Some patients choose ongoing maintenance treatments because of recurrent relapse when ECT is discontinued. These patients and their outpatient treaters are instructed to report any early signs of relapse, as an adjustment of the treatment schedule to include a few closely spaced treatments can often prevent relapse (103).

Substantial evidence supports the efficacy of continuation or maintenance ECT treatment in preventing relapse (103–105). One recent study examined long-term follow-up of chronically depressed patients who had responded to an acute course of ECT. At two years, those who received continuation ECT with antidepressant treatment had a survival rate without relapse or recurrence of 93%, compared to 52% for those on antidepressant treatment alone (104). Another study found that 1-year relapse rates for patients with psychotic depression dropped from 95% to 42% following the institution of continuation ECT for these patients at their facility (105).

Psychosocial Maintenance

In examining data regarding the effectiveness of pharmacologic or ECT maintenance treatment, the contribution of psychosocial factors should not be ignored. Treatment interventions such as individual psychotherapy, group therapy, social day programs, increased family involvement, or a move to a more suitable home environment are often combined with ECT and enhance its effectiveness. The collaborative involvement of a psychotherapist, day program, or geriatric care manager is likely to synergize with ECT maintenance treatment to produce an optimal outcome over an extended course of treatment.

SUMMARY

ECT is a powerful treatment that should be considered as an option in geriatric patients with mood disorders when other therapeutic options have failed, or when the illness is so severe that delay in treatment can be life-threatening. As with any serious treatment, the risks and potential benefits need to be reviewed carefully with the patient and family. Elderly patients can present with medical or neurologic problems that put them at somewhat higher risk with ECT, but in most patients these problems can be managed safely. Furthermore, because these patients are also at significant medical risk from the depression itself, and may be more sensitive to the side effects of many antidepressants, the decision to not treat with ECT may in many cases present significant risk to the severely depressed geriatric patient.

NEUROTHERAPEUTIC TECHNIQUES

While ECT remains the gold standard therapy for TRD, several new somatic interventions have shown promise in patients who have failed multiple medication trials. Studies of the efficacy of these new therapies, often referred to as "neurotherapeutics" or "neuromodulation," have been carried out primarily in adult populations. Minimal data are available at this time to guide the use of these treatments for patients with bipolar mood disorders. Although further study in the elderly is needed, preliminary efficacy data for these interventions justifies their mention here.

Vagus Nerve Stimulation

Vagus nerve stimulation (VNS) is the first FDA-approved implanted device for the treatment of a psychiatric disorder. VNS treatment is administered using a pacemaker-like device that is surgically implanted in the left chest wall, where it delivers an electrical signal via an implanted lead that is wrapped around the left cervical vagus nerve. No portion of the device is in the brain, but because 80% of the fibers in the vagus nerve are afferent, intermittent stimulation of the vagus nerve provides chronic bilateral activation of brain circuits. The vagus nerve sends sensory information from the periphery to the brain, including the locus ceruleus (a major source of norepinephrine in the brain), the raphe nuclei (the main source of serotonin in the brain), and the nucleus tractus solitarius (106). Functional brain imaging studies indicate that VNS induces changes in regional cerebral blood flow that are similar to changes seen with antidepressant treatment (107–108).

The most common side effects resulting from VNS are voice alteration (reported by approximately 55% of patients), increased cough, dyspnea, laryngisimus, neck pain, dysphagia, and paresthesia. Rare but serious adverse effects included cases of ventricular asystole when the device is tested during the implantation procedure in the operating room. However, no long-term negative outcomes resulted in these cases (109). Contraindications to VNS therapy include a history of bilateral or left cervical vagotomy and receiving diathermy.

Although the procedure was initially approved by the FDA in 2001 for treatment of epilepsy, it was soon noted that many of the patients treated with VNS experienced an improvement in mood. (110,111). Following multiple clinical trials, the FDA approved the use of VNS for TRD in 2005. The first of these clinical trials compared adjunctive VNS therapy to sham treatment in patients with TRD. All patients continued to receive treatment as usual (TAU) in addition to active VNS or sham VNS treatment. There were 112 patients in the active VNS treatment group, and 110 patients receiving sham VNS treatment for a period of 8 weeks. In this short-term study, VNS therapy failed to exhibit statistically significant efficacy (112). However, patients in both groups (a total of 205 patients) went on to receive open active adjunctive treatment with VNS therapy for one year. At one year, 27.2% of patients responded, and 15.8% met criteria for remission. In addition, the rates of response and remission doubled from 3 months to 12 months, suggesting that longer-term treatment may be required with VNS (113). Finally, the patients who had TRD receiving adjunctive VNS therapy during the 1-year follow-up study were compared with a matched group of 124 patients who had TRD and who received only TAU. The difference in response rates with VNS plus TAU (19.6%) versus TAU only (12.1%) was not statistically significant. There was, however, a statistically significant difference between remission rates with VNS therapy plus TAU (13.2%) and TAU alone (3.2%) (114).

Several questions have been posed in interpreting the data from the forementioned studies. First, could the long-term improvements be due to placebo effects? It is unlikely that placebo effects would occur in 20% to 35% of treatment-resistant, chronically ill patients and would increase over time. Rather, they would be expected to appear acutely and then wane over time. Second, could the resulting long-term improvement be naturally occurring? The waxing and waning of symptoms in depressive disorders is well established. However, the treatment resistant nature of the illness exhibited by the subjects in the studies in addition to evidence from multiple studies of long-term medication trials revealing a decrease rather than an increase in treatment efficacy over time, even in non-TRD patients, makes this unlikely. Hence, VNS appears to provide modest but sustained improvement in mood symptoms that cannot be accounted for by a placebo effect or the natural course of the depressive disorder itself.

VNS may be considered in individuals with both unipolar and bipolar, severe, chronic, recurrent depression that has not responded to at least four adequate antidepressant trials. The effects of VNS on rapid cycling bipolar disorder are still under investigation. No trials have specifically assessed efficacy in the geriatric population at present. Unlike other neurotherapeutic interventions mentioned in this chapter, VNS is not considered an acute treatment for affective disorders, but rather may present a viable long-term treatment option.

Repetitive Transcranial Magnetic Stimulation

Initially used by neurologists as a research instrument to assess central nerve conduction pathways, repetitive transcranial magnetic stimulation (rTMS) is slowly establishing itself as an efficacious tool in the acute treatment of major depressive disorder. Though currently approved for treatment of TRD in Canada, Australia, New Zealand, the European Union, and Israel, its use remains experimental in the United States.

In 2007, Neuronetics, Inc. submitted a premarket notification to the FDA, evaluating the safety and effectiveness of the NeuroStar(TM) rTMS System in a 3-phase clinical trial. The FDA panel stated that they "believed that the study data for the NeuroStar(TM) System did not establish a risk to benefit profile that was comparable to the risk to benefit profile of the predicate device, ECT, because effectiveness had not been demonstrated. The Panel agreed that the safety profile of the device was better than of ECT devices. Some Panel members believed that the device showed a signal of effectiveness and that it would be worth pursuing another study to demonstrate effectiveness."

There have now been multiple blinded, sham-controlled studies evaluating the efficacy of rTMS as a treatment for depression in adults, with many reporting that rTMS applied to the left dorsal lateral prefrontal cortex significantly improved MDD symptoms (115,116,117). However, due to numerous variations in how the procedure is performed as well as small sample sizes (the number of subjects included in studies ranged from 2 to 71), comparing studies is difficult. Of the seven published meta-analyses (118–124), six found that rTMS was effective for treating depression when compared with sham controls. Most studies were two weeks long. However, a few longer studies have suggested that a better outcome may be associated with longer treatment duration.

In a study of particular interest with respect to late-life depression, Jorge and colleagues (125) reported positive effects of rTMS on older patients with clinically defined vascular depression. Ninety-two patients were randomly assigned to receive active or sham rTMS of the left dorsolateral-prefrontal cortex. In experiment 1, at a total cumulative dose of 12,000 pulses, the sham group showed a 13.6% decrease in HAMD-17 scores compared with a 33.1% decrease in the group receiving rTMS Response rates were 6.7% in the sham group as compared to 33.3% in the active treatment group. Remission rates were 6.7% and 13.3%, respectively. In experiment 2, a higher dose of rTMS produced more significant results. At a total cumulative dose of 18,000 pulses, response rates were 6.9% in the sham group and 39.4% in the active rTMS group. Remission rates were 3.5% and 27.3%, respectively. Older age and smaller frontal gray matter volumes correlated with a poorer response to rTMS.

The rTMS device works by emitting a rapidly alternating current that passes through a small coil placed over the patient's scalp. This generates a magnetic field that induces an electric field in underlying areas of the brain (usually the prefrontal cortex). Ionic currents are generated and neuronal depolarization occurs. This focal stimulation that does not result in a seizure or require anesthesia differs from the global stimulation induced by ECT. Several neuroimaging studies have found abnormal metabolism or perfusion in the prefrontal cortex of patients with major depressive disorder (126,127), a neuroanatomic region easily accessible by rTMS. rTMS is believed to exert its effects on depressive disorders by altering regional cerebral blood flow in the prefrontal cortex and other brain structures involved in modulating mood, such as the anterior cingulate, thalamus, and the periinsular cortex.

Although additional studies are warranted in the geriatric population, rTMS seems to offer a potentially effective treatment option for mood disorders with no significant cognitive or cardiac sequelae. The most common adverse effects of the procedure were headache and neck pain, which were also reported by subjects undergoing sham treatment. A rare but serious side effect, noted on eight occasions, was seizures. These were attributed to stimulation of the primary motor cortex using settings outside the currently published guidelines or due to the use of seizure threshold lowering medications.

Deep Brain Stimulation

Used for more than a decade as a treatment for Parkinson disease, Deep Brain stimulation (DBS) has recently spurred the interest of the medical community as a therapeutic option for TRD after it was noted to provoke depressive and manic states in individuals without psychiatric illness (128). Early theories suggested that the antidepressant effect of DBS was related to repeated stimulation leading to inactivation of overactive voltage-dependent ion channels and thus reduction in impulse generation, coinciding with marked reduction in local cerebral blood flow on PET. Although initial studies involved stimulation of the subthalamic nucleus and internal globus pallidus, the subgenual cingulated region (Brodman area 25) has been the recent focus of DBS in depressed patients, due to its connections to the brainstem, insula, hypothalamus, orbitofrontal, cingulate, and medial prefrontal cortices, all of which have been implicated in leading to various depressive symptoms. Decreased activity in Brodman area 25 has also been reported in responders to ECT, rTMS, SSRIs, and ablation surgeries.

In 2005, Mayberg et al. performed an open pilot trial in six TRD patients. They implanted DBS bilaterally in the white matter fibers connecting to Brodman area 25 (subgenual cingulate gyrus), and used the generators to essentially cause a focal ablation of function. After stimulation for six months, while still on medications, three of six patients had remitted and an additional one met criteria for response. The study results suggest that disrupting focal pathologic activity in limbic-cortical circuits using electrical stimulation of the subgenual cingulate white matter can effectively reverse symptoms in otherwise treatment-resistant depression (129). Despite Mayberg's promising results, remission rates more than 50% appear to be uncommon.

The most common side effects reported are associated with the implantation procedure itself and include infection of implantation site, skin erosion, subcutaneaous seroma, intracerebral hematoma, and extension cable discomfort. However, more concerning questions have been raised by Burkhard et al. who reported six cases of completed suicide over a 9-year period in 140 patients with movement disorders treated with DBS (130). Five had a history of severe depression and four were on medication or being seen by a psychiatrist at the time of death.

DBS is still considered experimental and is not FDA approved for the treatment of psychiatric disorders. Although data is available regarding treatment efficacy and safety in geriatric movement disorders, little evidence exists as to the treatment's efficacy in geriatric affective disorders. Further studies will shed light, too, on the relative effectiveness of DBS in comparison to ECT.

Ablative Limbic System Surgery

The mere mention of psychosurgery can conjure up nightmarish images of repressive mind control. Because frontal lobotomy was administered without adequate empirical support or appropriate assessment for a period during the mid-twentieth century, many current elders recall the harmful effects this procedure produced as a result of misguided use at the height of its popularity, during its period of inappropriately widespread use.

Nonetheless, modern day neurosurgical interventions, including anterior cingulotomy, anterior capsulotomy, subcaudate tractotomy, and limbic leucotomy use craniotomy and gamma knife techniques to create target lesions in specifically defined regions of the brain. There is considerable evidence from neuroimaging studies that areas within the anterior cingulate cortex are functionally and structurally abnormal in patients with major depressive disorder. Strategically placed lesions, therefore, appear to target and modify function within such regions.

Depending on response criteria, response rates have been reported to range from 35% to 70% over a period of several weeks to months (131–135). However, to date, studies have focused on younger adult rather than elderly subjects. Common adverse effects present after surgery include headache, nausea, and edema, and are usually transient. More rare but serious side effects may include cerebral hemorrhage or infarct, cognitive deficits, deficit in emotion-recognition accuracy, seizures, infection, urinary difficulties, and weight gain.

SUMMARY

While these novel neurotherapeutic techniques have not yet proven themselves to be as effective as ECT for the treatment of severe late-life depression, they offer hope for those unresponsive to ECT or unable or unwilling to have ECT. Also, they offer important and fascinating information about the neuroanatomy and neurobiology of depression. This information may lead to advances not only in our treatment of depression but in our understanding of the illness, which in turn could lead to the improved overall care of the depressed elderly person.

REFERENCES

1. Schulz R, Beach SR, Ives DG, et al. Association between depression and mortality in older adults: The Cardiovascular Health Study. Arch Intern Med 2000; 160(12):1761–1768.
2. Penninx BW, Geerlings SW, Deeg DJ, et al. Minor and major depression and the risk of death in older persons. Arch Gen Psychiatry 1999; 56(10):889–895.
3. Lee Y, Choi K, Lee YK. Association of comorbidity with depressive symptoms in community-dwelling older persons. Gerontology 2001; 47(5):254–262.
4. Milic CT. Age as a suicide risk factor. Vojnosanit Pregl 2000; 57(2):191–195.
5. Lloyd L, Armour PK, Smith RJ. Suicide in Texas: A cohort analysis of trends in suicide rates, 1945- 1980. Suicide Life Threat Behav 1987; 17(3):205–217.
6. Katz IR, Simpson GM, Curlik SM, et al. Pharmacologic treatment of major depression for elderly patients in residential care settings. J Clin Psychiatry 1990; 51(suppl):41–47; discussion 48.
7. Peabody CA, Whiteford HA, Hollister LE. Antidepressants and the elderly. J Am Geriatr Soc 1986; 34(12):869–874.
8. Tew JD, Jr, Mulsant BH, Haskett RF, et al. Acute efficacy of ECT in the treatment of major depression in the old-old. Am J Psychiatry 1999; 156(12):1865–1870.

9. Manly DT, Oakley SP, Jr, Bloch RM. Electroconvulsive therapy in old-old patients. Am J Geriatr Psychiatry 2000; 8(3):232–236.
10. Gormley N. ECT should be treatment option in all cases of refractory depression. Bmj 1998; 316(7126):233.
11. O'Connor MK, Knapp R, Husain M, et al. The influence of age on the response of major depression to electroconvulsive therapy: A C. O.R.E. Report. Am J Geriatr Psychiatry 2001; 9(4):382–390.
12. Rao V, Lyketsos CG. The benefits and risks of ECT for patients with primary dementia who also suffer from depression. Int J Geriatr Psychiatry 2000; 15(8):729–735.
13. Grant JE, Mohan SN. Treatment of agitation and aggression in four demented patients using ECT. J ECT 2001; 17(3):205–209.
14. Ujkaj M, Forester B, Seiner SJ, et al. Safety and efficacy of Electroconvulsive Therapy (ECT) for the treatment of agitation and other behavioral complications of dementia. Poster Presentation. American Association for Geriatric Psychiatry Meeting, Orlando, FL. March 16, 2008.
15. Coryell W. The treatment of psychotic depression. J Clin Psychiatry 1998; 59(suppl 1):22–27; discussion 28–29.
16. Coryell W. Psychotic depression. J Clin Psychiatry 1996; 57(suppl 3):27–31; discussion 49.
17. Iwanami A, Oyamada S, Shirayama Y, et al. Algorithms for the pharmacotherapy psychotic depression. Psychiatry Clin Neurosci 1999; 53(suppl):S45–S48.
18. Petrides G, Fink M, Husain MM, et al. ECT remission rates in psychotic versus nonpsychotic depressed patients: A report from CORE. J ECT 2001; 17(4):244–253.
19. Parker G, Roy K, Hadzi-Pavlovic D, et al. Psychotic (delusional) depression: A meta-analysis of physical treatments. J Affect Disord 1992; 24(1):17–24.
20. Flint AJ, Rifat SL. The treatment of psychotic depression in later life: A comparison of pharmacotherapy and ECT. Int J Geriatr Psychiatry 1998; 13(1):23–28.
21. Cummings JL, Masterman DL. Depression in patients with Parkinson's disease. Int J Geriatr Psychiatry 1999; 14(9):711–718.
22. Glue P, Costello MJ, Pert A, et al. Regional neurotransmitter responses after acute and chronic electroconvulsive shock. Psychopharmacology 1990; 100(1):60–65.
23. Fall PA, Ekman R, Granerus AK, et al. ECT in Parkinson's disease. Changes in motor symptoms, monoamine metabolites and neuropeptides. J Neural Transm Park Dis Dement Sect 1995; 10(2–3):129–140.
24. Moellentine C, Rummans T, Ahlskog JE, et al. Effectiveness of ECT in patients with parkinsonism. J Neuropsychiatry Clin Neurosci 1998; 10(2):187–193.
25. Fall PA, Granerus AK. Maintenance ECT in Parkinson's disease. J Neural Transm 1999; 106(7–8):737–741.
26. Wengel SP, Burke WJ, Pfeiffer RF, et al. Maintenance electroconvulsive therapy for intractable Parkinson's disease. Am J Geriatr Psychiatry 1998; 6(3):263–269.
27. Rummans T. Medical indications for electroconvulsive therapy. Psychiatric Annals 1993; 23(1):27–32.
28. Mann S, Caroff S. Electroconvulsive therapy of the lethal catatonia syndrome: Case report and review. Convuls Ther 1990; 6(3):239–247.
29. Fink M. Toxic serotonin syndrome or neuroleptic malignant syndrome? Pharmacopsychiatry 1996; 29(4):159–161.
30. Trollor JN, Sachdev PS. Electroconvulsive treatment of neuroleptic malignant syndrome: A review and report of cases. Aust N Z J Psychiatry 1999; 33(5):650–659.
31. Mukherjee S, Sackeim HA, Schnur DB. Electroconvulsive therapy of acute manic episodes: A review of 50 years' experience. Am J Psychiatry 1994; 151(2):169–176.
32. Devanand DP, Polanco P, Cruz R, et al. The efficacy of ECT in mixed affective states. J ECT 2000; 16(1):32–37.
33. Ciapparelli A, Dell'Osso L, Tundo A, et al. Electroconvulsive therapy in medication-nonresponsive patients with mixed mania and bipolar depression. J Clin Psychiatry 2001; 62(7):552–555.

34. Satlin A, Liptzin B. Diagnosis and treatment of mania. In: Salzman C, ed. Clinical Geriatric Psychopharmacology. Baltimore, MD: Williams and Wilkins, 1998:310.
35. Small JG, Small IF, Milstein V, et al. Manic symptoms: An indication for bilateral ECT. Biol Psychiatry 1985; 20(2):125–134.
36. Black DW, Winokur G, Nasrallah A. Treatment of mania: A naturalistic study of electroconvulsive therapy versus lithium in 438 patients. J Clin Psychiatry 1987; 48(4):132–139.
37. Daly JJ, Prudic J, Devanand DP, et al. ECT in bipolar and unipolar depression: Differences in speed of response. Bipolar Disord 2001; 3(2):95–104.
38. Serby M. Manic reactions to ECT. Am J Geriatr Psychiatry 2001; 9(2):180.
39. Abrams R. The mortality rate with ECT. Convuls Ther 1997; 13(3):125–127.
40. Avery D, Winokur G. The efficacy of electroconvulsive therapy and antidepressants in depression. Biol Psychiatry 1977; 12(4):507–523.
41. Coppen A. Lithium in unipolar depression and the prevention of suicide. J Clin Psychiatry 2000; 61(suppl 9):52–56.
42. Philibert RA, Richards L, Lynch CF, et al. Effect of ECT on mortality and clinical outcome in geriatric unipolar depression. J Clin Psychiatry 1995; 56(9):390–394.
43. Zielinski RJ, Roose SP, Devanand DP, et al. Cardiovascular complications of ECT in depressed patients with cardiac disease. Am J Psychiatry 1993; 150(6):904–909.
44. Rice EH, Sombrotto LB, Markowitz JC, et al. Cardiovascular morbidity in high-risk patients during ECT. Am J Psychiatry 1994; 151(11):1637–1641.
45. Welch C, LJ D. Cardiovascular Effects of ECT. Convuls Ther 1989; 5(1):35–43.
46. Eagle KA, Brundage BH, Chaitman BR, et al. Guidelines for perioperative cardiovascular evaluation for noncardiac surgery. Report of the American College of Cardiology/American Heart Association Task Force on Practice Guidelines. Committee on Perioperative Cardiovascular Evaluation for Noncardiac Surgery. Circulation 1996; 93(6):1278–1317.
47. Applegate RJ. Diagnosis and management of ischemic heart disease in the patient scheduled to undergo electroconvulsive therapy. Convuls Ther 1997; 13(3):128–144.
48. Frasure-Smith N, Lesperance F, Talajic M. Depression following myocardial infarction. Impact on 6-month survival. JAMA 1993; 270(15):1819–1825.
49. Frasure-Smith N, Lesperance F, Talajic M. Depression and 18-month prognosis after myocardial infarction. Circulation 1995; 91(4):999–1005.
50. Castelli I, Steiner LA, Kaufmann MA, et al. Comparative effects of esmolol and labetalol to attenuate hyperdynamic states after electroconvulsive therapy. Anesth Analg 1995; 80(3):557–561.
51. Zvara DA, Brooker RF, McCall WV, et al. The effect of esmolol on ST-segment depression and arrhythmias after electroconvulsive therapy. Convuls Ther 1997; 13(3):165–174.
52. Dolinski S, Zvara D. Anesthetic considerations of cardiovascular risk during electroconvulsive therapy. Convuls Ther 1997; 13(3):157–164.
53. The Practice of Electroconvulsive Therapy. Recommendations for Treatment, Training, and Privileging: A Task Force Report of the American Psychiatric Association, 2nd ed. Washington, D.C.: American Psychiatric Association, 2001:30–40.
54. Petrides G, Fink M. Atrial fibrillation, anticoagulation, and electroconvulsive therapy. Convuls Ther 1996; 12(2):91–98.
55. Alexopoulos GS, Nasr H, Young RC, et al. Electroconvulsive therapy in patients on anticoagulation. Can J Psychiatry 1982; 27(1):46–8.
56. Mehta V, Mueller PS, Gonzalez-Arriaza HL, et al.Safety of electroconvulsive therapy in patients receiving long-term warfarin therapy. Mayo Clin Proc 2004; 79(11):1396–401.
57. Wingate BJ, Hansen-Flaschen J. Anxiety and depression in advanced lung disease. Clin Chest Med 1997; 18(3):495–505.
58. Devanand DP, Decina P, Sackeim HA, et al. Status epilepticus following ECT in a patient receiving theophylline. J Clin Psychopharmacol 1988; 8(2):153.
59. Rasmussen KG, Zorumski CF. Electroconvulsive therapy in patients taking theophylline. J Clin Psychiatry 1993; 54(11):427–431.
60. Stewart JT. Prolongation of ECT-induced seizures with theophylline. J Am Geriatr Soc 1996; 44(4):475.

61. Brimacombe JR, Berry AM. Cricoid pressure. Can J Anaesth 1997; 44(4):414–425.
62. de Carle AJ, Kohn R. Electroconvulsive therapy and falls in the elderly. J ECT 2000; 16(3):252–257.
63. Milo TJ, Kaufman GE, Barnes WE, et al. Changes in regional cerebral blood flow after electroconvulsive therapy for depression. J ECT 2001; 17(1):15–21.
64. Henry ME, Schmidt ME, Matochik JA, et al. The effects of ECT on brain glucose: A pilot FDG PET study. J ECT 2001; 17(1):33–40.
65. Meyer J. Importance of ischemic damage to small vessels in experimental cerebral infarction. J Neuropathol Exp Neurol 1958; 17:571–585.
66. Welch C. ECT in medically ill patients. In: C CE, ed. The Clinical Science of Electroconvulsive Therapy. Washington, D.C.: American Psychiatric Press, Inc., 1993:167–182.
67. Murray GB, Shea V, Conn DK. Electroconvulsive therapy for poststroke depression. J Clin Psychiatry 1986; 47(5):258–260.
68. Weintraub D, Lippmann SB. Electroconvulsive therapy in the acute poststroke period. J ECT 2000; 16(4):415–418.
69. Currier MB, Murray GB, Welch CC. Electroconvulsive therapy for post-stroke depressed geriatric patients. J Neuropsychiatry Clin Neurosci 1992; 4(2):140–144.
70. Miller AR, Isenberg KE. Reversible ischemic neurologic deficit after ECT. J ECT 1998; 14(1):42–48.
71. Salaris S, Szuba MP, Traber K. ECT and intracranial vascular masses. J ECT 2000; 16(2):198–203.
72. Patkar AA, Hill KP, Weinstein SP, et al. ECT in the presence of brain tumor and increased intracranial pressure: Evaluation and reduction of risk. J ECT 2000; 16(2):189–197.
73. Mattingly G, Baker K, Zorumski CF,et al. Multiple sclerosis and ECT: Possible value of gadolinium-enhanced magnetic resonance scans for identifying high-risk patients. J Neuropsychiatry Clin Neurosci 1992 Spring; 4(2):145–151.
74. Rasmussen KG, Keegan BM. Electroconvulsive therapy in patients with Multiple sclerosis. J ECT 2007; 23(3):179–180.
75. Pirl WF, Roth AJ. Diagnosis and treatment of depression in cancer patients. Oncology (Huntingt) 1999; 13(9):1293–1301; discussion 1301–1292, 1305–1296.
76. Blewett AE, Kareem O. ECT in a patient with psychotic retarded depression, metastatic hepatic cancer, and esophageal varices. J ECT 2000; 16(3):291–294.
77. Beale MD, Kellner CH, Parsons PJ. ECT for the treatment of mood disorders in cancer patients. Convuls Ther 1997; 13(4):222–226.
78. Hochberg F, Pruitt A, Neoplastic diseases of the central nervous system. In: BE Wilson JD, Isselbacher KJ, Petersdorf RG, Martin JB, Fauci AS, Root RK, eds. Harrison's Principles of Internal Medicine. New York, NY: McGraw-Hill, Inc., 1991:2014.
79. Weeks D, Freeman CP, Kendell RE. ECT: III: Enduring cognitive deficits? Br J Psychiatry 1980; 137:26–37.
80. Frith CD, Stevens M, Johnstone EC, et al. Effects of ECT and depression on various aspects of memory. Br J Psychiatry 1983; 142:610–617.
81. Calev A, Nigal D, Shapira B, et al. Early and long-term effects of electroconvulsive therapy and depression on memory and other cognitive functions. J Nerv Ment Dis 1991; 179(9):526–533.
82. Taylor JR, Tompkins R, Demers R, et al. Electroconvulsive therapy and memory dysfunction: Is there evidence for prolonged defects? Biol Psychiatry 1982; 17(10):1169–1193.
83. Sackeim HA, Prudic J, Fuller R, et al. The cognitive effects of electroconvulsive therapy in community settings. Neuropsychopharmacology 2007; 32(1):244–254.
84. Brodaty H, Berle D, Hickie I, et al. "Side effects" of ECT are mainly depressive phenomena and are independent of age. J Affect Disord 2001; 66(2–3):237–245.
85. Rubin EH, Kinscherf DA, Figiel GS, et al. The nature and time course of cognitive side effects during electroconvulsive therapy in the elderly. J Geriatr Psychiatry Neurol 1993; 6(2):78–83.
86. Stoudemire A, Hill CD, Morris R, et al. Improvement in depression-related cognitive dysfunction following ECT. J Neuropsychiatry Clin Neurosci 1995; 7(1):31–34.

87. Stoudemire A, Hill CD, Morris R, et al. Cognitive outcome following tricyclic and electroconvulsive treatment of major depression in the elderly. Am J Psychiatry 1991; 148(10):1336–1340.
88. Shapira B, Tubi N, Drexler H, et al. Cost and benefit in the choice of ECT schedule. Twice versus three times weekly ECT. Br J Psychiatry 1998; 172:44–48.
89. McAllister DA, Perri MG, Jordan RC, et al. Effects of ECT given two vs. three times weekly. Psychiatry Res 1987; 21(1):63–69.
90. Fromm-Auch D. Comparison of unilateral and bilateral ECT: Evidence for selective memory impairment. Br J Psychiatry 1982; 141:608–613.
91. Rosenberg J, Pettinati HM. Differential memory complaints after bilateral and unilateral ECT. Am J Psychiatry 1984; 141(9):1071–1074.
92. Sackeim HA, Prudic J, Nobler M, et al. Ultra-brief pulse ECT and the affective and cognitive consequence of ECT. J ECT 2001; 17:77. abstract.
93. Loo C, Sheehan P, Pigot M, et al. A report on mood and cognitive outcomes with right unilateral ultrabrief pulsewidth (0.3 ms) ECT and retrospective comparison with standard pulsewidth right unilateral ECT. J Affect Disord 2007; 103(1–3):277–281. Epub 2007, Aug 16.
94. Kim SW, Grant JE, Rittberg BR, et al. Decreased memory loss associated with right unilateral ultra-brief pulse wave ECT. Minn Med 2007; 90(1):34–35.
95. Sackeim HA, Haskett RF, Mulsant BH, et al. Continuation pharmacotherapy in the prevention of relapse following electroconvulsive therapy: A randomized controlled trial. JAMA 2001; 285(10):1299–1307.
96. Wijkstra J, Nolen WA, Algra A, et al. Relapse prevention in major depressive disorder after successful ECT: A literature review and a naturalistic case series. Acta Psychiatr Scand 2000; 102(6):454–460.
97. Sackeim HA, Prudic J, Devanand DP, et al. The impact of medication resistance and continuation pharmacotherapy on relapse following response to electroconvulsive therapy in major depression. J Clin Psychopharmacol 1990; 10(2):96–104.
98. Nolen WA, Haffmans PM, Bouvy PF, et al. Monoamine oxidase inhibitors in resistant major depression. A double-blind comparison of brofaromine and tranylcypromine in patients resistant to tricyclic antidepressants. J Affect Disord 1993; 28(3):189–197.
99. Thase ME, Frank E, Mallinger AG, et al. Treatment of imipramine-resistant recurrent depression, III: Efficacy of monoamine oxidase inhibitors. J Clin Psychiatry 1992; 53(1):5–11.
100. Parker G, Hadzi-Pavlovic D, Hickie I, et al. Psychotic depression: A review and clinical experience. Aust N Z J Psychiatry 1991; 25(2):169–180.
101. Robinson DG, Spiker DG. Delusional depression. A one-year follow-up. J Affect Disord 1985; 9(1):79–83.
102. Flint AJ, Rifat SL. Two-year outcome of psychotic depression in late life. Am J Psychiatry 1998; 155(2):178–183.
103. Fox HA. Extended continuation and maintenance ECT for long-lasting episodes of major depression. J ECT 2001; 17(1):60–64.
104. Gagne GG, Jr, Furman MJ, Carpenter LL, et al. Efficacy of continuation ECT and antidepressant drugs compared to long-term antidepressants alone in depressed patients. Am J Psychiatry 2000; 157(12):1960–1965.
105. Petrides G, Dhossche D, Fink M, et al. Continuation ECT: Relapse prevention in affective disorders. Convuls Ther 1994; 10(3):189–194.
106. George MS, Post RM, Ketter TA, et al. Neural mechanisms of mood disorders. Curr Rev Mood Anxiety Disorders 1997; 1:71–83.
107. Zobel A, Joe A, Freymann N, et al. Changes in regional cerebral blood flow by therapeutic vagus nerve stimulation in depression: An exploratory approach. Psychiatry Res 2005; 139:156–179.
108. Conway CR, Sheline YI, Chibnall JT, et al. Cerebral blood flow changes during vagus nerve stimulation for depression. Psychiatry Res 2006; 146:179–184.
109. Tatum WO, IV, Moore DB, Stecker MM, et al. Ventricular asystole during vagus nerve stimulation for epilepsy in humans. Neurology 1999; 52:1267–1269.

110. Elger G, Hoppe C, Falkai P, et al. Vagus nerve stimulation is associated with mood improvements in epilepsy patients. Epilepsy Res 2000; 42:203–210.
111. Harden CL, Pulver MC, Ravdin LD, et al. A pilot study of mood in epilepsy patients treated with vagus nerve stimulation. Epilepsy Behav 2000; 1:93–99.
112. Rush AJ, Marangell LB, Sackeim HA, et al. Vagus nerve stimulation for treatment-resistant depression: A randomized-controlled acute phase trial. Biol Psychiatry 2005; 58:347–354.
113. Rush AJ, Sackeim HA, Marangell LB, et al. Effects of 12 months of vagus nerve stimulation in treatment-resistant depression: A naturalistic study. Biol Psychiatry 2005; 58:355–363.
114. George MS, Rush AJ, Marangell LB, et al. A one-year comparison of vagus nerve stimulation with treatment as usual for treatment-resistant depression. Biol Psychiatry 2005; 58:364–373.
115. Berman RM, Narasimhan M, Sanacora G, et al. A. randomized clinical trial of repetitive transcranial magnetic stimulation in the treatment of major depression. Biol Psychiatry 2000; 47:332–337.
116. Avery DH, Holtzheimer PE, Faxaz W, et al. A controlled study of repetitive transcranial magnetic stimulation in medication-resistant major depression. Biol Psychiatry 2006; 59:187–194.
117. Herwig U, Lampe Y, Juenglig FD, et al. Add-on rTMS for treatment of depression: A pilot study using stereotaxic coil-navigation according to PET data. J Psychiatr Res 2003; 37:267–275.
118. Aare T, Dahl AA, Johansen JB, et al. Efficacy of repetitive transcranial magnetic stimulation in depression: A review of the evidence. Nord J Psychiatry 2003; 57:227–232.
119. Burt T, Lisanby H, Sackeim H. Neuropsychiatric applications of transcranial magnetic stimulation: A meta-analysis. Int J Neuropsychopharmacol 2002; 5:73–103.
120. Couturier JL. Efficacy of rapid-rate repetitive transcranial magnetic stimulation in the treatment of depression: A systematic review and meta-analysis. J Psychiatry Neurosci 2005; 30:83–90.
121. Holtzheimer PE, Russo J, Avery DH. A meta-analysis of repetitive transcranial stimulation in the treatment of depression. Psychopharmacol Bull 2001; 35:149–169.
122. Kozel F, George MS. Meta-analysis of left prefrontal repetitive transcranial magnetic stimulation (rTMS) to treat depression. J Psychiatr Pract 2002; 8:270–275.
123. Martin JLR, Barbanoj-Rodriguez M, Schlaepfer T, et al. Transcranial magnetic stimulation for treating depression. Br J Psychiatry 2003; 182:480–491.
124. McNamara B, Ray JL, Arthurs OJ, et al. Transcranial magnetic stimulation for depression and other psychiatric disorders. Psychol Med 2001; 31:1141–1146.
125. Jorge R, Moser D, David J, et al. Treatment of vascular depression using repetitive transcranial magnetic stimulation. Archives Gen Psychiatry 2008; 65(3):268–276.
126. Steele JD, Currie J, Lawrie SM, et al. Prefrontal cortical functional abnormality in major depressive disorder: A stereotactic meta-analysis. J Affect Disord 2007; Epub ahead of print.
127. Soares JC, Mann JJ. The functional neuroanatomy of mood disorders. J Psychiatr Res 1997; 31:393–432.
128. Mandat TS, Hurwitz T, Honey CR. Hypomania as an adverse effect of subthalamic nucleus stimulation: Report of two cases Acta Neurochir 2006; 148:895–897.
129. Mayberg HS, Lozano AM, Voon V, et al. Deep brain stimulation for treatment-resistant depression. Neuron 2005; 45:651–660.
130. Burkhard PR, Vingerhoets FJ, Berney A, et al. Suicide after successful deep brain stimulation for movement disorders. Neurology 2004; 63:2170–2172.
131. Dalgleish T, Yiend, Bramham J, et al. Neuropsychological processing associated with recovery from depression after stereotactic subcaudate tractotomy. Am J Psychiatry 2004; 161:1913–1916.
132. Dougherty DD, Baer L, Cosgrove GR, et al. Prospective long-term follow-up of 44 patients who received cingulotomy for treatment-refractory obsessive-compulsive disorder. Am J Psychiatry 2002; 159:269–275.

133. Cosgrove GR, Rauch SL. Stereotactic cingulotomy. Neurosurg Clin N Am 2003; 14:225–235.
134. Greenberg BD, Price LH, Rauch SL, et al. Neurosurgery for intractable obsessive-compulsive disorder and depression: Critical issues. Neurosurg Clin N Am 2003; 14:199–212.
135. Montoya A, Weiss AP, Price BH, et al. Magnetic resonance imaging-guided stereotactic limbic leucotomy for treatment of intractable psychiatric disease. Neurosurgery 2002; 50:1043–1049.

17 Psychotherapy for Late-Life Mood Disorders

Francesca Cannavo Antognini

Geriatric Psychiatry Program, McLean Hospital, Belmont, and Department of Psychiatry, Harvard Medical School, Boston, Massachusetts, U.S.A.

Benjamin Liptzin

Department of Psychiatry, Baystate Health, Springfield, and Department of Psychiatry, Tufts University School of Medicine, Boston, Massachusetts, U.S.A.

Back in the 1920s, Sigmund Freud presented his position on psychoanalysis with older adults:

> Near and above the fifties, the elasticity of the mental processes on which the treatment depends is as a rule lacking—old people are no longer educable, and on the other hand, the mass of material to be dealt with would prolong the duration of the treatment indefinitely (1).

As outmoded as this view may seem during our time, when so many adults enjoy decades of vigorous and productive life beyond their 50s, many psychotherapists are still reluctant to work with older adults. However, in the context of an increasing average life span and a growing number of "graying" baby boomers, interest in geriatric mental health is appropriately spreading and the number of geriatric clinicians is expected to increase. There are compelling reasons to encourage psychotherapists to treat older patients. In addition to the surge in the elderly population that will create greater demand for skilled geriatric psychotherapists, there is considerable evidence that psychotherapy is acceptable and efficacious in treating a range of psychiatric conditions in older adults. For late life depression, the value of psychotherapy is particularly supported.

DEVELOPMENTAL CONSIDERATIONS

Older adulthood is a stage that presents unique developmental tasks. Colarusso and Nemiroff (2) have outlined these tasks as: dealing with the aging process in the body; adjusting to increasing awareness of limitation and death; coping with illnesses or death of friends and loved ones; dealing with changes in sexual drive and activity; adjusting to markedly altered relationships with parents, young adult children, and maturing spouse; assessment of career accomplishment and recognition that not all personal goals will be reached; and planning for retirement. In the parlance of self-psychology, older adults who fail to accept the transformations and losses of the aging self are at risk for self-fragmentation, depression, and anxiety (3), the avoidance of which requires substantial psychological reserve, drawing in part on having successfully passed through previous life stages:

> The elderly self is a self that has adapted, not adjusted, to its somatic limitations ... (and) to the limitations imposed by the cultural institutions in the family, on the job, and in the reactions of the culture toward aging ... unique values and unique ambitions that are particular to this specific group of aged persons who have passed through the described stages mark the person as a

> member of the elderly group in the culture to which he or she belongs ... the badge signifying membership ... is not age, but rather the fact that one has undergone the self transformations that mark one as elderly ... (3, p. 5).

In their later years, Erikson et al. (4) emphasized the importance of wisdom in successfully negotiating the challenges of aging:

> The elder is challenged to draw on a life cycle that is far more nearly completed than yet to be lived, to consolidate a sense of wisdom with which to live out the future, to place him- or herself in perspective among those generations now living, and to accept his or her place in an infinite historical progression ... wisdom is detached concern with life itself in the face of death itself. It maintains and learns to convey the integrity of experience, in spite of the decline of bodily and mental functions (p. 56).

For Erik Erikson, the successful outcome of this stage of life was "ego integrity or 'the acceptance of one's own and only life cycle as something that had to be and that, by necessity, permitted of no substitutions'" (5). The unsuccessful outcome is despair. Unresolved developmental issues from even earlier in life (e.g., basic trust vs. mistrust) can and may need to be addressed in order to deal with the challenges and problems of late life, including, at the extreme, suicidal ideation and behavior (6).

PSYCHOTHERAPY'S EFFICACY IN THE TREATMENT OF GERIATRIC DEPRESSION

Psychotherapy has become well established as a treatment for depression in the past three decades. It is generally acknowledged that the efficacy of cognitive behavior therapy (CBT) is comparable to that of medication in alleviating mild-to-moderate depression (7,8), but combined therapy is more effective for severe recurrent depression (9). One comprehensive literature review confirmed generally greater improvement for nongeriatric-depressed patients receiving combined treatments when compared with those receiving drug treatment alone (10). Moreover, when antidepressant treatment exceeded 12 weeks, the addition of psychotherapy was found to result in lower rates of patient dropout. Throughout the 1980s and 1990s there were few such studies with depressed older adults. In an early study, each of the three forms of psychotherapy alone (behavioral, cognitive, and brief psychodynamic) significantly delayed the recurrence of depression in older adults (11). In studies from 1974 to 1998 behavior therapy, CBT and psychodynamic approaches were significantly more effective for geriatric depression than placebo medication, with response rates comparable to those observed with antidepressants (12). A combination of interpersonal psychotherapy and nortriptyline was correlated with lower recurrence rates than either treatment alone over a 3-year period (13).

In 2001, an expert panel endorsed psychotherapy as a first-line treatment for minor geriatric depression, recommending the addition of antidepressants after 3 months if there has been improvement (14). For geriatric major depression, a combination of antidepressants and psychotherapy was recommended, with medication alone as another first-line strategy. A more recent expert panel (15) recommended individual CBT as a key component of overall care (including medication when appropriate) for community-dwelling older adults with clinical depression at all levels of severity, based on results of a large-scale review of the literature (16). Contemporaneously, another group of researchers integrated and analyzed the results of 89 controlled studies of treatments focused on acute geriatric major depression (37 studies) and mixed depressive disorders (52 studies) (17). On clinician-rated measures of depression, 66.3% of those receiving pharmacotherapy and 72.4% of those who received psychotherapy showed above average improvement. For self-rated depression, 64.8% of the medicated patients and 69.2% of those receiving psychotherapy showed above average improvement. An analysis of the percentage of patients in remission revealed consistent findings. When responsiveness by level of depression was analyzed, pharmacotherapy and psychotherapy were similarly effective in decreasing observer rated major depression; however, when studies also included patients with minor depression and/or dysthymia, the effect of psychotherapy was larger. Finally, this meta-analysis revealed that "the effect of CBT on clinician-rated depression was greater than the effects of other forms of psychotherapy, SSRIs, other drugs and all medications combined" (p. 1498).

PSYCHOTHERAPY AS A TREATMENT OPTION: EXTERNAL AND INTERNAL BARRIERS

Despite demonstrated efficacy, the actual utilization of psychotherapy by older depressed adults is low. Only 25% of 2025 depressive episodes identified in a survey of Medicare data were treated with psychotherapy (18). A strong positive correlation emerged between educational level and psychotherapy use, and there was less consistent use of psychotherapy when the sole provider was a psychiatrist. Depressed older patients may initially seek help from a primary care clinician and may not be referred for psychosocial treatments for a variety of reasons including the primary care clinician's limited awareness of psychotherapy's efficacy or of available referral resources. Even in mental health settings, there is a tendency for prescribing clinicians and patients to focus on pharmacotherapy and this sometimes results in a treatment plan that fails to address the developmental or psychosocial issues for which psychotherapy may be of value.

In treating older adults, it is essential to consider contextual and cohort–based effects, as "... working with someone from another cohort is like working with someone from another culture" (19, p. 930). The people considered "old" today were born, roughly, between 1908 and 1943. Although this 35-year span encompasses two generations, the entire cohort was impacted by catastrophic world events that affected virtually every household: the Great Depression and World War II. Self-reliance was a major coping strategy during the Great Depression (20). Perhaps this accounts for the well-known fact that older adults of this cohort tend to express distress indirectly or somatically or attribute psychiatric symptoms to somatic causes. An older patient recommended for psychotherapy may feel that psychotherapy will take too long and that "I'm too old to change." Moreover, today's older adults remember the stigma of mental illness that prevailed during an era when psychotic patients were treated surgically or confined indefinitely in large public mental institutions. Geriatric clinicians will observe that their patients eschew references to "psychotherapy", preferring the term "counseling," with its implications of advice or coaching rather than treatment.

While cohort-specific inhibition about engaging in psychotherapy will fade as the psychotherapeutically savvy baby boomers enter their geriatric years, some purely age-related issues will continue to make the therapeutic process challenging for the older patient. Older adults with mood disorders tend to have coexisting physical ailments and they often present with unexplained somatic symptoms (21,22). Considerable psychotherapeutic time may be required initially to address and explore these complaints. In addition, hearing loss may make communication more difficult, requiring the therapist to speak clearly and slowly, while maintaining eye contact with the patient. Furthermore, short-term memory deficits may interfere with retention between sessions and require frequent repetition of material, perhaps contributing to the sobering observation that the patience of the older adult in therapy may exceed that of the therapist (23).

THE "GEROTHERAPIST" AND THE PATIENT: ENGAGING AND TREATING THE OLDER ADULT

Many older adults come to a psychotherapist at the behest of a family member, and the therapist's first contact may therefore be with someone other than the patient (24). The perceived stigma of seeing a mental health professional (25) may further complicate matters. The patient may feel wary of the clinician sitting behind the desk who may be no older than his or her grandchild. Furthermore, the therapist may harbor ageist attitudes and biases, owing in part to the influence of experiences with parents or grandparents. Some personal therapists may feel discouraged or even impotent when treating with a patient whose life seems to be in decline: "attempting to treat a life in decline is a blow to our medical narcissism" (26). Because so many older adults nowadays are segregated into senior centers, assisted living facilities, and nursing homes, les-experienced therapists may have an impression of older adults based primarily on family relationships (27) and feel compelled to "act and do, rather than to (simply) be with the patient" (26, p. 54). It is important for the therapist to grant the patient his/her expertise in living and aging. Especially with respect to cohort issues, "the therapist must have a willingness to use one's own ignorance constructively to learn from the client about the client's experience" (19, p. 930).

The "empathic diagnosis" is a thorough assessment of the older patient's functioning in all areas of the self, from self-worth to self-values (3). The development of the therapeutic alliance provides gradual restitution of the equilibrium of self. This requires the creation of a safe haven for the patient to self-disclose and develop the trust necessary to incorporate the therapist's validation. Older patients benefit not only from the caring of the therapist, but also from re-acquaintance with their own ability to care for another person through caring gestures toward the therapist, such as educating the young therapist about historical events through which they have lived (28). "If the therapist accepts the existential view of humans as always in a state of 'becoming', of being in a state of crisis without despairing, then a therapist can work with any cohort" (29, p. 92).

EMPIRICALLY VALIDATED THERAPIES AND ADAPTATIONS FOR OLDER ADULTS

The results of a number of empirical studies support the efficacy of four different psychotherapeutic approaches to the treatment of geriatric depression: psychodynamic psychotherapy, cognitive behavior therapy (CBT), and, more recently, interpersonal therapy (IPT) and problem-solving therapy (PST). While some studies demonstrate the efficacy of one approach over another, other studies show comparable efficacy across all four approaches (30).

Interpersonal therapy (31) has as its premise that depression is "a state of illness that plays itself out in the interpersonal sphere of the patient, regardless of whether it stems from a biological or genetic vulnerability or from psychological or psychosocial stressors" (32). IPT for older adults is in part based on the finding that older depressed patients have poorer outcomes after leaving the hospital when relationships with a spouse or adult child are strained (33). IPT has four foci: grief, role conflict, role transition, and interpersonal deficits, and has proven successful with depressed older adults when combined with antidepressant medication (34–37). A recent comparison study gave maintenance IPT no advantage over supportive clinical management in preserving health-related quality of life for older adults recovering from depression (38). Nonetheless, IPT offers an approach which would seem appealing to older adults in that it is time limited (16–20 sessions), focused on the present, and emphasizes action rather than exploration and insight (39).

The premise of PST is that depression results when deficits in problem solving lead to ineffective coping in times of stress. Trials of PST adapted for depressed older adults reported significantly greater results than reminiscence therapy (RT) in relieving depressive symptoms, although both produced improvement (40). PST has also served as a viable treatment for patients with major depression with impaired executive function, who could not benefit from pharmacological intervention (41). Severely depressed older adults in a home care setting, too, have been treated successfully with brief PST (42).

As the finitude of life becomes increasingly clear, "older individuals may become more reflective, more aware of life's vicissitudes, and have an increased need to get on with living" (43, p. 229). Psychodynamic psychotherapy "help(s) the individual to understand and make sense of these vicissitudes, in order to get on with living" (43, p. 229). In contrast to Freud's earlier formulation, the current view is that the defenses become more malleable as we age (44). The psychodynamic process can provide an examination of aspects of current relationships, such as those with grown children, that recapitulate old-life themes. "In the client's attempt to satisfy need gratification or to establish and maintain satisfying relationships, he or she typically acts in ways that unintentionally elicit repetition of past traumatic experiences and disappointments" (45, p. 936). This is illustrated in the following brief reconstruction of a psychodynamic intervention with a 72-year old widow, Ms. R, admitted to the hospital with agitated depression and passive suicidal ideation a few months after bypass surgery:

Patient: "My kids keep telling me to go walking every day for my heart, but I just don't feel like it . . . and I feel guilty that I keep letting them down. How can I be so ungrateful . . . I'm becoming such a burden.

Therapist: Wasn't there a time when you were there for your children?

Patient: I was their mother; it was my job. I tried to give them what I missed out on.

Therapist: Such as?

Patient: Well (pause) . . . my mother got so depressed after my father left. She would stay in bed for days. I did all I could to help but I was so young. When my brothers went off to war it was just me and her.

Therapist: How did her depression affect her caretaking of you?

Patient: I tried to stay out of her way. She was always telling me how good I was and how I'd make a great wife and mother someday.

Therapist: How about when you just behaved like a child?

Patient: I don't remember misbehaving. Actually it would have been unthinkable. (laugh)

Therapist: How so?

Patient:	She might have given up on me . . . thought less of me, I don't know.
Therapist:	So it was hard to just be a kid and risk having her not feel as good about you as she did when you did as you were told.
Patient:	Yes, but if she weren't depressed it all would have been different.
Therapist:	I wonder if your experience of your mother's depression is having some impact on your view of your own depression.
Patient:	What do you mean?
Therapist:	Well, I have two thoughts. One is that you might worry that your depression is causing the same pain for your children that your mother's depression caused for you. And secondly, you may fear that if you don't follow the advice of your children, they will give up on you, just as you feared your mother might, if you disobeyed or misbehaved.
Patient:	Maybe I'm being a little hard on myself. Is that what you're thinking?

Brief psychodynamic therapy has been found to be effective in alleviating depression, although it has not been shown superior to CBT (11,46,47).

Cognitive behavior therapy proposes that depression and anxiety derive from maladaptive thought patterns that the patient can work toward changing. Cognitive change, more technically termed cognitive restructuring, is accomplished through exploring and modifying maladaptive thoughts through "collaborative empiricism" between patient and therapist (48). Assertiveness, social skills training, and behavioral scheduling are among the interventions used to modify dysfunctional behaviors generated by maladaptive thinking. A number of studies have found that CBT is comparable to pharmacotherapy in treating depression (7). With minor modifications, the efficacy of CBT for depression in late life is gaining increasing support (49,50). The combination of CBT with pharmacotherapy has been shown in certain elderly depressed populations to have advantages over antidepressants alone (47), and some expert panels (see previous section) recommend CBT alone as a first-line treatment for geriatric depression not accompanied by dementia or psychosis. As and, as noted earlier, a large-scale meta-analysis of studies with older depressed patients found CBT more effective than all other treatments combined. In a recent review of five randomized, controlled trials, CBT-treated older adults fared significantly better than waiting list controls based on clinician-rated outcomes for depression (51) and the findings were particularly robust for major depression. Given the empirically validated efficacy of CBT for geriatric depression, new variants of CBT for older adults are emerging in the psychiatric literature that integrate cognitive behavioral techniques with other approaches, including gerodynamic behavior therapy (GBT) (see section, toward an integrative approach: gerodynamic behavior therapy) and mindfulness-based cognitive therapy (MBCT) (52), which combines cognitive behavioral techniques with elements of mindfulness-based therapies such as meditation for recurring geriatric depression.

A number of modifications can make CBT more elder friendly (53,54). For example, one of the typical psychological barriers to CBT in late-life depression is the familiar maladaptive cognition that "I'm too old to change." Challenging this resistance by presenting the patient with evidence to the contrary is an important component in the early stages of treatment (54,55). Additional strategies for adapating CBT to the needs of older adults include evaluating the patient on a measure of cognitive functioning such as the Folstein Mini Mental

State exam (56) to assess the need for greater use of repetition and rehearsal of new information, using large-type handouts to compensate for visual acuity impairment, encouraging the patient to audiotape sessions in order to aid memory and counteract the effect of reduced auditory acuity on comprehension, and pausing periodically during sessions to summarize information (57).

The following is a cognitive–behavioral reformulation of the concerns presented by Ms. R, the patient previously introduced, demonstrating identification of maladaptive cognitions amenable to examination and revision:

Patient: "My kids call and tell me to go to the gym, I'm not ready but I feel guilty about letting them down.
Therapist: What do you tell yourself after those conversations?
Patient: That I don't want to do it, but they won't be happy if I don't.
Therapist: And if they're not happy?
Patient: Well . . . they might say, "she's hopeless" and give up on me. How can I keep letting them down? I'm such a burden.
Therapist: So not following their suggestions makes you a burden?
Patient: Well, they keep checking. Soon they're going to get tired of worrying.
Therapist: Do you have a thought that keeps you from telling them you're not ready to do what they suggest?
Patient: They'd be mad. 'Don't bite the hand that feeds', my mother always said.
Therapist: What do they say when you tell them you didn't go to the gym?
Patient: They sigh; they sound worried.
Therapist: But not angry.
Patient: No. I avoid their calls lately. And then I feel about guilty that.
Therapist: Do you think you would you feel less guilt if, rather than avoiding their calls, you told them you're not ready to do what they suggest?
Patient: I can't get myself to be, well, assertive. I just agree, and then hide.
Therapist: Let's assume they do get angry. What would happen then?
Patient: Well, then I'd really be alone.
Therapist: Sounds pretty final—if they get angry, they will be gone.
Patient: Well, they might get fed up with me . . . (pause) as you know, my mother was depressed; she always expected a lot. And now it's my kids.
Therapist: So maybe you're telling yourself: "If I say no, I'll be letting them down, just like I might have let Mom down if I'd said no to her".
Patient: Yeah, something like that, I guess.
Therapist: Can you think of a more useful thought that would help you tell your children that you need to do things in your own time?
Patient: Gee, that sounds great, Doctor, when you say it. But I don't know if I can.
Therapist: You remember that we have often talked about how depression involves a feeling of helplessness, and how assertiveness helps depression.
Patient: Yes.
Therapist: So, do you think it might make sense to be assertive in this situation as well, so that your depression can be helped? And of course if you feel better, your children may not pressure you as much.

Patient: (chuckling) true.
Therapist: So what can you tell yourself when they tell you what to do?
Patient: Well . . . first, I guess, I could tell myself that it's important to be assertive so I can feel less depressed. And then, that they probably won't really be angry, but if they are, I'll survive—I guess (laugh). And maybe if I clear the air I won't feel so guilty if I don't do the stuff they want me to do. Sounds good right now in the office . . . actually, I don't think it would turn out so bad.

TOWARD AN INTEGRATIVE APPROACH: GERODYNAMIC BEHAVIOR THERAPY

Older adults who prefer to focus on the present rather than the past may reject the psychodynamic approach because they fear it will force them to dwell on disappointments or unresolved conflicts that are not central to current concerns. Others may find CBT dry or pedantic, a risk for this approach when it is implemented mechanically, for example, by inexperienced therapists or by those who rely excessively on treatment manuals. Our approach to psychotherapy attempts to steer between these hazards by integrating aspects of psychodynamic and cognitive behavior therapies. This approach, which is called "gerodynamic behavior therapy" (GBT) (58), examines the impact of relevant aspects of a patient's history while working in the "here-and-now" using CBT and other techniques to modify "outmoded" or "obsolete" maladaptive cognitions and behaviors, providing a foundation for ongoing change. The GBT therapist emphasizes to the patient that the purpose of exploring historical factors is not to assign blame, but to facilitate understanding and insight.

Viewing the case of Ms. R. through the integrative perspective of GBT, a psychotherapist would explore the patient's recollections of childhood experiences with a depressed mother with a view toward fostering an understanding of her current maladaptive assumptions about her own children. Techniques from CBT, IPT, or PST would then be employed to modify the counterproductive beliefs and expectations arising from her history, allowing her the freedom to explore new behaviors.

SPECIALIZED TREATMENT MODALITIES

Group Therapy

Group therapy, often the psychosocial treatment of choice on inpatient units, given its promotion of peer support as well as its more efficient use of resources, is an effective form of treatment for depression in older adults (59–62). Group treatment affords depressed older adults the "re-motivation" to combat loneliness and facilitate relationships, the enhancement of self-esteem through realization that many problems of aging are universal, and the emotional catharsis of safely expressing anger, self-pity, guilt, feelings of failure, or other affective and existential concerns (63). Addressing these issues is especially important in inpatient units, where group therapy can help patients cope with the feelings of isolation and hopelessness triggered by severe depression or other psychiatric illness. The group affirms the universality of problems which may seem unique and shameful, thus mitigating the stigma associated with depression, and may provide a therapeutic alternative more appealing than meeting individually with a "shrink." The older adult, perhaps as a form of rationalization, often perceives group therapy as an educational experience, even referring to the group as a "class." The politeness of this cohort presents fewer challenges for the group therapist and other group members. For example, older adults are more tolerant of group "monopolists," trusting that their turn will come if they wait (23, p. 225).

It is increasingly common in treatment facilities for group therapy to be the primary mode of psychosocial intervention rather than serving as an adjunct to individual therapy, and group therapists must revise their format and goals accordingly. "Contact work" (64), that is, serial focus on each individual within the context of the group, is given a more central role in the group process and other group members are invited to offer feedback to the patient whose turn it is to be "on." Every member is given the opportunity to benefit from the focus of the group, an objective that in large groups requires considerable skill on the part of the therapist to redirect patients and set limits.

Groups with a specifically cognitive behavioral focus have become a popular modality for treating late-life depression on inpatient units. In group CBT, a "lecturette" on a particular topic may precede serial contact work (64). The topic may be a theme universal to older depressed patients such as coping with transitions, loss, aging or family issues. The lecturette is followed by contact work that employs modification of maladaptive cognitions in order to help patients cope more successfully. During contact work, patients may share completed homework or simply explore their thoughts and experiences regarding the chosen topic, while other members of the group offer feedback.

Reminiscence therapy (RT) is a form of group therapy undertaken almost exclusively with older adults. Also called "life review therapy," it can be effective for late-life depression (65). Based on the premise that reviewing one's life can result in an enhanced sense of identity and accomplishment, patients are asked to recall and share meaningful experiences. A structured modification of RT for depressed older inpatients, "retrospective focus therapy" (RFT) (58), reacquaints patients with their strengths by having them recall and share challenging life events that they dealt with successfully. The patients' strengths are thereby validated as enduring personality traits that can be invoked even during depressive episodes. This fosters hope, decreases "learned helplessness" (66), and enhances self-esteem and identity—achievements helpful for any depressed patient and perhaps of special value with patients in an early state of cognitive decline.

Couple Therapy

Couple therapy has received relatively little attention in the literature as a treatment for older adults. The need for couple therapy may emerge during the treatment process of one spouse. The older couple in such cases is often dealing with change, perhaps of crisis proportions, that derives from the illness of one of the partners or from other life transitions. Expectations must change, including perhaps cherished hopes for the long-awaited retirement years, especially when a spouse's illness imposes a lifestyle increasingly limited to activities of caretaking and domestic maintenance (67). Meaningful patterns of interaction may break down, for example, when retirement of a spouse results in greatly increased time together at home (68). Furthermore, the need for one spouse to adapt to the other's illness may accentuate longstanding difficulties, which have been dealt with over the years in a dysfunctional but relatively stable equilibrium (69).

It is most useful for couple therapy to begin with an assessment of the couple's strengths, the couple's perceptions and handling of the current problem, and the couple's external social resources. The evaluative phase can also be therapeutic in emphasizing the longevity of the relationship as a sign of success and strength. Persistence of a relationship for 50 years implies that a powerful force in support of continuation exists, regardless of how dysfunctional the couple's relationship may appear to the observer—or even to the couple itself! In the context of this focus, successful coping mechanisms are identified and explored. It is appropriate to point out that a breakdown has occurred and to explore how situational changes have contributed, while respecting the stability of the long term relationship and avoiding blame of either member of the couple. Once the couple in therapy can move beyond blame and unite into a team focused on addressing a shared problem, true change can begin. The therapist should then proceed to work on the problem at hand and avoid the temptation to change longstanding patterns. The old adage, "don't fix what's not broken" is a good general rule in treating elderly couples (69); in doing otherwise the therapist risks losing the alliance and ultimately, the couple.

As a final word, it is important to note that depression is often accompanied by impairment of a couple's sexual relationship, yet this difficulty may remain unspoken unless an attempt is made to elicit it. Such couples may be referred by a primary care physician; however, the sexual dysfunction, although deeply troubling to the couple, may be difficult for them to discuss openly, and equally difficult for the much younger therapists to address, given generational boundaries. Yet sexual difficulties are unfortunately quite common in patients who have specific illnesses such as diabetes or postprostate surgery or who are taking medications which may affect libido, for example, antidepressants or antihypertensives. While discussion of this important aspect of couple therapy with older adults is beyond the scope of this chapter, the reader is referred to a sensitive and informative work by Helen Singer Kaplan, who underscores the need for attention to this often neglected dimension of the older couple's relationship:

> Though it is widely believed that sex no longer matters as an individual gets older, the opposite is often true. Sex may become more important in a person's life with the passage of time because sexuality is among the last of the pleasure giving biological processes to deteriorate. It is a potentially enduring source of emotional well-being at a time when more and more losses must be accepted and few and fewer gratifications remain available (70, p. 37).

Family Therapy

Within the limited literature on family therapy with older adults, several authors have addressed the needs of families in which a depressed older adult is the identified patient. Didactic and psychoeducational approaches have been used by some therapists, while others have focused on intervening in the family system by identifying their both the problem and the resources for its solution (67). Special considerations include recognition of the longstanding nature of interactional patterns of the family and the influence of cohort differences in values such as views regarding the provision of long-term care. When possible, the participation of the older patient in family sessions is important even when physical or cognitive impairment make involvement more difficult. Presenting common family themes with depressed older adults include marital discord, conflicted relationships with adult children, caregiver burden, or difficulty coping with major transitions or losses such as the move to a long-term care facility or the death of a spouse. Family therapy is rarely initiated by the older patient, but is often sought by a grown child, spouse, individual therapist or other involved treater. This is not surprising, as the final stage of the family cycle is the time, following the "launching" of grown children, during which adults recognize and respond to the growing dependence of their own parents (71). Adult children may be in denial about an elderly parent's decline; to recognize it means facing role changes and acknowledging their own mortality as they move closer to becoming the "Omega generation" (72), that is, the next in line to die. Family interventions during this stage typically include revision of expectations and facilitation of "filial maturity," whereby a grown child may be forced to "take the reins" and adjust to a role reversal (71). Clearly, this role redefinition presents great difficulty for many older adults who must relinquish some degree of autonomy and self-reliance as they allow their children increasing amounts of control. It can be helpful for members of both generations to share with each other their discomfort in a safe therapeutic context, as this facilitates a common ground on which to build mutual coping strategies and communication.

Guilleard (67) discusses the inherent therapeutic value of a thoughtful family evaluation, presenting four stages of assessment with the family of an older adult (73): (1) identification of past history, future possibilities, and hopes and fears; (2) identification of family structure and boundaries; (3) identification of family communication patterns; and (4) discovery of "hidden dynamics" which are creating, maintaining or intensifying the problem(s). Where the older adult is the identified patient, "indirect techniques" described by Benbow and colleagues (74) include circular questioning, positive reframing, restraining change, and employing paradox, while "direct techniques" include genogram interpretation, communication work, advice giving, and recommendations. Arguing for further research to assess systemic approaches with older adults, Guilleard (67) stresses "indirect techniques" as the essence of family therapy, where the goal is to foster change, as opposed to family work, where the goal is more simply to inform and advise the family.

SPECIAL APPLICATIONS OF GERIATRIC PSYCHOTHERAPY

The Depressed Adult with Generalized Anxiety

Anxiety symptoms are very frequently described by people over 65 years age, and generalized anxiety disorder (GAD) has been estimated by some investigators to be about as common as major depression in this age group (75). Few studies have focused on psychological treatments for geriatric anxiety, despite the fact that older adults consume a disproportionate share of anxiolytic medications whose side effects include not only tolerance and withdrawal but also a cluster of symptoms that are especially dangerous for the elderly: cognitive slowing, drowsiness, impaired coordination, and falling (76). Studies have demonstrated the efficacy of CBT for older patients with GAD (76–78). Protocols for the treatment of GAD typically include psychoeducation, self-monitoring, relaxation training, exposure with systematic desensitization, and cognitive restructuring. CBT is combined with medication in some studies, and it has also been shown helpful in reducing dependence on anxiolytics (79). One study showed both supportive therapy and CBT to be effective in decreasing anxiety in a sample of older adults with GAD (80) with a trend toward greater improvement for those subjects receiving supportive therapy. Two extensive protocols developed for older adults with anxiety have shown promising results. CALM (81) includes, in addition to the standard components (above), sleep hygiene, pain management and problem solving skills to address worry. Another protocol provides a manual for CBT for geriatric patients with GAD (76).

Any clinician working with older adults in psychiatric inpatient settings has observed the frequent comorbidity of major depression and intense anxiety symptoms. Inpatient group interventions, which include meditation and relaxation training, appear helpful, with the caveat that some modification is necessary to allow for cohort and aging factors. In our experience, relaxation training that attempts to teach diaphragmatic breathing can be confusing or off-putting for an older adult who has been breathing the same way for 70 years or longer. Rather, a directive that introduces deep breathing by drawing an analogy between filling the lungs with air and inflating two balloons seems easier to accept. Also, as some researchers note (78), the standard muscle relaxation practice of tightening and release may be uncomfortable for older adults with arthritis, stiffness, and other painful conditions. Having the patient simply notice muscular tension and then relax the muscle on exhaling may be an effective alternative. Finally, guided imagery, if used, should be kept simple and tailored to the cohort—for example the image of relaxing in a comfortable armchair or a garden might be a more familiar and accessible image for the older adult than basking in the sun by the surf.

The Bipolar Older Adult

Many geriatric psychotherapists would agree that the psychotherapeutic techniques shown effective with unipolar depressed older adults appear applicable to those whose depression is in the context of a bipolar disorder. Unfortunately and surprisingly, no psychotherapeutic approaches have as yet been empirically validated specifically with geriatric bipolar patients. This is particularly lamentable in light of observations that psychotherapy can support adherence to a medication regimen that defers recurrence of further episodes. Nonadherence among relapsing bipolar patients may be as high as 75% (82), and the complicated medication regimens that reflect elderly patients' combined medical and psychiatric treatment needs put them at high risk for nonadherence (83).

Researchers have attempted to define the psychotherapeutic factors that produce a favorable change in adherence or compliance in younger bipolar patients, and many of these are directly applicable to the treatment of older patients as well. Adherence problems can be addressed with psychoeducation about bipolar disorder and therapeutic assistance in grieving the loss of the healthy self (84). Stress and disruptions of circadian rhythms or sleep have also been identified as potent triggers of bipolar relapse (85) and interventions have been developed to teach bipolar patients techniques for monitoring and managing stress (86,87). Findings from family studies that have lowered relapse rates in bipolar individuals by reducing the level of negative "expressed emotion" (EE) in their family environments (88) have relevance for bipolar older adults who are treated in a hostile or critical manner by their families or caregivers.

Although individual psychotherapy with an acutely manic patient is generally ineffective in controlling symptoms, family interventions often prove useful at this stage and can be adapted easily for use with the families of manic older adults. A unique aspect of work with such families is the need, in cases where bipolar episodes have recurred over many years, to address the stressfulness of adult children's longstanding and current struggles with a bipolar parent. In contrast to work with younger families, psychoeducation of a manic older adult's family takes into account the frequent medical factors or associated cognitive symptoms more commonly associated with mania occurring in this age group.

Between episodes or during a depressive phase, group therapy models developed for unipolar depressed older adults might be considered for bipolar patients as well. Like the unipolar patient, the older bipolar patient may benefit from group therapy that addresses medication compliance, illness management, and stress reduction. In leading such a group, the therapist may face difficulties in maintaining the delicate balance between redirecting and validating patients recovering from mania or hypomania and still experiencing flight of ideas or pressured speech. As the therapist focuses intently on the content of each patient's communication and responds with feedback that may include both verbal comments and nonverbal cues to assist in limit setting and redirecting, the other group members follow suit, providing the newly stabilized patient with a context of acceptance and support while modeling appropriate modes of communication. Individual psychotherapy becomes increasingly feasible as the patient stabilizes further and graduates to a partial hospital or outpatient setting. An "empathic diagnosis" (3) (see section, the "gerotherapist" and the patient: engaging and treating the older adult) would inform the cognitive behavioral and problem-solving components of an integrative form of psychotherapy, gerodynamic behavior therapy (GBT) (58), adapted for geriatric bipolar disorder.

The adaptation of gerodynamic behavior therapy for bipolar disorder (termed here GBT-B) offers preventive strategies modified for the older adult and incorporating stress management and maintenance of consistent circadian rhythms through behavioral scheduling, "bi-directional mood monitoring" (monitoring highs and lows), and reparative measures to deal with the psychological, interpersonal, and practical aftermath of the depressive or manic episode through thought recording and journaling. Consistent with standard GBT, GBT-B examines historical variables that might have contributed to the patient's denial of illness or resistance to treatment, then uses behavioral techniques to address current maladaptive thoughts that enhance the risk for treatment nonadherence and recurrent episodes.

The Older Suicidal Patient

People aged 75 years or older are more likely to complete a suicide attempt and die than people in any other age group (89,90). The older patient with suicidal ideation is often seen on an emergency basis and perhaps admitted for inpatient care. Of course, he or she may also present in an outpatient setting. Geriatric clinicians will observe that the experience of a depressive episode can in itself induce a "metadepression" resulting in suicidal ideation as the older patient fears that this depressive episode is part of a final descent to the "end of the road" and that their loss of functioning is permanent.

The patient with suicidal ideation presents a clinical crisis, and one that may be especially alarming for the less-experienced psychotherapist. Despite the strong inclination such a therapist might feel to rush into a "safety contract" with the patient, prematurely requesting a patient to guarantee that he or she will not commit suicide in the next 24 hours may reduce the therapists' anxiety more than the patient's actual risk. In contrast, allowing the patient time and support to express fully his/her intense emotional pain or "psychache" (91), and attempting to "empathize with the patient's pain experience to such a point that [the psychotherapist] can 'see' why suicide is the only alternative" (92, p. 173) may initially relieve the patient, set the stage for a more thorough and accurate assessment of "safety," and ultimately strengthen the therapeutic alliance. The psychological factor which correlates most strongly with suicide potential, an extreme sense of hopelessness (93–95), is all too common among older people, who face irreversible decline and loss as they age (96). The patient's communication of these feelings to a therapist is a form of reaching out, however feeble, and an indication of some degree of hope, however small, that there may be an alternative solution. Caring for the older suicidal patient "consists of the imperative 'do something' and also the imperative 'be there' which implies 'being with the other person'" (90, p. 379). At the same time, the therapist must walk the delicate line between empathic understanding of the patient's despair and collaborative exploration of reasons for continued survival. The following excerpt from a psychotherapy session with a 68-year-old widow hospitalized after overdosing on Lorazepam on the anniversary of her husband's death illustrates the balance between empathy and the development of an alliance around shared problem solving:

Patient: I was fine for awhile. Everyone stopped in—the kids, Sam's sister. I didn't have to lift a finger for the funeral. For awhile, they all called. I got invited by our friends. Then there was the financial stuff to deal with. Sam always loved good times, and he was so much fun to be around. Everyone loved him, but he wasn't much of a planner. So I spent time talking to lawyers, accountants . . . there was so much to do.

Therapist: So you're saying that in the first few months after his death, you had a lot of support from family and friends. And settling the finances kept you busy for quite some time also.

Patient: Yes, but that's all over now. My children are busy with their own lives. Sam's family I don't hear from much any more. And the friends . . . I'm just a fifth wheel now, the odd person out with no husband. So whom do I have? Nobody called last Sunday, his anniversary. That was the last straw. Nobody remembered. Nobody cared if I was dead or alive.

Therapist: You must have felt very alone. Did you think of calling someone yourself?

Patient: I shouldn't have to. They know I've had anxiety and depression. They just don't care. Now that I'm in the hospital they're all concerned. But it's too late. I don't want to go on.

Therapist: I imagine that you must on some level feel pretty angry at your family.

Patient: Well . . . upset, I suppose. Wouldn't you be? But they have their own lives. Their kids are more important than an old lady (crying). How can anyone possibly understand? It's no use.

Therapist: You feel you don't matter any more, your life doesn't matter any more.

Patient: Yes! . . . that's exactly how I feel.

Therapist: I don't know what your pain feels like, because I'm not in your shoes, but I'd like to try to understand, so that we can work together to help you feel better. You've taken a good first step in sharing your thoughts and feelings so honestly today. Together, you and I and the

> rest of your team will work toward finding a solution that you'll come to see as preferable to ending your life. We don't know what that is yet, but it will become clearer as we work together.

Notice that the therapist models for the patient some expression of helplessness and anger—two powerful contributors to suicidal behavior. The therapist also reduces the patient's profound sense of aloneness through a number of "we" statements, and attempts to empower the patient through reinforcement of her ability to express her feelings. Finally, the promise of a better "solution" gives the patient a sense of hope. In subsequent sessions, this patient might be asked to list some things she has to live for. The therapist can and should assume a very proactive stance in this, as the patient herself may be at a loss. It is also important to educate the patient about the effect of a successful suicide on other family members, in particular the risk that close relatives or descendants may learn to view suicide as an acceptable solution to life's difficulties and consider ending their own lives in this way. To reduce the risk of engendering guilt feelings in an already depressed patient, it is important to emphasize with the patient that his or her suicide attempt was not completed. The enduring lesson for the patient's family will depend less on the uncompleted attempt and more on constructive problem solving.

Richman (97), discussing psychotherapy with families of the suicidal elderly, emphasizes the importance of understanding suicidal behavior in the context of a family's approach to problem solving: "To understand suicide we must explore at least three generations, especially how the family deals with loss and bereavement ... suicidal events may be inseparable from the relationships between the generations ... unresolved mourning can usually be traced back to at least three generations in depression and suicide prone families" (p. 655). Richman cites Stengel (98) in underscoring the importance of the family's response to a suicidal gesture, noting that the outcome of a suicidal act depends upon its consequences: "If it (the suicidal gesture) brings people closer, no further suicidal or other self destructive behavior will take place. If nothing changes, or if the situation becomes worse, the result is further suicidal behavior and completed suicides" (p. 653). In families where a suicide was completed, placing surviving family members at increased risk for similar behavior (99), family treatment can have an especially important role.

Aaron Beck, the "father" of CBT who, with his colleagues, developed the Beck Hopelessness Scale to assess suicide potential in adults (95), is a strong proponent of CBT in the treatment of suicidal ideation. In Beck's schema, feelings of hopelessness derive from negative thought patterns such as "catastrophic thinking" and "overgeneralization" in coming to maladaptive and inaccurate conclusions about his/her situation. This can occur at any age, but older adults, with their vulnerability to a variety of losses, are particularly at risk. Through a therapeutic process of examining the evidence for their conclusions, patients can begin to question their negative thinking, generate more realistic thoughts and thereby reduce their feelings of hopelessness.

The Depressed Older Adult with a Personality Disorder

Patients with personality disorders present special challenges to the psychotherapeutic process, discussion of which could easily fill a large volume. Yet, the importance of personality disorder cannot be overlooked in a discussion of depression, as researchers have shown that a history of depression in an older adult is associated with a greater prevalence of personality disorder (100). In older adults with comorbid personality disorder and major depressive disorder, pharmacotherapy combined with a modified form of Linehan's (101) dialectical behavior therapy (DBT) for older adults has been shown significantly more effective than medication alone (102). As adapted for use with older adults, DBT extends its focus on cognitive, affective, and behavioral functioning to emphasize problem solving, accepting reality, relating to others, and maintaining a sense of self (103). Older adults with personality disorders are more isolated, partly because of poor social skills and partly because of burnout in their social networks (24). Estrangement from grown children is not uncommon and may increase the risk of suicide. Such patients require longer term psychotherapy that may alternate between crisis prevention and the development of more adaptive behaviors (24).

It should be remembered that in treating the personality disordered older adult with depression, the goal is not to "cure" the personality disorder but to treat the depression. The therapist must achieve a balance between providing genuine empathy, maintaining neutrality and firm boundaries, and carefully structuring the therapy around clear, concrete goals. Personality disordered patients can ultimately develop a strong, healthy therapeutic alliance when they discover that the therapist has the strength to remain neutral and objective. Careful monitoring of the therapeutic alliance will allow negotiation of early mistrust and hostility and preparation later for termination, which the patient may experience as a painful loss. For many older patients, infrequent but consistent follow-up contact serves a stabilizing and protective function (24).

The Depressed Older Adult with Cognitive Impairment

While the literature is replete with behavioral and pharmacotherapeutic approaches for the management of symptoms associated with advanced dementia, less guidance is available regarding psychotherapy with depressed patients in the early stages of cognitive decline. Anxiety about functional impairment often accompanies the depressive symptoms in such patients and support is needed in working through a progressive loss and in addressing the practical consequences of diminished capability.

Teri and Thompson (104) have developed a program of cognitive behavioral interventions for the treatment of depression in early Alzheimer's patients. They outline a set of guidelines for cognitive therapy for patients with mild impairment, and behavioral interventions for patients with moderate-to-severe impairment. In the earlier stage of impairment, patients identify and record maladaptive cognitions that increase feelings of hopelessness and helplessness, such as ruminations about the future or magnification of current deficits. Patients work with the therapist to challenge these thoughts and explore adaptive alternatives, such as focusing on remaining capabilities rather than deficits and staying grounded in the present. Patients rate their feelings before and after generating adaptive thoughts, which affords a sense of control and accomplishment. For more severe impairment, the focus is on increasing the frequency of pleasant experiences for the patient. As the patient declines further, caregivers are increasingly included in the therapeutic process to facilitate implementation of the plan. While this approach may seem simplistic, it actually involves a thorough analysis of behaviors and situations that maintain the patient's depression.

In group therapy, "here and now" experiences can build coping strategies in patients despite the presence of mild-to-moderate cognitive impairment (105). For example, if one patient loses the thread of a problem being discussed, she may experience support and relief by asking other group members to report similar difficulties with remaining on track. Some researchers stress the adaptive denial in patients with progressive dementia however, and caution therapists to be mindful about the consequences of breaking through such denial (105).

Modified forms of individual and group psychotherapy can offer support even to patients with more severe degrees of cognitive impairment. Validation therapy (106) offers a selection of nonverbal techniques to help the cognitively impaired patient express and process feelings and needs triggered by intact remote memory, while resolution therapy (107) employs empathic listening to help the patient identify feelings in the here-and-now, while modifying the environment, if possible, to accommodate to the patient's needs. These approaches share the goal of reducing the "excess disability" that depression adds to cognitive impairment (108).

CROSS-CULTURAL CONSIDERATION IN PSYCHOTHERAPY WITH OLDER ADULTS

In addition to the "cultural" differences between successive generations already noted, treatment of depressed geriatric patients and their families must take into account cross-cultural concerns that arise when an elder's youth was spent not only in a different era but also in a different country with contrasting values and attitudes toward the aged. In a comparison of Korean American and Caucasian American caregivers, for example, obligation, affection, and reciprocity, for example, were endorsed by all subjects as important motivational responses, while respect for parents, family harmony, and filial sacrifice were given much greater value by the Korean American caregivers (109). Culture, which has been defined as "the totality of learned, socially transmitted behavior of a group that emerges from its members' interpersonal interactions" (110, p. 132), unavoidably influences the ways in which people perceive the problems associated with aging and the way in which they seek solutions (111).

Culturally transmitted values, or their dissolution, become of particular importance when treating newly arrived and first generation Americans. Many ethnic groups share characteristics that may affect the older adult's engagement in a psychotherapeutic process, such as mistrust of the dominant culture, greater reliance upon religious institutions, reverence for parents and grandparents as sources of wisdom and teachers of culture and oral history, and strong family bonds, which keep problem solving within the family (110). These culturally specific issues naturally affect the older adult's comfort with divulging personal problems, expectations of adult children, and readiness to accept physical care from an outsider or within a psychiatric or long-term care facility. Individuals as well as regional mores differ, however, so the clinician must take care to avoid overgeneralizing assumptions about the behavior and values of large but varied ethnic groups. For example, the concept of "filial piety" in the Asian culture (110), that is, the expectation that grown children will honor and respect their parents, is expressed differentially in Japan, China, and Korea. Similarly, beliefs and practices differ significantly between various tribes of Native Americans (110). Thus, the clinician must not only become educated about variation between specific cultural groups, but also appreciate how the role-specific transmitted values mingle with individual experience, needs, and expectations. The clinician can gain such knowledge and insight by seeking education directly from the patient or family. The following case example underscores the importance of this:

> Ms. P., an Asian American older adult, was attending a partial hospitalization program for treatment of depression. After moving from another state to live with her grownup daughter in her rural home, Ms. P. had become increasingly lonely and overworked, as she spent her days in the house cleaning and cooking while her daughter was at work. The therapist attempted to work with Ms. P. on directly communicating to her daughter her need for transportation, and her desire to cut back a bit on the household chores. However, Ms. P. could not bring herself to have the recommended "talk" with her daughter, and furthermore could not explain why. During the treatment of this patient, the therapist attended a lecture on cross-cultural issues with patients. Suspecting that cultural factors might be at play, the therapist in the next session gently explored the reasons for the patient's reluctance to talk with her daughter, offering some speculations from what she had learned. Encouraged by the therapist's genuine interest, the patient informed the therapist that in her particular culture, the grownup child assuming the caretaking role became the authority; it was therefore inappropriate for Ms. P. to "challenge" her daughter. Moreover, the patient admitted that she had not wanted to share this information with the therapist because it would also be inappropriate to challenge another caretaker, the Doctor; to do so would undermine the therapist's authority. Thus, the patient had felt stymied, both with her daughter and with her therapist. As a result of this discussion, the therapist arranged a family meeting with mother and daughter, in which communication was gently and sensitively facilitated between parent and grownup child, with productive results.

CONCLUDING REMARKS

This chapter has attempted to acquaint the reader with the importance and viability of psychotherapy as an integral component in the treatment of older adults with psychiatric conditions, and to familiarize clinicians with some special issues of aging that affect psychotherapeutic process and outcome. Comfort and knowledge in treating older patients will attain even greater value as the geriatric population continues to account for a growing percentage of our total population. Aging "baby boomers," who have reached maturity during an era of greater openness, psychological sophistication, and reduced stigmatization of mental illness, are likely to demand greater availability of skilled geriatric psychotherapists. As we treat today's older adults and prepare for an even larger geriatric population's needs, we must keep in mind that older adults, no less than younger adults, can use psychotherapy to gain insight and problem solve about issues both universal and unique, enhance their engagement in a social network, modify their thoughts and behaviors, and continue their emotional growth and change during a stressful and complex but potentially rich stage of life.

REFERENCES

1. Freud S. On Psychotherapy. Collected Papers. Translated by London BJ. Richmond, England, U. K.: Hogarth Press, 1924; 258.
2. Colarusso CA, Nemiroff RA. Clinical implications of adult developmental theory. Am J Psychiatry 1987; 144:1263–1270.

3. Muslin HL. The Psychotherapy of the Elderly Self. New York, NY: Brunner/Mazel Inc., 1992.
4. Erikson EH, Erikson JM, Kivnick HQ. Vital Involvement in Old Age. New York, NY: W. W. Norton & Company Inc., 1989.
5. Erikson EH. Childhood and Society. New York, NY: W. W. Norton & Company Inc., 1950:232.
6. Liptzin B. Psychotherapy with the elderly: An Eriksonian perspective. J Geriatric Psychiatry 1985; 18:183–202.
7. McGinn LK. Cognitive behavioral therapy of depression: Theory, treatment and empirical status. Am J Psychother 2000; 54:257–261.
8. DeRubeis FJ, Hollon SD, Amsterdam JD, et al. Cognitive therapy vs medications in the treatment of moderate to severe depression. Arch Gen Psychiatry 2005; 62:409–416.
9. Thase ME, Greenhouse JB, Frank E, et al. Treatment of major depression with psychotherapy or psychotherapy–pharmacotherapy combinations. Arch Gen Psychiatry 1997; 54:1009–1015.
10. Pampallona S, Bollini P, Tibaldi G, et al. Combined pharmacotherapy and psychological treatment for depression: A systematic review. Arch Gen Psychiatry 2004; 61:714–719.
11. Thompson LW, Gallagher D, Breckenridge JS. Comparative effectiveness of psychotherapies for depressed elders. J Consult Clin Psychol 1987; 55:385–390.
12. Gerson S, Belin TR, Kaufman A, et al. Pharmacological and psychological treatments for depressed older patients: A meta-analysis and overview of recent findings. Harv Rev Psychiatry 1999; 7:1–28.
13. Reynolds CF III, Frank E, Perel JM, et al. Nortriptyline and interpersonal psychotherapy as maintenance therapies for recurrent major depression. J Am Med Assoc 1999; 281:39–45.
14. Alexopoulos GS, Katz IR, Reynolds CF III, et al. Pharmacotherapy of depressive disorders in older patients. Postgraduate Medicine: Special Report, 2001.
15. Steinman LE, Frederick JT, Prohaska T, et al. Late Life Depression Special Interest Project Panelists. Recommendations for treating depression in community based older adults. Am J Prev Med 2007; 33:175–181.
16. Frederick JT, Steinman LE, Prohaska T, et al. Late Life Depression Special interest Project Panelists. Community-based treatment of late life depression an expert panel-informed literature review. Am J Prev Med 2007; 33:222–249.
17. Pinquart M, Duberstein PR, Lyness JM. Treatments for later-life depressive conditions: A meta-analytic comparison of pharmacotherapy and psychotherapy. Am J Psychiatry 2006; 163:1493–1501.
18. Wei W, Sambamoorthi U, Olfson M, et al. Use of psychotherapy for depression in older adults. Am J Psychiatry 2005; 162:711–717.
19. Knight BG. The scientific basis for psychotherapeutic interventions with older adults: An overview. JCLP/In Session: Psychothe Pract 1999; 55:927–934.
20. Tice CI, Perkins K. Mental Health Issues and Aging. Pacific Grove, CA: Brooks/Cole, 1996.
21. Drayer RA, Mulsant BH, Lenze EJ, et al. Somatic symptoms of depression in elderly patients with medical comorbidities. Int J Geriatr Psychiatry 2005; 20:973–982.
22. Sheehan B, Banerjee S. Review: Somatization in the elderly. Int J Geriatr Psychiatry 1999; 14:1044–1049.
23. Finkel SI. Group psychotherapy in later life. In: Myers WA, ed. New Techniques in the Psychotherapy of Older Patients. Washington, DC: American Psychiatric Press, 1991:223–244.
24. Zarit SH, Zarit JM. Mental Disorders in Older Adults. New York, NY: Guilford Press, 1998.
25. Snowden M, Steinman L, Frederick J. Treating depression in older adults: Challenges to implementing the recommendations of an expert panel. Prev Chronic Dis 2008; 5(1). http://www.cdc.gov/pcd/issues/2008/jan/07_0154.htm
26. Garner J. Psychotherapies and older adults. Aust N Z J Psychiatry 2003; 37:538–552.

27. Newton NA, Jacobowitz J. Transferential and countertransferential processes in therapy with older adults. In: Duffy M, ed. Handbook of Counseling and Psychotherapy with Older Adults. New York, NY: Wiley, 1991:21–40.
28. Kivnik HQ, Kafka A. It takes two: Therapeutic alliance with older clients. In: Duffy M, ed. Handbook of Counseling and Psychotherapy with Older Adults. New York, NY: Wiley, 1999; 122.
29. Brody CM. Existential issues of hope and meaning in late life therapy. In: Duffy M, ed. Handbook of Counseling and Psychotherapy with Older adults. New York, NY: Wiley & Sons, 1999:91–106.
30. Niederebe G. Psychosocial treatments with depressed older adults. Am J Geriatr Psychiatry 1996; 4(Suppl. 1):566–578.
31. Klerman GL, Wiseman MM. New applications of interpersonal psychotherapy. Washington, D.C.: American Psychiatric Press Inc., 1993.
32. Miller MD, Frank E, Cornes C, et al. The value of maintenance interpersonal psychotherapy (IPT) in older adults with different IPT foci. Am J Geriatr Psychiatry 2003; 11:97–102.
33. Zweig RA, Hinrichsen GA. Factors associated with suicide attempts by depressed older adults. Am J Psychiatry 1993; 150:1687–1692.
34. Reynolds CF III, Frank E, Dew MA, et al. Treatment of 70+ year olds with recurrent major depression. Am J Geriatr Psychiatry 1999; 7:64–66.
35. Reynolds CF III, Frank E, Houck PR, et al. Which elderly patients with remitted depression remain well with continued interpersonal psychotherapy after discontinuation of antidepressant mediation? Am J Psychiatry 1997; 154:958–962.
36. Reynolds CF III, Frank E, Kupler DJ, et al. Treatment outcome in recurrent major depression: A post hoc comparison of elderly ("young old") and midlife patients. Am J Psychiatry 1996; 153:1288–1292.
37. Reynolds CF III, Frank E, Perel JM, et al. Treatment of consecutive episodes of major depression in the elderly. Am J Psychiatry 1994; 151:1704–1743.
38. Dembrovski AY, Lenze EJ, Dew MA, et al. Maintenance treatment of old age depression preserves health-related quality of life: A randomized, controlled trial of paroxetine and interpersonal psychotherapy. J Am Geriatr Soc 2007; 55:1325–1332.
39. Markowitz JC. Is IPT time-limited psychodynamic psychotherapy? J Psychother Pract Res 1998; 7:185–195.
40. Arean PA, Perri MG, Nezu AM, et al. Comparative effectiveness of social problem-solving therapy and reminiscence therapy as treatments for depression in older adults. J Consult Clin Psychol 1993; 6:1003–1010.
41. Alexopoulos GS, Raue P, Arean P. Problem solving therapy vs supportive therapy in geriatric major depression with executive dysfunction. Am J Geriatr Psychiatry 2003; 11:46–52.
42. Gellis ZD, McGinty J, Horowitz A, et al. Problem-solving therapy for late-life depression in home care: A randomized field trial. Am J Geriatr Psychiatry 2007; 15:968–978.
43. Leigh R, Varghese F. Psychodynamic psychotherapy with the elderly. J Psychiatr Pract 2001; 229–237.
44. Myers WA. Psychoanalytic psychotherapy and psychoanalysis with older patients. In: Myers WA, ed. New Techniques in the Psychotherapy of Older Patients. Washington, D.C.: American Psychiatric Press Inc., 1991.
45. Nordhus IH, Nielsen GH. Brief dynamic psychotherapy with older adults. JCLP/In Session: Psychother Pract 1999; 55(8):935–947.
46. Gallagher-Thompson D, Thompson LW. Psychotherapy with older adults in theory and practice. In: Bonger B, Beutler B, eds. Comprehensive Textbook of Psychotherapy. New York, NY: Oxford University Press 1994; 357–379.
47. Arean PA, Cook BL. Psychotherapy and combined psychotherapy/pharmacotherapy for late life depression. Biol Psychiatry 2002; 52:293–303.
48. Beck AT, Rush J, Shaw B, et al. Cognitive therapy of depression. New York, NY: Guilford Press, 1974.
49. Scogin F, McElreath L. Efficacy of psychosocial treatments for geriatric depression: A quantitative review. J Couns Clin Psychol 1994; 62:69–74.

50. Teri L, Gallagher-Thompson D. Cognitive–behavioral interventions for treatment of depression in Alzheimer's patients. Gerontologist 1991; 31:413–416.
51. Wilson K, Mottram P, Vassilas C. Psychotherapeutic treatments for older depressed people. Cochrand Database Syst Rev 2008; 1:CD004853.
52. Smith A, Graham L, Senthinathan S. Mindfulness-based cognitive therapy for recurring depression in older people: A qualitative study. Aging Ment Health 2007; 11:346–357.
53. Pinquart M, Duberstein PR, Lyness JM. Treatments for later-life depressive conditions: A meta-analytic comparison of pharmacotherapy and psychotherapy. Am J Psychiatry 2006; 163:1493–1501.
54. Garner J. Psychotherapies and older adults. Aust N Z J Psychiatry 2003; 37:538–552.
55. Thompson LW, Gantz F, Florscheim M, et al. Cognitive behavioral therapy for affective disorders in the elderly. In: Myers WA, ed. New Techniques in the Psychotherapy of Older Patients. Washington, D.C.: American Psychiatric Press Inc., 1991:3–20.
56. Folstein M, Folstein S, McHugh P. "Mini-Mental State"—A practical method for grading the cognitive state of patients for the clinician. J Psychiat Res 1975; 12:189–198.
57. Dick-Sisken L. Cognitive behavioral therapy with older adults. The Behavior Therapist 2002; open forum, special series, January: 3–6.
58. Antognini FC. Psychotherapy with depressed older adults. In: Ellison JM, Verma S, eds. Depression in Late Life: A Multidisciplinary Psychiatric Approach. New York, NY: Marcel-Dekker, 2003.
59. Finkel SI. Group psychotherapy in later life. In: Myers WA, ed. New Techniques in the Psychotherapy of Older Patients. Washington, D.C.: American Psychiatric Press, 1991.
60. Steuer JL, Mintz J, Hammen CL, et al. Cognitive–behavioral and psychodynamic group psychotherapy in treatment of geriatric depression. J Consult Clin Psychol 1984; 51:180–189.
61. Beutler LE, Scogin F, Kirkish P, et al. Group cognitive therapy and alprazolam in the treatment of depression in older adults. J Consult Clin Psychol 1987; 55:550–556.
62. Lewisohn PM, Munoz RF, Youngren MA, et al. Control Your Depression. New York, NY: Simon & Schuster, 1992.
63. Moberg P, Lazarus L. Psychotherapy of depression in the elderly. Psychiatr Ann 1990; 20:92–96.
64. Yost EB, Beutler LE, Corbishley MA, et al. Group Cognitive Therapy: A Treatment Approach for Depressed Older Adults. New York, NY: Pergamon Press, 1986.
65. Molinari V. Using reminiscence and life review as natural therapeutic strategies in group therapy. In: Duffy M, ed. Handbook of Counseling and Psychotherapy with Older Adults. New York, NY: Viking, 1999;154–165.
66. Seligman ME. Helplessness: On Depression, Development and Death. San Francisco, CA: Freeman, 1975.
67. Guilleard C. Family therapy with older clients. In: Woods RT, eds. Handbook of the Clinical Psychology of Ageing. Chichester, U.K.: Wiley, 1996:561–574.
68. Wyman MF, Gum A, Arean P. Psychotherapy with older adults. In: Agronin ME, Maletta GJ, eds. Principles and Practice of Geriatric Psychiatry. Philadelphia, PA: Lippincott Williams & Wilkins, 2004:177–198.
69. Rosowsky E. Couple therapy with long-married older adults. In: Duffy M, ed. Handbook of Counseling and Psychotherapy with Older Adults. New York, NY: Wiley, 1999:222–266.
70. Kaplan HS. Sex therapy with older patients. In: Myers W, ed. New Techniques in the Psychotherapy of Older Patients. Washington, D.C.: American Psychiatric Press, 1992:21–38.
71. Qualls SH. Realizing power in intergenerational family hierarchies: Family reorganization when older adults decline. In: Duffy M, eds. Handbook of Counseling and Psychotherapy with Older Adults. New York, NY: Wiley, 1999:228–241.
72. Hegestad GO. Demographic change and the life course: Some emerging trends in the family realm. Fam Relat 1988; 37:405–410.
73. Neidhardt ER, Allen JA. Family Therapy with the Elderly. London, U.K.: Sage, 1992.

74. Benbow SM, Marriott A, Morley M, et al. Family therapy and dementia: Review and clinical experience. International J Geriatr Psychiatry 1993; 8:717–725.
75. Wetherell JI, Gatz M, Craske MG. Treatment of generalized anxiety disorder in older adults. J Consult Clin Psychology 2003; 71:31–40.
76. Stanley MA, Diefenbach GJ, Hopko DR. Cognitive behavioral treatment for older adults with generalized anxiety disorder. Behav Modif 2004; 28:73–117.
77. Gorenstein EE, Papp LA. Cognitive behavior therapy for anxiety in the elderly. Curr Psychiatry Rep 2007; 9:20–25.
78. Ayers CR, Sorrell IT, Thorp SR, et al. Evidence based psychological treatments for late life anxiety. Psychol Aging 2007; 22:8–17.
79. Gerenstein EE, Kleber MS, Mohlman J, et al. Cognitive behavioral therapy for management of anxiety and medication taper in older adults. Am J Geriatr Psychiatry 2005; 13:901–909.
80. Stanley MA, Beck JG, Glasco JD. Treatment of generalized anxiety in older adults: A preliminary comparison of cognitive–behavioral and supportive approaches. Behav Ther 1996; 27:565–581.
81. Wetherell JL, Lenze EJ, Stanley MA. Evidence-based treatment of geriatric anxiety disorders. Psychiatr Clin North Am 2005; 28:871–896.
82. Post RM, Demicoff KD, Frye MA, et al. A history of the use of anticonvulsants as mood stabilizers in the last two decades of the 20th century. Neuropsychobiology 1998; 38:152–156.
83. Salzman C. Medication compliance in the elderly. J Clin Psychiatry 1995; 56(suppl.):18–22.
84. Miklowitz DJ, Frank E, George E. Bipolar Disorder: A Family Focused Approach. New York, NY: Guilford Press, 1997.
85. Ellicott AC, Hammon C, Gitlin M, et al. Life events in the course of bipolar disorder. Am J Psychiatry 1990; 147:1194–1198.
86. Basco MR, Rush AJ. Cognitive Behavioral Therapy for Bipolar Disorder. New York, NY: Guilford Press, 1996.
87. Frank E. Treating Bipolar Disorder: A Clinician's Guide to Interpersonal and Social Rhythm Therapy. New York, NY: Guilford Press, 2005.
88. Miklowitz DJ, Frank E, George EL. New psychosocial treatments for the outpatient management of bipolar disorder. Psychopharmacol Bull 1996; 32:613–621.
89. World Health Organization. Figures and facts about suicide. Technical Report. Geneva: WHO, 1999.
90. Vanlaere L, Bouckaert F, Gastmans C. Care for suicidal older people: Current clinical–ethical considerations. J Med Ethics 2007; 33:376–381.
91. Schneidman E. The Suicidal Mind. New York, NY: Oxford University Press, 1996.
92. Orbach R. Therapeutic empathy with the suicidal wish: Principles of therapy with suicidal individuals. Am J Psychother 2001; 55a:166–184.
93. Beck AT, Weissman A, Lester D, et al. The measurement of pessimism: The hopelessness scale. J Consult Clin Psychol 1974; 42:861–865.
94. Beck AT, Weishaar ME. Suicide risk assessment and prediction. Crisis 1990; 11:22–30.
95. Beck AT, Steer RA, Beck JS, et al. Hopelessness, depression, suicidal ideation, and clinical diagnosis of depression. Suicide Life Threat Behav 1993; 23:139–145.
96. McIntosh L, Santos JE, Hubbard RW, et al. Elder Suicide: Research, Theory and Techniques. Washington, D.C.: American Psychological Association, 1994.
97. Richman J. Psychotherapy with the suicidal elderly: A family oriented approach. In: Duffy M, ed. Handbook of Counseling and Psychotherapy with Older Adults. New York, NY: Wiley, 1999:650–661.
98. Stengel E. Suicide and Attempted Suicide. Baltimore, MD: Penguin, 1964.
99. Szantos K, Reynolds CF, Conwell Y, et al. High levels of hopelessness persist in geriatric patients with remitted depression and a history of attempted suicide. J Am Geriatr Soc 1998; 46:1401–1406.
100. Abrams RC, Alexopoulos GS, Young R. Geriatric depression and DSMIII-R personality criteria. J Am Geriatr Soc 1987; 35:383–386.

101. Linehan MM. Cognitive–Behavioral Treatment of Borderline Personality Disorder. New York, NY: Guilford Press, 1993.
102. Lynch TR, Cheavens JS, Cukrowicz KC, et al. Treatment of older adults with co-morbid personality disorder and depression: A dialectical behavior therapy approach. Int J Geriatr Psychiatry 2007; 22:702–703.
103. Lynch TR, Morse JQ, Mendelson T, et al. Dialectical behavior therapy for depressed older adults. Am J Geriatr Psychiatry 2000; 11:33–45.
104. Teri L, Thompson D. Cognitive behavioral interventions for the treatment of depression in Alzheimer's patients. Gerontologist 1991; 31:413–416.
105. Yale R. A Guide to Facilitating Support Groups for Newly Diagnosed Alzheimer's Patients. San Francisco, CA: Alzheimer's Association, Greater San Francisco Chapter, 1991.
106. Feil N. Validation: An empirical approach to the care of dementia. Clin Gerontol 1989; 8:89–94.
107. Stokes G, Goudie F. Counselling elderly people. In: Stokes G, Goudie F, eds. Working with Dementia. Bicester, U.K.: Winslow Press, 1990:181–190.
108. Reifler BV, Larson E. Excess disability in dementia of the Alzheimer's type. In: Light E, Lebowitz BD, eds. Alzheimer's Disease Treatment and Family Stress: Directions for Research. Rockville, MD: National Institute of Mental Health, 1989:363–397.
109. Sung TK. Cross cultural comparison of motivations for parent care: The case of Americans and Koreans. J Aging Stud 1994; 8:195–209.
110. Morales P. The impact of cultural differences in psychotherapy with older clients: Sensitive issues and strategies. In: Duffy M, ed. Handbook of Counseling and Psychotherapy with Older adults. New York, NY: Wiley, 1999:132–153.
111. Wong PT, Ujimoto KV. The elderly: their stress, coping and mental health. In: Lee LC, Zane NWS, eds. Handbook of Asian American Psychology. Thousand Oaks, CA: Sage, 1998:401–432.

18 Barriers to Treatment: Nonadherence to Medications in the Treatment of Mood Disorders in Later Life

Shunda M. McGahee

Healthcare for the Homeless, Massachusetts General Hospital, and Department of Psychiatry, Harvard Medical School, Boston, Massachusetts, U.S.A.

Lianne K. Morris-Smith

Health Sciences and Technology, Harvard Medical School, Boston, Massachusetts, U.S.A.

Helen H. Kyomen

McLean Hospital, Belmont, and Department of Psychiatry, Harvard Medical School, Boston, Massachusetts, U.S.A.

INTRODUCTION

Multiple and complex factors determine medication adherence and nonadherence. Adherence to a treatment regimen indicates a patient's observance of health care providers' therapeutic recommendations. These therapeutic recommendations may involve the use of medications, participation in psychotherapy and completion of assigned work between sessions, and lifestyle or behavioral changes (1). Inherent within this definition of adherence is the suggestion that good patients who care about their health take medications as prescribed and bad patients who do not care about their health are nonadherent to a medication regimen. Salient research shows that nonadherence to treatment results in greater morbidity and mortality associated with chronic psychiatric illness, causing poor treatment response, increased outpatient visits and psychiatric hospitalizations, decreased social supports, increased suicides and other violent behaviors, and rising health care costs (2). In the United States, of all medication-related hospitalizations, 33–69% have been attributed to poor medication adherence. The costs (direct and indirect) of medical and psychiatric nonadherence have been estimated at $100 billion per year (3,4).

Despite the health and financial costs to society due to treatment nonadherence, "adherence" often has little significance for patients. Rather, patients assess therapeutic benefits of prescribed medications by the tangible relief of suffering, convenience, low costs, and tolerability (5). Clinicians' objectives are similar, although "patient response," the behavioral reaction of the patient to treatment, rather than "disease response," the effect of the treatment on the signs and symptoms of the illness, may be a better indicator of adherence and efficacy (1). In this chapter, we will discuss patient, clinician, and medication-related factors that influence medication adherence and nonadherence (6).

PATIENT-RELATED FACTORS INFLUENCING MEDICATION ADHERENCE AND NONADHERENCE

Normal Physiologic Changes Associated with Aging

Treatment of mood disorders in the elderly requires attention to the normal physiologic changes that accompany aging. Most psychiatric medications are taken orally. Drug absorption, distribution, metabolism, and elimination, which are affected by aging, may affect drug efficacy and tolerability. Efficacy and tolerability, as perceived by the patient, affect adherence (7). As described in more detail in chapter 16, the predominant effect of aging on medication pharmacokinetics is to increase the plasma level and extend the duration of action of an administered medication on an elderly patient. Given the increased sensitivity to certain neurotransmitter effects and enhanced opportunities for drug interactions as a consequence of the multiple medications taken by an average elderly adult, the changes of aging carry a risk of decreasing efficacy, increasing adverse effects, and therefore reducing adherence.

Medication and Health Beliefs

Patient's attitudes, beliefs, and group norms all influence adherence in multiple important dimensions. The rate of nonadherence appears to be highest in patients who are receiving preventive treatment or who are asymptomatic, lower in patients with symptomatic chronic illness, and lowest for the acutely ill who are receiving time limited treatment regimens (8). The Health Belief Model proposes that medication adherence will be related to patients' beliefs about the seriousness of the disease, the likelihood that the medication will affect the disease, and the obstacles they encounter in taking their medication (9). If a clinician prescribes medications that are incongruent with a patient's beliefs or if the patient's family or community holds negative views about a specific illness and its treatment, patients may be unwilling to engage in treatment (10).

The stigmatization of psychiatric illnesses and their treatments are important sources of nonadherence, as would be predicted by this model. Studies regarding patient beliefs about depression and its treatment reveal the following: Givens et al. (11) explored attitudes toward antidepressants in a sample of community dwelling depressed elders. Four themes emerged: fear of addiction, resistance to viewing depression as a medical illness, concern that antidepressants will prevent feelings of natural sadness, and prior negative experiences with medications for depression. The side effects and discontinuation syndrome associated with some antidepressants could certainly be mistaken for an indication that these medications induce dependence or "addiction." Additional themes associated with attitudes toward antidepressant use include fearing that their use implies psychologic weakness, obstructs the capacity to experience genuine sadness, or increases the risk of losing control. Further, older adults often attributed symptoms of depression to the aging process itself, to the loss of loved ones, or to age-related physical illness, and thus were less willing to accept medication and treatment (11). The work of Karasz (12) showed that when patients attributed depression to social or interpersonal causes, they were less willing to view their condition as requiring medication. But when seen as a medical disorder, there was a greater sense of severity and need to seek care (12). Furthermore, treatment adherence is a dynamic process, influenced on a daily basis by situational factors and subject to constant negotiation and renegotiation (13).

Psychiatric Diagnosis

Few studies have focused on medication nonadherence in the elderly, particularly in those with mood disorders. DiMatteo et al. (14) found that depression was the strongest predictor of patient nonadherence to medical treatment. Major depressive disorder, which affects up to 4% of community dwelling elders (2), is associated with adherence-reducing pessimism, apathy, forgetfulness, and social withdrawal. Depressive symptoms that fall below the threshold of a diagnosis of major depressive disorder are far more common and can have similar effects on adherence. In addition, elderly persons with depression had higher rates of cognitive impairment (15) that can diminish adherence through forgetfulness, confusion, or misunderstanding of treatment instructions. In patients with bipolar disorder, which accounts for a significant proportion of geriatric psychiatry inpatient, outpatient, and psychiatric emergency diagnoses, cognitive impairment is also a common finding among affected older adults. Approximately 50% of the older adults with bipolar disorder show substantial cognitive impairment on global cognitive screening measures (16,17). In addition to the impulsivity and denial that characterize hypomania and mania, cognitive changes may add confusion or forgetfulness that undermine treatment adherence. The great importance of nonadherence among bipolar patients was highlighted by a chart review of elderly bipolar inpatient admissions. During a 5-year follow-up period, approximately 45% of these patients' admissions were attributed to medication nonadherence (18).

Personality Traits

Attempts to identify personality traits that predict behavior may be useful when considering treatment nonadherence (6). Gabbard (19) suggested that problems with medication adherence could be formulated psychodynamically, considering issues such as resistance, transference, or core beliefs. Ciechanowski et al. (20) proposed that attachment theory may be helpful in understanding how the quality of early caregiving influences an individual's perceptions about and engagement in subsequent relationships, including treatment relationships. Within a primary care setting, diabetic patients were given questionnaires to determine attachment style. Information on glycemic control, medical comorbidity, and adherence to medication and clinic appointments was also collected. Patients who exhibited dismissive attachment perceived the quality of communication with their provider as poor and had significantly higher hemoglobin glycosylation, suggesting decreased treatment adherence (20). Using a descriptive framework to explore the effects of personality traits on adherence behavior, Wiebe and Christensen (21) suggested application of the Five Factor Model of personality, which includes neuroticism, extraversion, assertiveness, openness, agreeableness, and conscientiousness. When the Five Factor Model was applied to elderly dialysis patients, conscientiousness was the personality trait descriptor most closely associated with adherence behavior (22).

CLINICIAN-RELATED FACTORS INFLUENCING MEDICATION ADHERENCE AND NONADHERENCE

Knowledge of and Adherence to Clinical Guidelines

Practice guidelines, available for many diseases, offer systematic suggestions for improving clinical decision making. Many guidelines include suggestions for increasing patient adherence. McGlynn et al. (23) reported on the quality of healthcare delivered to adults in the United States for preventive and acute care of 30 conditions. For treatment of each condition, quality assessment tools were developed from established national guidelines and the medical literature. Additionally, a 49-member multispecialty expert panel reviewed the validity of the indicators proposed by the assessment tool. Alcohol dependence was the only psychiatric illness included. Of the 6712 participants, analysis of care delivered showed participants received only 54.9% of what would be considered quality care. Underuse of guideline was frequently observed and recommended care was not received by 46.3% of assessed subjects (23). These findings raise an important question: Would clinician adherence to treatment guidelines increase patient adherence to therapeutic recommendations, thereby decreasing morbidity, mortality, and cost associated with the chronic treatment of psychiatric and medical illness? Yet, clinicians' clinical decision making is not based solely on an algorithm of symptoms. Physician adherence can be a sensitive issue: "Many physicians resent or even resist scrutiny of the unique prerogative to prescribe, since it symbolizes the essence of their physicianship" (24).

In a retrospective study of physician noncompliance with length of hospital stay for low-risk chest pain patients, Ellrodt et al. (25) reported on reasons for increased hospital length of stay. Reasons included inaccurate classification of patient risk due to the sensitivities, specificities and predictive values of guidelines. Other factors that decreased the utility of the guidelines included patients' changes in clinical status, inefficiency of the hospital/health care systems, and outright physician refusal. Individual patient profiles must be considered when interpreting clinical guidelines (25,26).

Mood disorder treatment in the elderly, and particularly treatment of bipolar patients, is addressed by a very limited number of treatment guidelines (27). Colenda et al. (28) compared clinical practice, clinical guidelines, and treatment outcomes in depressed geriatric patients, using a national psychiatric practice research network to follow the course of treatment of depression over a 12-week study period. Major depressive disorder was diagnosed in 84% of patients; 90% received psychotropic medication and over 75% received antidepressants prescribed in a way that was largely consistent with usual clinical guidelines for dosing and given class of medication. Improvement as measured by the Clinicians' Global Impression of Change (CGI) occurred in 90% of treated patients. The Global Assessment of Functioning (GAF) mean score, initially measured at 47.5, rose to a mean score of 61. Limitations of this research included the impressionistic measurement of improvement and limitations on data regarding symptom remission. Further study will be needed to demonstrate whether there are specific therapeutic benefits which result from adherence to clinical guidelines for psychiatric illness (28).

Effect of Physician Specialty

Several studies have demonstrated that provider specialty can influence outpatients' adherence to antidepressant treatment. Robinson et al. (29) have shown that "receipt of mental health specialty care" was the single greatest predictor of high-quality antidepressant management. Lewis et al. (30) reported the consistent finding that the rate of early antidepressant discontinuation was lower in patients treated by a psychiatrist (30). Bambauer et al. (31) indicated that patients treated by a psychiatrist refill an initial antidepressant prescription more often than those treated by primary care physicians, but once patients are on antidepressant therapy, the rates of nonadherence during treatment do not differ between psychiatrists' and primary care physicians' patients (31,32).

Although Depression Care Management programs such as PROSPECT are demonstrating high levels of engagement among depressed primary care patients, treatment by a psychiatrist has been shown more likely to be adequate than primary care "treatment as usual." Treatment by nonpsychiatric specialists too is associated with low adherence rates. This may reflect the relative lack of psychiatric training and greater time constraints of nonpsychiatric specialists. Alternatively, patients who seek help from psychiatrists may be more likely to comply with treatment (33). Better adherence was associated with treatment by the collaborative care of multiple providers and older patient age (34). Without collaborative treatment and communication between the treaters, medication adherence is dramatically declined.

When mood disorders are treated by primary care clinicians, factors that can contribute to nonadherence to treatment include lack of knowledge and training in psychiatry, reluctance to inquire about patients' psychologic states, and time limits for visits (32).

Communication

Effective communication with patients who require an appropriate level of information regarding diagnosis and treatment should be given in order to help the patient feel confident about their treatment regimen. Patient adherence to drug regimens and doses has been positively correlated with their level of understanding of the drug and with use of compliance aids (for example, pill organizers). More effective and comprehensive communication of the purpose and risks of medications and the use of compliance aids may improve adherence rates, particularly important for older persons living alone or with cognitive problems related to their illness. Clinicians can contribute to patients' poor adherence by prescribing complex regimens, failing to explain the benefits and side effects of a medication adequately, not giving consideration to the patient's lifestyle or the cost of the medications, and having poor therapeutic relationships with their patients. The patients' ability to pay is paramount and copayments, deductibles, benefits, and drug prices all need to be addressed (35–37). Clinicians have technical knowledge about psychiatric illness and medications and provide clinically relevant knowledge to patients. Personal and cultural experiences help patients conceptualize ideas about their illness and develop preferences for treatment, including the extent and type of side effects which they will tolerate. Patient perspectives provide clinicians with the information needed to individualize treatment (38).

DRUG-RELATED FACTORS INFLUENCING MEDICATION ADHERENCE AND NONADHERENCE

Polypharmacy and Complicated Medication Regimens

Many older adults have multiple chronic medical illnesses. Psychiatric illness increases the likelihood that medical comorbid disorders will be present. Medication interventions to treat disease and prolong life have increased significantly. The increasing polypharmaceutical treatment of the elderly may explain why the 11.7% of the U.S. population that is 65-year-old or more makes use of 31% of prescription medications (39). This figure does not include the use of over the counter medications, nutritional supplements, and herbal remedies. Healthcare providers contribute to polypharmacy by poor coordination of care with other treaters and failure to review an accurate consolidated medication list. The likelihood of drug redundancy, drug errors, and adverse effects increases exponentially with the number of prescriptions. In aged patients, the less complicated the drug regimen, the greater the chance for medication adherence (40).

Side Effects

Treatment of mood disorders commonly includes, but is not limited to, prescription of antidepressants, often a selective serotonin reuptake inhibitor, tricyclic antidepressant, antipsychotic (typical or atypical), mood stabilizer, or psychostimulant. Among the side effects of these medications, which are discussed in greater detail in chapter 16, hyponatremia resulting from syndrome of inappropriate secretion of antidiuretic hormone (SIADH) appears to occur more commonly in elderly than in young patients (41). Unlike those treated with selective serotonin reuptake inhibitors, elderly patients taking tricyclic antidepressants may experience peripheral and central anticholinergic effects such as constipation, urinary retention, delirium, and cognitive dysfunction as well as the antihistaminergic effects of sedation and antiadrenergic effects of postural hypotension (42). Regarding antipsychotic medications, atypical agents have a lower incident of movement disorders and have been proposed for treatment of both psychotic depression and for augmentation of antidepressants in nonpsychotic patients with treatment resistant depressive symptoms (43). Mood stabilizers such as the anticonvulsants are a standard treatment approach with patients who are manic. Lithium carbonate, though possessed of significant side effects such as interference with cognitive functioning, is nonetheless one of the first line choices for maintenance treatment of geriatric bipolar patients and has an additional benefit in protecting partially against suicidality and recurrent depressive episodes. However, elderly patients, due to decreased glomerular filtration rate, poor nutrition, and a narrow therapeutic window, are at greater risk for lithium toxicity. Psychostimulants have the advantage of rapid onset of action so that response to treatment can be noted with the first several doses. Since cardiovascular illness is commonly seen in elderly patients with psychiatric illness and the predominant side effects of psychostimulants are palpations; tachycardia; and hypertension, caution and close monitoring are necessary for effective treatment.

CONCLUSION

Adherence to therapeutic recommendations plays a significant role in the overall success of the care of depressed elderly patients. The factors that determine adherence remain complex and multifaceted. Patients, their support systems, and their health care providers must consider these barriers to adherence and take proactive steps to achieve optimal collaborative and concordant patient care and treatment outcomes.

REFERENCES

1. Liang MH. Compliance and quality of life: Confessions of a difficult patient. Arthritis Care Res 1989; 2(3):S71–S74.
2. Zubenko GS, Mulsant BH, Sweet RA, et al. Mortality of elderly patients with psychiatric disorders. Am J Psychiatry 1997; 154(10):1360–1368.

3. Noncompliance with medications. An Economic Tragedy with Implications for Health Care reform. Baltimore, MD: Task Force for Compliance, 1993.
4. Osterberg L, Blaschke T. Adherence to medication. NEJM 2005; 353(5):487–497.
5. Hughes CM. Medication non-adherence in the elderly: How big is the problem? Drugs Aging 2004; 21(12):793–811.
6. Vermeire E, Hearshaw H, Van Royen P. Patient adherence treatment: Three decades of research. A comprehensive review. J Clin Pharm Therapeut 2001; 26:331–342.
7. Merle L, Laroche M, Dantoine T, et al. Predicting and preventing adverse drug reactions in the very old. Drugs Aging 2005; 22(5):375–392.
8. Christensen AJ, Johnson JA. Patient adherence with medical treatment regimens: An interactive approach. Current Directions in Psychol Sci 2002; 11(3):94–97.
9. Becker M. The health belief model and personal health behavior. Health Edu Monogr 1974; 2:324–473.
10. Britten N, Stevenson F, Gafaranga J, et al. The expression of aversion to medicines and general practice consultation. Soc Sci Med 2004; 59:1495–503.
11. Givens JL, Datto CJ, Ruckdeschel K, et al. Older patient's aversions to antidepressants: A qualitative study. J Gen Intern Med 2006; 21(2):146–151.
12. Karasz A. Cultural differences in conceptual models of depression. Soc Sci Med 2005; 60:1625–1635.
13. Elliott RA, Ross-Degnan D, Adams AS, et al. Strategies for coping in a complex world: Adherence behavior among older adults with chronic illness. Soc Gen Internal Med 2007; 22:805–810.
14. DiMatteo MR, Lepper HS, Croghan TW. Depression is a risk factor for noncompliance with medical treatment: A meta-analysis of the effects of anxiety and depression on patient adherence. Arch Intern Med 2000; 160:2101–2107.
15. Birrer RB, Vemuri SP. Depression in their life: A diagnostic and therapeutic challenge. Am Fam Physican 2004; 69(10):2375–82.
16. Sajatovic M, Blow FC, Kales HC. Age comparison of treatment adherence with antipsychotic medications among individuals with bipolar disorder. Inter J Geri Psychiatry 2007; 22(10):992–998.
17. Depp CA, Lebowitz BD, Patterson TL, et al. Medication adherence skills training for middle-aged and elderly adults with bipolar disorder: Development and pilot study. Bipolar Disord 2007; 9:636–645.
18. Lehmann SW, Rabins PV. Factors related to hospitalization in elderly manic patients with early and late onset bipolar disorder. Int J Geriatr Psychiatry 2006; 21:1060–1064.
19. Gabbard GO, Kay J. The fate of integrated treatment: What ever happened to the biopsychosocial psychiatrist. Am J Psych 2001; 158:1956–1963.
20. Ciechanowski PS, Katon WJ, Russo JE, et al. The patient provider relationship: Attachment theory and adherence treatment in diabetes. Am J Psychiatry 2001; 158:29–35.
21. Wiebe JS, Christensen AJ. Patient adherence in chronic illness: Personality and coping in context. J Pers 1996; 64:815–835.
22. Christensen AJ. Patient-by-treatment context interaction in chronic disease: A conceptual framework for the study of patient adherence. Psychosom Med 2000; 62:435–443.
23. McGlynn EA, Asch SM, Adams J, et al. The quality of healthcare delivered to adults in the United States. NEJM 2003; 348(26):2635–2645.
24. Blackwell B. Treatment adherence: A contemporary overview. Psychosomatics 1979; 20(1):27–35.
25. Ellrodt AG, Conner L, Riedinger M, et al. Measuring and improving physician compliance with clinical practice guidelines. Ann Intern Med 1995; 122:277–282.
26. Grimshaw JM, Russell IT. The effect of clinical guidelines on medical practice: A systematic review of rigorous evaluations. Lancet 1993; 342:1317–1322.
27. Corghan TW, Hanna MP, Kennedy S, et al. The effects of adherence to antidepressant treatment guidelines on relapse and recurrence of depression. Arch Gen Psychiatry 1998; 55:1128–1132.

28. Colenda CC, Wagenaar DB, Mickus M, et al. Comparing clinical practice with guidelines recommendations for the treatment of depression in geriatric patients. Am J Geriatr Psychiatry 2003; 11(4):448–458.
29. Robinson RL, Long SR, Chang S, et al. Higher cost and therapeutic factors associated with adherence to NCQA HEDIS antidepressant medication management measures: Analysis of administration claims. J Mang Care Pharm 2006; 12:43–54.
30. Lewis E, Marcus SC, Olfson M, et al. Patient's early discontinuation of antidepressant prescriptions. Psychiatr Serv 2004; 55:494.
31. Bambauer KZ, Safran DG, Ross-Degnan D, et al. Depression and cost related medication non-adherence and medicare beneficiaries. Arch Gen Psychiatry 2007; 64:602–608.
32. Bambsuer KZ, Soumerai SB, Adams AS. Provider and patient characteristics associated with antidepressant non-adherence: The impact of provider specialty. J Clin Psychiatry 2007; 68(6):867–873.
33. Martin LR, Williams SL, Haskard KB, et al. The challenge of patient adherence. Ther Clin Risk Manag 2005; 1(3):189–199.
34. Andreasen BF, Damsgaard EM. Drug therapy in the elderly: What doctors believe in what patients actually do. Br J Clin Pharmacol 2001; 51:615–622.
35. Gellad WF, Haas JS, Safran DG. Race/ethnicity and non-adherence to prescription medications among seniors: Results of a national study. J Gen Intern Med 2007; 22(11):1572–1578.
36. Kyomen HH, Gottlieb GL. The cost of psychotropic drug use for the elderly. In: Salzman C, ed. Clinical Geriatric Psychopharmacology, 4th ed. Philadelphia, PA: Lippincott Williams & Wilkins, 2005:49–60.
37. Kyomen HH, Gottlieb GL. Financial issues in the delivery of geriatric psychiatric care. In: Sadock BJ, Sadock VA, eds. Comprehensive Textbook of Psychiatry / VIII, Vol. 2. Philadelphia, PA: Lippincott Williams & Wilkins, 2005:3775–3782.
38. Stevenson FA, Barry CA, Britten N, et al. Doctor-patient communication about drugs: The evidence for shared decision making. Soc Sci Med 2000; 50:829–840.
39. Rollason V, Vogt N. Reduction of polypharmacy in the elderly: A systematic review of the role of the pharmacist. Drugs Aging 2003; 20(11):817–832.
40. Ownby RL, Hertzog C, Crocco E, et al. Factors related to medication adherence in memory disorder clinic patients. Aging Mental Health 2006; 10(4):378–385.
41. Solai LK, Mulsant BH, Pollock BG. Selective serotonin reuptake inhibitors for late-life depression. Drugs Aging 2001; 18(5):355–368.
42. Sajatovic M, Madhusoodanan S, Cononcea N. Managing bipolar disorder in the elderly: Defining the role of the newer agents. Drugs Aging 2005; 22(1):39–54.
43. Finkel S. Pharmacology of antipsychotic in the elderly: A focus on aytpicals. JAGS 2004; 52:S258–S265.

19 Late-Life Depression and Bipolar Disorder: Factors Affecting Long-Term Prognosis and Maintenance Treatment Outcomes

Julie A. Kmiec and Ariel Gildengers

Advanced Center for Interventions and Services Research for Late-Life Mood Disorders, Department of Psychiatry, University of Pittsburgh, School of Medicine, Pittsburgh, Pennsylvania, U.S.A.

Robert C. Young

Department of Psychiatry, Weill Medical College of Cornell University, White Plains, New York, U.S.A.

Charles F. Reynolds III

Advanced Center for Interventions and Services Research for Late-Life Mood Disorders and the John A. Hartford Center of Excellence in Geriatric Psychiatry, Department of Psychiatry, University of Pittsburgh, School of Medicine, Pittsburgh, Pennsylvania, U.S.A.

INTRODUCTION: PUBLIC HEALTH SIGNIFICANCE OF MAJOR DEPRESSION AND BIPOLAR DISORDER IN LATER LIFE

As the proportion of elderly persons grows, concerns about geriatric mental health become increasingly more pertinent to public health. In the year 2000, unipolar depression was the fourth leading contributor to the global burden of illness-related disability, according to the World Health Organization (1). Moussavi (2) analyzed data from the World Health Organization's World Health Survey which studied adults, aged 30 years or older, in 60 countries and found the 1-year prevalence of major depression was 3.2%, which is similar to the prevalence of other chronic illnesses such as angina (4.5%), arthritis (4.1%), asthma (3.3%), and diabetes (2%). Furthermore, those who had chronic physical diseases were more likely to have comorbid depression and those with depression and one or more chronic physical diseases had the worst decrement in health compared to angina, arthritis, asthma, and diabetes (2). In the United States, late life depression affects a significant number of community dwelling elders and an even higher number of those residing in long-term care facilities (see Chapter 3).

Many primary care providers admit that one of the most challenging problems in their practices is the treatment of geriatric depression. Geriatric depression is prevalent, persistent, and disabling, but minimal case finding takes place and therefore many patients remain undiagnosed. A recent study by Tai-Seale et al. (3)

showed that in primary care practices where 50% of patients answered a questionnaire in such a way as to indicate depression, discussions of mental health occurred during only 25% of visits and then only for an average of two minutes. Absent correct identification of depression, clinicians may attribute depressive symptoms such as weight loss, sleep impairment, and fatigue to physical illness instead of depression. Even when depression is correctly diagnosed, patients usually receive no or at best inadequate treatment (4). Common errors include observing rather than treating the patient, prescribing ineffective (i.e., too low) dosages of antidepressant medication, or discontinuing treatment at first signs of remission, thereby failing to prevent recurrence.

Depression in old age is strongly linked to increased utilization of health care services, thereby costing the healthcare system almost twice as much to treat depressed versus nondepressed elders (5,6). When compared to nondepressed geriatric patients, depressed elderly patients make almost twice the number of medical visits (5,7), take more medications, undergo more laboratory and imaging studies, and utilize more specialty consultations even after controlling for medical comorbidity (7). For example, in the year following a cerebrovascular accident, patients with poststroke depression had significantly more inpatient days and outpatient visits than those who were not depressed (8). Additionally, depressive symptoms in medically hospitalized elderly patients are correlated with an increased rate of readmission in the six months following discharge (9). In addition to direct costs of depression, there are indirect costs such as informal caregiving that is provided by relatives to depressed elderly patients living at home. If formal caregivers were hired, the estimated national cost for this care would be $9 billion per year (10).

Since depression exacts high societal and financial costs, investigators have identified risk factors for depression in an effort to determine which groups could be appropriate targets for depression prevention. They found that female sex, low educational level, the presence of two or more chronic illnesses, a small social network, and experiencing functional limitations and depressive symptoms increased the likelihood of developing a depressive episode (11). A study examining the clinical benefits of preventive intervention is now underway (12).

Geriatric depression has not only financial costs; if left untreated it can result in death from suicide or medical causes. The reported suicide rate for those 60 and older was 14/100,000 in 2004–2005. White males 75 years of age and older have a higher suicide rate (38/100,000) than any other group, often using firearms to end their lives (13). Most elderly suicides are strongly linked to depression. A study in 1989 showed that depression is a predictor of suicide among the "old-old" such that among those 75 years of age and older, 60% to 75% of those who committed suicide had diagnosable depression. A majority of these patients had seen their primary care physician the month before committing suicide, and 39% had seen their physician the previous week (14). Fifteen years later, a study of elderly suicide attempters found that a majority of patients had seen their primary care physician within the last year, yet depression was only diagnosed after the attempt (15). Even more unfortunate is that a suicide attempt does not always lead to adequate treatment of depression (16). In an attempt to determine how best to treat depressed and suicidal elderly, the Prevention of Suicide in Primary Care Elderly: Collaborative Trial (PROSPECT) study found that when a treatment algorithm was employed [physician education, involvement of a depression care manager, and treatment with either an SSRI, interpersonal psychotherapy (IPT), or a combination] suicidal ideation decreased more quickly than in patients undergoing usual primary care treatment (17).

Depression also contributes to the risk of death from causes other than suicide in elderly patients. In medically hospitalized patients, those with six or more depressive symptoms had an increased mortality rate for up to three years after discharge (56%) than those with five or fewer symptoms (40%) after adjusting for age, illness, and functioning (18). In nursing home patients, major depressive disorder increases the likelihood of mortality by 59%, independent of previous physical health (19). More recently, data from PROSPECT were analyzed to test whether depression care management was associated with a decrease in mortality secondary to depression. Depressed geriatric patients who were in PROSPECT's intervention group were 50% less likely to die in the following five years than patients in usual care practices (20). In addition to increased mortality, depression may also lead to comorbid problems such as anxiolytic or alcohol dependence, cognitive impairment, physical disabilities, medical symptoms, and loss of functioning. In fact, one study found depression to be as debilitating as advanced coronary artery disease (21).

Not only can depression trigger other problems and diseases, but chronic medical illness is also highly correlated with the onset of depression (22). Of the elderly residing in the community, depression affects one in four of those with chronic medical illness versus one in ten medically healthy elderly (23). The combination of depression and medical illness can amplify the negative effects of each, particularly on disability. For further discussion of the relationship between depression and medical illnesses, refer to Chapter 11.

The prevalence of bipolar disorder (BD) in the elderly ranges from 0.1% to 0.4%. Although much attention is paid to treatment of mania, depression is the more common mood state in BD. As with unipolar depression, bipolar depression increases the risk of suicide. In a study of bipolar I and II individuals by Valtonen et al. (24), 61% had suicidal ideation when surveyed (64% of these were depressed), and only 20% reported that they had no suicidal behavior during their lifetime. Clearly acute treatment of depressive episodes in BD is important and requires vigilance for suicidal behavior, but no less important is the prevention of future episodes via maintenance therapy.

Acute and maintenance treatment options for bipolar depression, as noted in Chapter 4, differ from those used in unipolar depression, as mood stabilizers are often the first-line treatment rather than antidepressants. Acute and maintenance treatment of elderly patients with BD, due to a lack of controlled trials in this population, are based upon extrapolation from data gathered in mixed-age groups. Findings from mixed age group studies are problematic as elderly patients have different treatment needs due to age-related changes such as increased medical comorbidities and pharmacokinetic changes discussed in Chapter 11.

MANAGING DEPRESSION IN OLD AGE: THE NEED FOR CONTINUATION AND MAINTENANCE TREATMENT

The public health context of late life mood disorders and their severe disease burden underscore the need to take a long-term view of managing mood disorders in later life. Though geriatric depression is both serious and widespread among the aging population, data on treatment success provide reasons to be optimistic. The effectiveness of acute treatment of major depressive disorder is reviewed in

Chapter 15. Chapter 4 discusses acute treatment of bipolar states. Here we will focus on data describing the effects of maintenance treatment.

Despite current evidential support for maintenance therapies, many physicians fail to provide the necessary therapies or they choose to end treatment prematurely once the patient has achieved remission (25). Without continuation or maintenance therapy there is a high rate of relapse and recurrence (26–28). Any gains that are achieved as a result of the depression's remission, such as in overall well-being, social functioning, and the impact of emotional states on social functioning, can be lost (29). Therefore, research in the field of geriatric mental health has focused on how to effectively prevent depression from recurring and following a chronic course (27).

One of the landmarks in the study of maintenance treatment in late life depression was the 1999 report by Reynolds et al. (26), who measured the value of IPT and/or antidepressant medication in preventing recurrence of depressive episodes. In 180 depressed elderly depressed subjects, acute treatment with nortriptyline and weekly IPT sessions was administered. Those who remitted entered continuation therapy for 16 weeks, which consisted of the remission-achieving dosage of nortriptyline combined with twice monthly IPT sessions. All patients completing continuation therapy without relapse were then randomly assigned to one of four maintenance therapies: (1) medication clinic with nortriptyline; (2) medication clinic with placebo; (3) monthly IPT and nortriptyline; or (4) monthly IPT with placebo. The combination maintenance treatment of nortriptyline and monthly IPT sessions produced the best outcome, with only a 20% recurrence rate during the three years of maintenance therapy as compared to recurrence rates of 40% with nortriptyline monotherapy, 65% with IPT monotherapy, and 90% with placebo.

While tricyclic antidepressants (TCAs) like nortriptyline are often successful in acute and maintenance phases of treatment, they lack certain advantages of the selective serotonin re-uptake inhibitors (SSRIs). They are more toxic in overdose, not as well tolerated by some patients, may require monitoring of blood levels, and are regarded by many primary care physicians as more complicated to prescribe and monitor. Since many older depressed patients are treated acutely with an SSRI, it is therefore important to understand the value of SSRI maintenance therapy.

The first study using an SSRI for maintenance therapy in the elderly was reported in 2002 by Klysner et al. (30). After patients 65 years of age and older recovered from depression on citalopram and underwent a 16-week continuation phase, they entered a 48-week maintenance phase in which they were randomized to placebo or citalopram (the same dose they had been on during the continuation phase). Patients who were in the placebo group had a significantly higher rate of recurrence (67%) than those in the citalopram group (32%). Based on the hazard ratio, the risk for recurrence was three times higher for those on placebo. Furthermore, those on citalopram remained well significantly longer than those on placebo (53.8 vs. 30.3 weeks, respectively). Similar results were found in a 24-week study of continuation pharmacotherapy using escitalopram (31). In contrast, a 2-year maintenance study failed to find a difference between sertraline and placebo in time to recurrence (32).

To look at long-term maintenance treatment using an SSRI and IPT, a clinical trial similar to the nortriptyline-IPT study already described (26) was performed using paroxetine (28). The 195 subjects included in this study, however, were on average 10 years older than those in the nortriptyline-IPT study, with an average

age of 77 years. After patients had remitted on paroxetine and weekly IPT for three consecutive weeks during the acute phase of treatment, they began continuation treatment for 16 weeks, consisting of the same dose of paroxetine but decreasing IPT sessions to twice monthly. Those who stayed well were then randomly assigned to one of four maintenance conditions which lasted until depression recurred or for two years, whichever came first: (1) paroxetine plus clinical management; (2) paroxetine plus IPT; (3) placebo plus IPT; or (4) placebo plus clinical management. The time from randomization to recurrence of depression varied between groups, such that patients taking paroxetine had a lower recurrence rate (37%) than those taking placebo (58%). Unlike results in the nortriptyline-IPT study, patients in the antidepressant and IPT condition did not have a lower rate of recurrence when compared to those on paroxetine with supportive clinical management.

It has been shown that SSRIs and TCAs have equal efficacy in the acute phase of treatment of depression (33). This is also believed to be the case in continuation and maintenance phases. While further studies may be needed to verify that view, the results of one open trial comparing paroxetine and nortriptyline over 18 months of continuation and maintenance treatment showed similarly low rates of recurrence in subjects taking nortriptyline (10%) and subjects taking paroxetine (16%) (34).

Many elderly patients have comorbid medical conditions that require them to be on several concurrent medications to maintain their physical health. Therefore, some may wish to treat their depression only briefly with medication or without medication at all. Hence, it is important to ascertain whether some patients may remain in remission with psychotherapy alone. A study by Dew et al. (35) looked at the initial recovery patterns of depressed elderly patients and how these may be used to choose which maintenance therapies would be best suited for each patient. Only patients with a rapid, complete response to acute treatment with both IPT and nortriptyline remained well with maintenance IPT monotherapy. Taylor et al. (36) also examined this question and concluded that patients who had a milder depression at the commencement of treatment and had fewer residual symptoms upon remission were able to maintain their recovery with IPT alone.

DETERMINING THE PARAMETERS OF CONTINUATION AND MAINTENANCE TREATMENT

Continuation and maintenance therapy are the keys to achieving full and long-lasting remission and durable recovery. A survey of academic geriatric psychiatrists found that the majority of experts recommend continuing treatment for one year if the patient has had a single lifetime episode, but two years or longer with a history of two or more episodes (37). For continuation and maintenance treatment, the experts surveyed strongly recommended using doses found effective during acute treatment, i.e., "the dose that gets you well keeps you well"(38). The most recent recommendations from the RAND ACOVE project (39) (Assessing the Care of the Vulnerable Elderly) state that after a depressed elderly patient responds to an antidepressant, he or she should remain on the same dose of that medication for *at least* six months. Though most agree that continuation therapy should continue for at least 6–12 months following remission, researchers have yet to reach a consensus regarding the amount of time that maintenance treatment should be continued. Perhaps the most important finding from Reynolds et al. (28) was that patients in their *first* lifetime episode of depression benefited from 2-year maintenance treatment with paroxetine, as demonstrated by the significantly lower recurrence rate of those on maintenance paroxetine (27%) versus those on placebo (56%). In light of these newer findings, current recommendations regarding continuation and maintenance treatment after the first episode of depression may need reexamination and revision. Antidepressant treatment for at least two years, and maybe even lifetime treatment, should be considered to prevent further depressive episodes.

To place the issue in a broader medical context, it is useful to consider the evidence-based medicine measure of effect size termed number needed to treat (NNT). The NNT refers to the number of individuals who must be offered a treatment in order to achieve one response that cannot be explained on the basis of placebo effect. We found that to prevent a recurrent episode of depression, the NNT is 4, which means that only four people needed to be maintained on paroxetine as compared to placebo in order to achieve one extra remission that was attributable to the effect of the paroxetine (28). In other medical specialties, preventative guidelines are adopted even when the NNT is much less favorable than this one. For example, for an elderly person with known coronary artery disease, the NNT with a statin in order to prevent a vascular event, such as a myocardial infarction or cerebrovascular accident, over five years is 28 (40).

PREDICTORS AND MODERATORS OF MAINTENANCE PHARMACOTHERAPY RESPONSE IN OLD AGE

Just as there are factors that predict a poor response to acute treatment (see references 41,42 for a full review) such as co-occurring anxiety (43,44) and low self-esteem (44), there are characteristics that may influence susceptibility to relapse or recurrence during maintenance treatment. These include the age at first onset of depression (25,45), the number of lifetime episodes (46), the rate of response to pharmacotherapy (35), the current age of the depressed patient (47), the extent of coexisting medical burden (28), comorbid anxiety (43), and the quality of the patient's sleep (48). Also of consideration is the role of executive functioning on the success of maintenance therapy. Results of studies examining this relationship are varied. While Alexopoulos et al. (49,50) found that increased executive dysfunction was associated with a shorter time to relapse or recurrence of depression, Butters et al. (51) found that deficits in executive functioning were not correlated with time to relapse or recurrence of depression.

The risk of developing chronic depression increases with each subsequent relapse (46), therefore investigators have tried to determine if age at onset of depression is related to relapse and recurrence. A study by Brodaty et al. (45) reported that patients experiencing their first episode of depression before 60 years of age were more likely to experience recurrent episodes than those who had their first depressive episode later in life. In contrast, two studies found that age of onset was not an important factor in determining those who remain well, relapse during continuation treatment, or experience a recurrence during the first year of maintenance therapy (52,53).

Age at onset of depression has also been postulated to be related to time to recovery, but these results have also been mixed. First, Alexopolous et al. (25) found that late age at onset best predicted slow recovery, nonrecovery, and chronicity. Then Reynolds et al. (52) found that early-onset patients took an average of five to six weeks longer to achieve remission than their late-onset counterparts. Most recently, Kozel et al. (53) found no difference in recovery time based on age at onset.

The mixed findings regarding the age of onset of depression may be due to anything from the difference in methodology of the studies to the heterogeneity of the pathophysiology of major depressive disorder. Regardless, these discordant findings do lead to one conclusion and that is that all patients, irrespective of the age they first became depressed, are at risk for a recurrence of depression and vary in the amount of time they take to recover.

Reynolds et al. (28) showed that depression is harder to treat in the elderly than in patients in mid-life, as elderly patients took longer to get well and had a higher rate of relapse during continuation treatment than younger patients. Since there is a difference in response between middle-age patients versus geriatric patients, it has been hypothesized that there may also be a differential response to treatment within the elderly population. This does not appear to be the case with acute treatment, however. Gildengers et al. (55) divided elderly patients into three subgroups based on age (young-old: 60–70 years; middle-old: 71–76 years; and old-old: 77–95 years) and found that the old-old patients were just as responsive to acute antidepressant treatment as the young-old patients. Reynolds et al. (47) reported similar results as there was no difference in response to acute treatment between patients 60 to 69 years of age and those 70 and older after controlling for medical comorbidities. However, during the first year of a 3-year maintenance phase, patients 70 and older had a significantly higher rate of recurrence (61%) than patients aged 60 to 69 years (30%).

Although elderly depressed patients of all ages have the potential to be successfully treated, the most effective long-term treatment for each age group may vary. Once a patient has remitted during acute phase treatment, the major challenge is recurrence prevention. Because we found that patients aged 70 years and older were twice as likely to have a recurrence during the first year of maintenance treatment as those 60 to 69 years old (47), we addressed the need to find effective treatment strategies to prevent recurrence in the middle- and old-old. In our study, monotherapy with either nortriptyline or IPT was effective in preventing recurrence among patients 60 to 69 years of age. In patients aged 70 years and older, however, a combination of treatments was necessary to prevent recurrence as more than half experienced a recurrence of depression when assigned to either monotherapy, compared to less than one-third of the patients assigned to combination therapy (55).

Occasionally patients on antidepressant monotherapy (typically an SSRI) require augmentation with a medication from another class (e.g., bupropion, lithium, nortriptyline) due to lack of or an inadequate response. These patients can recover, but may do so more slowly than those who do not require augmentation (56). Once patients become well using an augmentation strategy, the utility of remaining on more than one medication may come into question. Alexopoulos et al. (57) attempted to answer this question using citalopram augmented with risperidone. Depressed elderly patients who entered the study took citalopram during the acute phase of treatment. Patients who did not respond continued in the acute phase, receiving citalopram augmented with risperidone. Those who responded to this treatment entered the continuation phase of the study in which they were randomized to remain on (1) the same doses of citalopram and risperidone or (2) the same dose of citalopram plus placebo. In terms of time to recurrence, the resulting trend approached statistical significance. Those who continued to receive risperidone augmentation remained well longer than patients who received placebo augmentation (105 days vs. 57 days). Additional support for the continuation of an augmenting medication following treatment response comes from a 1996 report by Reynolds et al. (58). Patients who responded to nortriptyline and an adjunctive medication (lithium, perphenazine, paroxetine, or a combination of these) had a higher relapse rate following the withdrawal of the augmenting medication compared to those patients who achieved a response without augmentation.

MAINTENANCE ELECTROCONVULSIVE THERAPY IN OLD AGE

In patients whose depression is medication-resistant, electroconvulsive therapy (ECT) may be a treatment option. The use of ECT is described in detail in Chapter 16 of this book. If patients respond to acute ECT, maintenance ECT (m-ECT) may be considered to prevent recurrence. To our knowledge, no prospective randomized controlled studies of m-ECT have been done with unipolar depressed elderly patients. However, both prospective and retrospective studies of continuation and maintenance ECT in the treatment of depressive episodes in patients with major depressive disorder, BD, and schizoaffective disorder include elderly patients and will be reviewed here. In a randomized prospective 6-month study following a successful acute course of ECT, there was no difference in time to relapse when comparing patients receiving continuation ECT versus those receiving pharmacotherapy (59) which is similar to the findings of a study by Swoboda et al. (60). However, a retrospective case controlled study of acute ECT responders continued on ECT with pharmacotherapy (c-ECT) or pharmacotherapy alone reported somewhat different results. Results of this study showed that the 2-year survival rate for the c-ECT patients was 93% versus 52% for pharmacotherapy only patients, and 73% versus 18% after five years, respectively. The mean survival time for c-ECT patients was 6.9 years compared to 2.7 years for the pharmacotherapy only patients (61). Although results regarding time to relapse or recurrence differ between studies, several studies show that patients who receive m-ECT have a lower number of rehospitalizations and hospital days (60,62).

MARKERS OF VULNERABILITY TO RECURRENCE

When treating depression, sleep quality needs to be monitored due to its relationship to rates of recurrence. Poor sleep quality in late life depression predicts a less successful response to maintenance treatment regardless of type of treatment. When assigned to IPT, only 30% of subjects with poor sleep quality remained depression-free for one year compared to 90% of good sleepers (63). Furthermore, residual sleep disturbance as measured by the Pittsburgh Sleep Quality Index after recovery from depression predicted recurrence (48). Treating insomnia complaints as part of the general management of depression in old age is important in achieving and sustaining remission. Often this is done with pharmacotherapy but several studies have shown that cognitive behavioral therapy is more likely to lead to sustained improvement in sleep (64–66).

Additionally, both pretreatment and residual anxiety are important factors in acutely treating depression and maintaining remission. Andreescu et al. (43) found that patients who had high levels of comorbid anxiety took longer to respond to acute treatment with paroxetine. During maintenance treatment the time to recurrence was similar for those treated with paroxetine versus placebo when the patients had high levels of pretreatment anxiety. Furthermore, residual anxiety is predictive of recurrence even after controlling for treatment with paroxetine versus placebo (48).

In summary, depression in later life is often a relapsing and recurrent illness, with a strong tendency to chronicity. Hence, patients, family members, and clinicians need to consider strategies that prevent a chronic course of illness. Expectations regarding treatment need to be discussed with both the patient and family so they understand that while the chances of remission are high, depressive symptoms cannot be alleviated in just a few weeks and treatment may take months to be fully effective. It is also important to convey that time to remission may be prolonged in patients with a recurrent depression, "double" depression (major depressive episodes superimposed upon dysthymia), severe index episodes, coexisting anxiety, heavy medical burden, and positive family history. Available treatments including TCAs, SSRIs, psychotherapy, and ECT, alone and in combination, can effectively prevent relapse, recurrence, and chronicity in many patients.

CONTINUATION/MAINTENANCE TREATMENT IN PATIENTS WITH BD

Since patients with BD, including the aged, are at risk for repeated mood episodes requiring treatment, continuation and maintenance pharmacotherapy is as critical an issue in bipolar depression. There are only a handful of reports regarding the long-term treatment of elderly BD patients.

Information concerning long-term treatment is mainly derived from reports involving naturalistic lithium treatment in mixed-age samples. Table 1 presents seven studies that included at least 10 elderly BD patients each. In aggregate, these studies involved 240 elders with BD. Stone found no decrease in rehospitalizations among patients treated with lithium carbonate after discharge compared to patients who did not receive lithium treatment (67). Gildengers et al. (68) found that even though patients experienced a good acute response to lithium, divalproex, and other mood-stabilizing agents, sustained euthymia was the exception among patients receiving maintenance treatment over two years of follow-up. In contrast, Lepkifker et al. (69) found that half of patients with BD and major depressive disorder treated with lithium had no relapse while in maintenance treatment. In a double-blind, placebo-controlled study comparing lithium and lamotrigine for maintenance treatment of elders with BD type I, Sajatovic et al. (70) found that lithium delayed time-to-intervention for mania, while lamotrigine delayed time-to-intervention for depression over 18 months. These studies provide evidence of the need for ongoing management of aged patients with BD, and preliminarily suggest the benefit of maintenance treatment with lithium, divalproex, and lamotrigine. Further studies are clearly needed in this area.

There is no current consensus regarding the dosing of maintenance mood stabilizers during continuation or maintenance treatment of late-life BD patients. The 240 patients in the seven reports presented in Table 1 were treated with lithium at concentrations of 0.5–1.1 mEq/L.

Of note, studies in mixed-age patients have suggested that lithium treatment can have an anti-suicide effect (71). While patients with BD are at increased risk for suicide (72), minimal research has addressed the issue of suicide in elders with BD. One important contribution to this area is by Lepkifker et al. (69), who reported a significant reduction of suicidal risk associated with lithium maintenance treatment.

Nonsuicide mortality rates upon follow-up of manic elders are greater than those of elders with major depressive disorder (73). No information is available regarding effect of psychiatric interventions on mortality in BD elders.

TABLE 1 Long-Term Lithium Treatment and Affective Status in Older Adult and Elderly BD Patients

Study	Design	*N*	Age mean (range) yr	Dx	Drug	Dose mean (range) mg/d	Mean Serum Level (range) mEq/L	Outcome measures	Duration	Results	Comments
Van der Velde[75]	R	12	67 (60–74)	BD, manic	Li	NA (900–2100)	NA (0.6–2)	Recurrence of affective episodes	3 yr after acute inpatient phase.	2 /12 (17%) had no recurrence in 1 year	Younger patients (*n* = 63; age 17–59 yr) remained better during follow-up.
Hewick et al.[77]	R	46	NA (50–84)	BD (82%) MDD (9%) Other (9%)	Li	NA (NA)	NA (0.5–1.5)	Global rating (0–3)	After >3 mo of treat-ment	13/46 (28%) of older patients "not optimally controlled" vs. 6/36 (17%) of younger patients	"Not optimally controlled" defined as global rating greater than 0. Older patients had lower Li level than younger patients (*n* = 36; 21–49 yr).
Murray et al.[76]	P	37	NA (60–78)	BD (*n* = 25) MDD (*n* = 12)	Li	NA (NA)	NA (NA)	Global rating (0–3)	2 yr	Trend for more severe and prolonged mania in elders	Similar Li levels in elders and younger patients (*n* = 129; age 21–59 yr); 69% of patients on Li for at least 12 mo.

Stone[67]	R	87	70.3 (65—82)	BD, manic	Li	NA (NA)	NA (NA)	Number of readmissions	Mean 3.2 yr	1.1 on Li ($n =$ 44) vs. 1.6 not on Li ($n =$ 43)	
Gildengers et al.[68]	P	31	71 (60–95)	BD	Li ($n =$ 17) Di ($n =$ 11)	657 (150–1500) 806 (250–1500)	0.67 (0.23–1) 66.1 (46–89)	Percentage of days well (HRSD and YMRS $\leq$ 10)	Median 398 days (range 20–735)	Mean percentage of "well days" was 72.5%	Only three patients remained euthymic throughout study participation.
Sajatovic et al.[70]	P	67	61 (55–82)	BD	Li ($n =$ 34) LTG (n = 33)	750 240 (50–400)	(0.8–1.1) NA	Time-to-intervention for a Mood Episode	Up to 18 mo	Li significantly delayed time-to-intervention for mania. LTG significantly delayed time-to-intervention for a depressive episode.	
Lepkifker et al.[71]	R	60	65.2 (60–84)	BD ($n =$ 41) MDD ($n = 19$)	Li	NA (NA) NA (NA)	0.67 (0.4–0.8) 0.65 (0.4–0.8)	Annual recurrence rate	Up to 15 yr	41/60 (68%) had a "good outcome." Of all patients, 52.6% had no relapse while on Li (51% of patients with BD and 59% patients with MDD).	"Good outcome" defined as a decrease of at least 50% in the annual rate of recurrences during Li treatment.

Outcome Measures: Global = 0, no conspicuous affective disturbance; 1, mild mania or depression; 2, moderate mania or depression; 3, severe mania or depression.
HRSD = Hamilton Rating Scale for Depression; YMRS = Young Mania Rating Scale
Abbreviations: R, retrospective; P, prospective; BD, bipolar disorder; MDD, major depressive disorder; Li, lithium; Di, divalproex; LTG, lamotrigine; NA, not available.

Clinical experience suggests that many elders with BD receive combined treatment with more than one psychotropic agent (68,70,74). The optimal duration of adjunctive agents, i.e., antidepressants or antipsychotic agents, after successful treatment is also not defined in aged BD patients.

MODIFIERS OF LONG-TERM OUTCOMES

As further data are gathered regarding the continuation and maintenance treatment of BD in later life, three variables have attracted attention as modifiers of long-term outcome: age, course of illness, and neurological status/cognitive impairment. These will be discussed in turn.

Age

There has been conflicting and limited evidence whether advanced age has adverse implications for long-term mood outcomes. The evidence that exists is confined to lithium treatment. Four of the studies listed in Table 1 included younger patients. While one of these indicated more recurrent mood episodes in elders (75), another (76) found only trends for greater manic psychopathology, but not more frequent hospitalizations, in elders compared to young patients. Interpretation of the third (77) report was confounded by differing lithium concentrations with age. Other studies of lithium maintenance treatment in mixed age populations that have examined age as a predictor have included few elders, or despite a wide age range did not report the numbers of elders in the sample; these reported no age effect on various outcome measures (78–81).

Course of Illness

In the naturalistic follow-up of geriatric mania by Stone (67), patients with a history of affective illness had a greater rate of recurrence. Schuroff et al. (80), on the other hand, reported a better outcome for lithium treatment in BD patients with illness onset after age 40 compared to those with earlier age at onset.

Neurological Status/Cognitive Impairment

Some studies indicate that neurological comorbidity and enduring cognitive impairments, despite control of mood symptoms, can each adversely affect long-term treatment outcomes. Shulman et al. (73) observed that patients with neurological comorbidity had a higher risk of psychiatric rehospitalization and institutionalization. In another study, cognitive deficits were associated with poor community living skills, deficits in performing activities of daily living, and placement in a nursing home (82). However, in a naturalistic, prospective study, elderly manic patients had an equal risk of relapse requiring hospitalization, regardless of the presence or absence of global cognitive impairment (83).

In summary, factors that alter acute treatment outcomes in elderly BD patients may also influence long-term treatment outcomes. Information on these issues derived from further controlled treatment trials is needed.

REFERENCES

1. World Health Organization. The world health report 2001—Mental Health: New Understanding, New Hope. http://www.who.int/whr/2001/en/index.html. 2001.

2. Moussavi S , Chatterji S, Verdes E, et al. Depression, chronic diseases, and decrements in health: Results from the World Health Surveys. Lancet 2007; 370(9590):851–858.
3. Tai-Seale M, McGuire T, Colenda C, et al. Two-minute mental health care for older patients: Inside primary care visits. J Am Geriatr Soc 2007; 55(12):1903–1911.
4. Joo JH, Solano FX, Mulsant BH, et al. Predictors of adequacy of depression management in the primary care setting. Psychiatr Serv 2005; 56(12):1524–1528.
5. Unutzer J, Patrick DL, Simon G, et al. Depressive symptoms and the cost of health services in HMO patients aged 65 years and older. A 4-year prospective study. JAMA 1997; 277(20):1618–1623.
6. Katon WJ, Lin E, Russo J, et al. Increased medical costs of a population-based sample of depressed elderly patients. Arch Gen Psychiatry 2003; 60(9):897–903.
7. Luber MP, Meyers BS, Williams-Russo PG, et al. Depression and service utilization in elderly primary care patients. Am J Geriatr Psychiatry 2001; 9(2):169–176.
8. Jia H, Damush TM, Qin H, et al. The impact of poststroke depression on healthcare use by veterans with acute stroke. Stroke 2006; 37(11):2796–2801.
9. Bula CJ, Wietlisbach V, Burnand B, et al. Depressive symptoms as a predictor of 6-month outcomes and services utilization in elderly medical inpatients. Arch Intern Med 2001; 161(21):2609–2615.
10. National Institute on Aging. Growing older in America: The health and retirement study. http://www.nia.nih.gov/ResearchInformation/ExtramuralPrograms/BehavioralAnd SocialResearch/HRS. htm
11. Smit F, Ederveen A, Cuijpers P, et al. Opportunities for cost-effective prevention of late-life depression: An epidemiological approach. Arch Gen Psychiatry 2006; 63(3):290–296.
12. Sriwattanakomen R, Ford AF, Thomas SB, et al. Preventing depression in later life: Translation from concept to experimental design and implementation. Am J Geriatr Psychiatry 2008; 16(6):460–468.
13. Center for Disease Control. WISQARS Injury Mortality Reports 1999–2005. http://webappa.cdc.gov/sasweb/ncipc/mortrate10_sy.html
14. Conwell Y, Nelson JC, Kim KM, et al. Depression in late life: Age of onset as marker of a subtype. J Affect Disord 1989; 17(2):189–195.
15. Suominen K, Isometsa E, Lonnqvist J. Elderly suicide attempters with depression are often diagnosed only after the attempt. Int J Geriatr Psychiatry 2004; 19(1):35–40.
16. Oquendo MA, Kamali M, Ellis SP, et al. Adequacy of antidepressant treatment after discharge and the occurrence of suicidal acts in major depression: A prospective study. Am J Psychiatry 2002; 159(10):1746–1751.
17. Bruce ML, Ten Have TR, Reynolds CF, et al. Reducing suicidal ideation and depressive symptoms in depressed older primary care patients: A randomized controlled trial. JAMA 2004; 291(9):1081–1091.
18. Covinsky KE, Kahana E, Chin MH, et al. Depressive symptoms and 3-year mortality in older hospitalized medical patients. Ann Intern Med 1999; 130(7):563–569.
19. Rovner BW. Depression and increased risk of mortality in the nursing home patient. Am J Med 1993; 94(suppl 5 A):19S–22S.
20. Gallo JJ, Bogner HR, Morales KH, et al. The effect of a primary care practice-based depression intervention on mortality in older adults: A randomized trial. Ann Intern Med 2007; 146(10):689–698.
21. Wells KB, Burnam MA. Caring for depression in America: Lessons learned from early findings of the Medical Outcomes Study. Psychiatr Med 1991; 9:503–519.
22. Evans DL, Charney DS, Lewis L, et al. Mood disorders in the medically ill: Scientific review and recommendations. Biol Psychiatry 2005; 58(3):175–189.
23. Reynolds CF, Kupfer DJ. Depression and aging: A look to the future. Psychiatr Serv 1999; 50(9):1167–1172.
24. Valtonen H, Suominen K, Mantere O, et al. Suicidal ideation and attempts in bipolar I and II disorders. J Clin Psychiatry 2005; 66(11):1456–1462.
25. Alexopoulos GS, Meyers BS, Young RC, et al. Recovery in geriatric depression. Arch Gen Psychiatry 1996; 53:305–312.

26. Reynolds CF, Frank E, Perel JM, et al. Nortriptyline and interpersonal psychotherapy as maintenance therapies for recurrent major depression: A randomized controlled trial in patients older than 59 years. JAMA 1999; 281(1):39–45.
27. Reynolds CF, Alexopoulos GS, Katz IR, et al. Chronic depression in the elderly: Approaches for prevention. Drugs Aging 2001; 18(7):507–514.
28. Reynolds CF, Dew MA, Pollock BG, et al. Maintenance treatment of major depression in old age. N Engl J Med 2006; 354(11):1130–1138.
29. Dombrovski AY, Lenze EJ, Dew MA, et al. Maintenance treatment for old-age depression preserves health-related quality of life: A randomized, controlled trial of paroxetine and interpersonal psychotherapy. J Am Geriatr Soc 2007; 55:1325–1332.
30. Klysner R, Bent-Hansen J, Hansen HL, et al. Efficacy of citalopram in the prevention of recurrent depression in elderly patients: Placebo-controlled study of maintenance therapy. Br J Psychiatry 2002; 19(1):29–35.
31. Gorwood P, Weiller E, Lemming O, et al. Escitalopram prevents relapse in older patients with major depressive disorder. Am J Geriatr Psychiatry 2007; 15(7):581–593.
32. Wilson KC, Mottram PG, Ashworth L, et al. Older community residents with depression: Long-term treatment with sertraline. Randomised, double-blind, placebo-controlled study. Br J Psychiatry 2003; 182:492–497.
33. Schneider LS. Treatment of depression in late life. Dialogues Clin Neurosci 1999; 1(2):113–124.
34. Bump GM, Mulsant BH, Pollock BG, et al. Paroxetine versus nortriptyline in the continuation and maintenance treatment of depression in the elderly. Depress Anxiety 2001; 13:38–44.
35. Dew MA, Reynolds CF, Mulsant B, et al. Initial recovery patterns may predict which maintenance therapies for depression will keep older adults well. J Affect Disord 2001; 65:155–166.
36. Taylor MP, Reynolds CF, Frank E, et al. Which elderly depressed patients remain well on maintenance interpersonal psychotherapy alone? Report from the Pittsburgh study of maintenance therapies in late-life depression. Depress Anxiety 1999; 10(2):55–60.
37. Alexopoulos GS, Katz I, Reynolds CF, et al. Pharmacotherapy of depressive disorders in older patients. In: Roberts WO, ed. Postgraduate Medicine Special Report. Minn, MN: McGraw-Hill Companies, 2001:1–86.
38. Reynolds CF, Perel JM, Frank E, et al. Three year outcomes of maintenance nortriptyline treatment in late-life depression: A study of two fixed plasma levels. Am J Psychiatry 1999; 156(8):1177–1181.
39. Nakajima GA, Wenger NS. Quality indicators for the care of depression in vulnerable elders. J Am Geriatr Soc 2007; 55 Suppl 2:S302–311.
40. Afilalo J, Duque G, Steele R, et al. Statins for secondary prevention in elderly patients: A hierarchical bayesian meta-analysis. J Am Coll Cardiol 2008; 51(1):37–45.
41. Whyte EM, Dew MA, Gildengers A, et al. Time course of response to antidepressants in late-life major depression: Therapeutic implications. Drugs Aging 2004; 21(8):531–554.
42. Whyte EM, Basinski J, Farhi P, et al. Geriatric depression treatment in SSRI nonresponders. J Clin Psychiatry 2004; 65(12):1634–1641.
43. Andreescu C, Lenze EJ, Dew MA, et al. Effect of comorbid anxiety on treatment response and relapse risk in late-life depression: Controlled study. Br J Psychiatry 2007; 190:344–349.
44. Saghafi R, Brown C, Butters MA, et al. Predicting 6-week treatment response to escitalopram pharmacotherapy in late-life major depressive disorder. Int J Geriatr Psychiatry 2007; 22(11):1141–1146.
45. Brodaty H, Harris L, Peters K, et al. Prognosis of depression in the elderly. A comparison with younger patients. Br J Psychiatry 1993; 163:589–596.
46. Keller MB, Lavori PW, Collins CE, et al. Predictors of relapse in major depressive disorder. JAMA 1983; 250:3299–3304.
47. Reynolds CF, Frank E, Dew MA, et al. Treatment in 70 +-year-olds with major depression: Excellent short-term but brittle long-term response. Am J Geriatr Psychiatry 1999; 7(1):64–69.

48. Dombrovski AY, Mulsant BH, Houck PR, et al. Residual symptoms and recurrence during maintenance treatment of late-life depression. J Affect Disord 2007; 103:77–82.
49. Alexopoulos GS, Meyers BS, Young RC, et al. Executive dysfunction and long-term outcomes of geriatric depression. Arch Gen Psychiatry 2000; 57(3):285–290.
50. Alexopoulos GS, Kiosses DN, Klimstra S, et al. Clinical presentation of the "depression-executive dysfunction syndrome" of late life. Am J Geriatr Psychiatry 2002; 10(1):98–106.
51. Butters MA, Bhalla RK, Mulsant BH, et al. Executive functioning, illness course, and relapse/recurrence in continuation and maintenance treatment of late-life depression: Is there a relationship? Am J Geriatr Psychiatry 2004; 12(4):387–394.
52. Reynolds CF, Dew MA, Frank E, et al. Effects of age at onset of first lifetime episode of recurrent major depression on treatment response and illness course in elderly patients. Am J Psychiatry 1998; 155(6):795–799.
53. Kozel FA, Trivedi MH, Wisniewski SR, et al. Treatment outcomes for older depressed patients with earlier versus late onset of first depressive episode: A sequenced treatment alternatives to relieve depression (STAR*D) report. Am J Geriatr Psychiatry 2008; 16(1):58–64.
54. Reynolds CF, Frank E, Kupfer DJ, et al. Treatment outcome in recurrent major depression: A post hoc comparison of elderly ("young old") and midlife patients. Am J Psychiatry 1996; 153(10):1288–1292.
55. Gildengers AG, Houck PR, Mulsant BH, et al. Course and rate of antidepressant response in the very old. J Affect Disord 2002; 69(1–3):177–184.
56. Dew MA, Whyte EM, Lenze EJ, et al. Recovery from major depression in older adults receiving augmentation of antidepressant pharmacotherapy. Am J Psychiatry 2007; 164(6):892–899.
57. Alexopoulos GS, Canuso CM, Gharabawi GM, et al. Placebo-controlled study of relapse prevention with risperidone augmentation in older patients with resistant depression. Am J Geriatr Psychiatry 2008; 16(1):21–30.
58. Reynolds CF, Frank E, Perel JM, et al. High relapse rate after discontinuation of adjunctive medication in elderly patients with recurrent major depression. Am J Psychiatry 1996; 153(11):1418–1422.
59. Kellner CH, Knapp RG, Petrides G, et al. Continuation electroconvulsive therapy vs. pharmacotherapy for relapse prevention in major depression: A multisite study from the consortium for research in electroconvulsive therapy (CORE). Arch Gen Psychiatry 2006; 63(12):1337–1344.
60. Swoboda E, Conca A, Konig P, et al. Maintenance electroconvulsive therapy in affective and schizoaffective disorder. Neuropsychobiology 2001; 43(1):23–28.
61. Gagne GG, Furman MJ, Carpenter LL, et al. Efficacy of continuation ECT and antidepressant drugs compared to long-term antidepressants alone in depressed patients. Am J Psychiatry 2000; 157(12):1960–1965.
62. Lim LM. A practice audit of maintenance electroconvulsive therapy in the elderly. Int Psychogeriatr 2006; 18(4):751–754.
63. Reynolds CF, Frank E, Houck PR, et al. Which elderly patients with remitted depression remain well with continued interpersonal psychotherapy after discontinuation of antidepressant medication? Am J Psychiatry 1997; 154(7):958–962.
64. Morin CM, Colecchi C, Stone J, et al. Behavioral and pharmacological therapies for late-life insomnia: A randomized controlled trial. JAMA 1999; 281(11):991–999.
65. Jacobs GD, Pace-Schott EF, Stickgold R, et al. Cognitive behavior therapy and pharmacotherapy for insomnia: A randomized controlled trial and direct comparison. Arch Intern Med 2004; 164(17):1888–1896.
66. Sivertsen B, Omvik S, Pallesen S, et al. Cognitive behavioral therapy vs. zopiclone for treatment of chronic primary insomnia in older adults: A randomized controlled trial. JAMA 2006; 295(24):2851–2858.
67. Stone K. Mania in the elderly. Br J Psychiatry 1989; 155:220–224.
68. Gildengers AG, Mulsant BH, Begley AE, et al. A pilot study of standardized treatment in geriatric bipolar disorder. Am J Geriatr Psychiatry 2005; 13(4):319–323.

69. Lepkifker E, Iancu I, Horesh N, et al. Lithium therapy for unipolar and bipolar depression among the middle-aged and older adult patient subpopulation. Depress Anxiety 2007; 24(8):571–576.
70. Sajatovic M, Gyulai L, CalabreseJR, et al. Maintenance treatment outcomes in older patients with bipolar I disorder. Am J Geriatr Psychiatry 2005; 13(4):305–311.
71. Tondo L, Hennen J, Baldessarini RJ. Lower suicide risk with long-term lithium treatment in major affective illness: A meta-analysis. Acta Psychiatr Scand 2001; 104(3):163–172.
72. Muller-Oerlinghausen B, Berghofer A, Bauer M. Bipolar disorder. Lancet 2002; 359(9302):241–247.
73. Shulman KI, Tohen M, Satlin A, et al. Mania compared with unipolar depression in old age. Am J Psychiatry 1992; 149(3):341–345.
74. Wylie ME, Mulsant BH, Pollock BG, et al. Age at onset in geriatric bipolar disorder: Effects on clinical presentation and treatment outcomes in an inpatient sample. Am J Geriatr Psychiatry 1999; 7(1):77–83.
75. Van Der Velde CD. Effectiveness of lithium carbonate in the treatment of manic-depressive illness. Am J Psychiatry 1970; 127(3):345–351.
76. Murray N, Hopwood S, Balfour DJ, et al. The influence of age on lithium efficacy and side-effects in out-patients. Psychol Med 1983; 13(1):53–60.
77. Hewick DS, Newbury P, Hopwood S, et al. Age as a factor affecting lithium therapy. Br J Clin Pharmacol 1977; 4(2):201–205.
78. Angst J, Weis P, Grof P, et al. Lithium prophylaxis in recurrent affective disorders. Br J Psychiatry 1970; 116(535):604–614.
79. O'Connell RA, Mayo JA, Flatow L, et al. Outcome of bipolar disorder on long-term treatment with lithium. Br J Psychiatry 1991; 159:123–129.
80. Abou-Saleh MT, Coppen A. The prognosis of depression in old age: The case for lithium therapy. Br J Psychiatry 1983; 143:527–528.
81. Schurhoff F, Bellivier F, Jouvent R, et al. Early and late onset bipolar disorders: Two different forms of manic-depressive illness? J Affect Disord 2000; 58(3):215–221.
82. Dhingra U, Rabins PV. Mania in the elderly: A 5–7 year follow-up. J Am Geriatr Soc 1991; 39(6):581–583.
83. Bartels SJ, Mueser KT, Miles KM. A comparative study of elderly patients with schizophrenia and bipolar disorder in nursing homes and the community. Schizophr Res 1997; 27(2–3):181–190.

Index